MASSAGE FOR THE HOSPITAL PATIENT
AND MEDICALLY FRAIL CLIENT

MASSAGE FOR THE HOSPITAL PATIENT AND MEDICALLY FRAIL CLIENT

GAYLE MacDONALD, MS, LMT

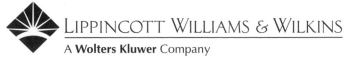

LIPPINCOTT WILLIAMS & WILKINS
A **Wolters Kluwer** Company

Philadelphia · Baltimore · New York · London
Buenos Aires · Hong Kong · Sydney · Tokyo

Editor: Pete Darcy
Development Editor: David Payne
Marketing Manager: Christen DeMarco
Project Editor: Jennifer D. Glazer
Indexer: Janet Perlman
Designer: Doug Smock
Artwork Director: Risa Clow
Photographer: Don Hamilton
Compositor: Maryland Composition
Printer: Courier Kendallville

Library of Congress Cataloging-in-Publication Data

MacDonald, Gayle, 1950-
  Massage for the hospial patient and medically frail client / Gayle MacDonald.
    p.;cm.
  Includes bibliographcal references and index.
  ISBN 0-7817-47058
  1. Massage therapy. 2. Hospital patients. I. Title.
  [DNLM: 1. Massage—nursing. 2. Complementary Therapies—nursing. 3. Inpatients. 4.
  Physical Therapy Techniqus—utilization. WB 537 M135m 2004]
  RM721.M217 2004
  615.8′22—dc22

                                                      2004048269

DEDICATION

Laura Koch—
    She quietly, without fanfare, brought us together with the creation of the Hospital-Based Massage Network.

PREFACE

Massage for the Hospital Patient and Medically Frail Client is a textbook for massage therapy students and bodywork practitioners. For those with no experience working in mainstream health care, this text will serve as an introduction to working in the hospital setting. For bodyworkers already employed or volunteering in a hospital, this book will serve as a reference manual and resource that will help them to expand the boundaries of massage within their setting or practice.

Additionally, this text will serve as a reference manual for bodyworkers who work with the medically frail outside the hospital setting. Massage has become so mainstream that practitioners now regularly encounter the medically frail in their private practice, at spas, chiropractic offices, clubs, health fairs, or special events, such as The Race for the Cure. With the knowledge from this book, bodyworkers will be able to continue massage sessions without missing a beat and even schedule appointments in the hospital.

The book will also prove useful in the following functions:

- As a guide for the student clinic for creating a safe massage plan for a wide variety of clients
- As a written resource around which schools can create a curriculum for hospital and medical massage courses
- As a guide to clinical decision making for hospitals, hospices, extended care facilities, and medical offices as they establish massage protocols, make referrals, or educate patients and family

APPROACH

My work is rooted in the pioneering efforts of Tedi Dunn, Marian Williams, and Karen Gibson; their grassroots manuals pointed the way for those who followed them. However, unlike these broadly focused manuals, which contain material on establishing a hospital massage program, writing proposals, funding possibilities, and rudimentary massage protocols, this text addresses the clinical picture only. It does not address financial issues, the ins and outs of establishing a hospital program, pathology, or instruction in massage techniques. Books that give guidance on those topics can be found in the Additional Resources list in Chapter 1.

This text answers the following questions:

- What knowledge and skills do practitioners need to safely administer massage to people who are experiencing ill health?
- What knowledge and skills are necessary when administering massage in healthcare settings, particularly the hospital?
- How might comfort-oriented massage be beneficial to the person who is ill?

A massage session with someone who is ill will be affected by the disease, the side effects of treatment, medical devices, and medications. This type of massage is not defined by new and special strokes so much as it is by the adaptations that must be made to the existing ones. Thus, it is the intent of this book to help therapists understand how to adapt the massage skills they already possess for use with these patients.

Nearly all touch disciplines can be adapted for acutely ill individuals. Some modalities, such as Reiki, Healing Touch, and Jin Shin Jyutsu®, are especially well suited for working with the seriously ill and require no changes. Others can be used with only minor adjustments, for example, Swedish massage and reflexology. But even more vigorous styles of bodywork, such as Shiatsu and trigger-point therapy, can be modified for these patients. Very few modalities are unworkable in this milieu. Thai massage, sports massage, and Rolfing come to mind. However, even aspects of these modalities are adaptable.

The majority of modifications to a massage session can be placed in one of three categories: **pressure considerations, site restrictions,** and **positioning adjustments.** These three classifications (discussed in Chapter 5) are at the heart of the book and provide a framework for performing intake with medical and nursing staff, organizing the patient's medical data, planning the massage session, and recording progress notes. This simple conceptual device can be applied to any area of the hospital, from cardiology to obstetrics to general medicine, making it easier for massage therapists to move from one area of specialty to another. Just as it is impossible these days for doctors and nurses to be highly knowledgeable in all specialties, the same is true for bodyworkers. The pressure, site, and position framework gives touch therapists a general tool to anchor them within this highly specialized world.

Massage for the Hospital Patient and Medically Frail Client concentrates much of the time on the period of hospitalization. However, the reader will be able to easily adapt the information to the client who is on an outpatient basis. The focus is on the use of massage as a comfort measure, which is presently the goal of most hospital massage programs. In the future, it is conceivable that the scope of hospital massage will expand to include the use of bodywork as a treatment for medical conditions. But, for now, as complementary modalities jostle to find their place within mainstream medicine and mainstream medicine readjusts to accommodate this new trend, the goal of creating comfort is a good starting place.

Providing comfort for massage therapists is also the aim of this book. Medical settings can be mystifying, uncomfortable places—a landscape of unfamiliar sights, sounds, and smells; foreign-looking machinery; and unknown procedures, rhythms, and customs. The unknown can contribute to the bodyworker feeling hesitant or fearful when approaching the patient. By becoming acquainted with the medical devices, medications, and diagnostic tests, and their relationship to massage, the therapist will be more comfortable. The practitioner can then relax with the patient who is beneath her hands, undistracted by the extraordinary landscape surrounding her.

DEFINING MASSAGE

Because definitions of "massage" can vary considerably and because of the special needs of the hospital patient and medically frail client, it is necessary to define how the term is used in this book. The following description of "massage," based on Karen Gibson's concept of *hospital-based massage therapy*, will be used as the central guiding force in this text (*Developing a Hospital-Based Massage Therapy Program*, 1992):

Massage is any skilled, systematic form of touch applied with sensitivity and compassion by professionally trained massage therapists with the specific intent of increasing comfort, complementing medical treatment, improving clinical outcomes, and promoting wholeness. *

---

*Note: The words "touch" and "bodywork" are used synonymously with "massage." Touch in this context means the skilled, systematic touch, such as a Reiki practitioner or Healing Touch therapist would apply, as opposed to the casual touch employed within greetings and goodbyes or straightening the bed covers and changing a dressing. The terms "therapist," "practitioner," and "bodyworker" also are used interchangeably and indicate the person administering skilled touch.

Also, because my roots are in the hospital, I refer most often to this arena when speaking about healthcare facilities. However, the terms nursing home, extended care facility, or rehabilitation center could just as easily be substituted for "hospital." The similarities are greater than the differences.

OVERVIEW

The first four chapters of this book provide background information essential to practicing massage in the hospital setting, including a brief history of hospital massage (Chapter 1), a review of the research regarding the benefits of massage (Chapter 2), how to adapt to hospital culture (Chapter 3), and infection control practices (Chapter 4).

The clinical material in Chapters 5 to 9 (covering the clinical framework, reasons for hospitalization, conditions and symptoms, medical devices and procedures, and medications, respectively) will be an invaluable complement during pathology instruction. Although this text makes no attempt to teach pathology, it trains bodyworkers how to make real-world adjustments to massage techniques when working with pathological conditions.

Chapters 10 to 12 provide information on the actual practice of massage in the hospital, including discussion of referrals, orders, and intakes, the massage session itself, and documentation. Chapter 13 concludes the book with accounts from numerous contributors on their "trailblazing" work in various settings within the hospital.

SPECIAL FEATURES

By its nature, a clinical textbook can seem formidable and inaccessible. Reading it may be a demanding ordeal. The task I set for myself in the writing and shepherding of this book was to convey the information in a scholarly yet warm tone, to bring together the two energies of this topic, the clinical nature of the medical setting with the heart and compassion of massage. The following features of the book help to accomplish this.

- *A Therapist's Journal.* People learn through and are inspired by stories. Anecdotes by experienced therapists and rank beginners have been liberally placed throughout the book.
- *Tips.* This feature conveys practical, down-to-earth suggestions about such things as lotion holders, acquiring medical devices for teaching purposes, or scheduling around diuretic medications, to name just a few.
- *Quotes.* Through these, the wisdom of those who have come before us is passed on.
- *Photos.* Images of therapists working with actual patients illustrate the concepts of the book in vivid, realistic detail.

- *Test Yourself.* These exercises and tests give the reader a chance to review the material presented in each chapter. Massage school instructors using the book as a text will find this a handy feature.
- *Of Special Interest.* These boxes highlight interesting facts and concepts related to the content.
- *Additional Resources.* At the end of each chapter, additional resources relevant to the material presented in each chapter, and not already listed in the References section, are compiled.

FINAL NOTE

Massage is more than a job or a profession for many touch therapists; it is a calling. No group of massage therapists feels more called than those who are drawn to work with the seriously ill. For them, I am pleased that there are greater and greater opportunities to fulfill their dream.

My students invariably start out with the expectation that their presence and touch will be a balm for patients who are hurting, tired, and dispirited. And it is. But little do the students realize that they too will be healed and transformed by the patients. I don't alert them to this possibility beforehand, for it is that instant when they make the discovery for themselves that is one of my most treasured moments and is why I love teaching hospital massage.

To say that I teach hospital massage is a misnomer. I hold the container in which the learning occurs. The patients, family, and the hospital itself are the true teachers. I am the guide, the cheerleader, the hand-holder, and the witness. This book is my way of guiding, supporting, and cheering on everyone who wants to give massage to those in the hospital setting or to the medically frail.

Gayle MacDonald

ACKNOWLEDGMENTS

This book is the result of teamwork. Every time I needed help, it was there—from massage therapists, nurses, doctors, students, my mother, friends, and LWW editors. The stories that bring the book to life came from all over the country—Carol Weinert and Tina Ferner (Ohio), Eileen Dolan, Jan Locke, Chad Wahjudi, and Jessica Glade (Oregon), Bambi Mathay (Massachusetts), Charlotte Versagi (Michigan), Lee Erman and Helen Campbell (California), Kim Howell (Arizona), and Dr. Judi Schmidt and Sue Lenander (Montana). A number of people filled in the gaps where my own knowledge was missing: Adela Basayne, Lisa Walters, Patti Cadolino, Toni Kline, Charlotte Versagi, Carole Osborne-Sheets, Mary Rose, Nicholas Kasovac, Diane Charmley, and Marybetts Sinclair. Thanks to Cheryl Chapman, Irene Smith, Tedi Dunn, and Mary Ann Finch for teaching me about professional generosity.

Nurses are my heroes. The care they give day in and day out is extraordinary. Many shared generously of their time and expertise—Janey Slunaker, Patty Wyman, and Doug Beal. Another group of nurses who are also massage therapists made special contributions: Judi Crooks, Lana Lyons, Lyndi Farmer, Linda Hughes, Janice Hein, Barbara Estes, Diane Charmley, Toni Kline, and Shelda Holmes. Thanks also to Dr. Miles Hassell and Dr. Anne Nedrow.

Heartfelt thanks to Patti Cadolino, Jan Locke, and Lee Erman who said, "Yes," every time I asked them to contribute "one more thing." Also, without the help of Marsha Coffman, Liz Davidson, Crystal Towne, Christine Montgomery, and Marcella MacDonald, this project wouldn't have come in on time, and my sanity would not have stayed intact. Joan Pinkert and Lois Curtin—thanks for literary and computer assistance. Don Hamilton—thanks for coming out of retirement to be a medical photographer one more time. Former students volunteered to be photographed while working with patients—Linda Abate, Monica Billingsly, Liz Davidson, Lisa Barck Garofalo, Alisa Goslin, Ken Graham, Alta Southwell, and Carol Tocher.

David Payne and Pete Darcy, my editors at LWW, have been simultaneously warm and professional—not always an easy task. Thanks to Ruth Werner for helping me keep perspective; Lonnie Howard, Tracy Walton, and Toni Creazzo for their personal and professional support; and also to Tracy Walton, the instigator and inspiration for this text.

To family and friends, apologies for the neglect you endured while I was absorbed in this effort. Thanks for being there for me even though I wasn't always there for you.

And, a final note to my students—through you I remember why this work is so important.

Gayle MacDonald

REVIEWERS

Lorraine Berté, RN, LMT
Faculty
Downeast School of Massage
Waldoboro, Maine

Mary Duquin, PhD
University of Pittsburgh
Pittsburgh, Pennsylvania

Cindy Varner, CMT
Tranquil Touch Therapeutic Massage
Orefield, Pennsylvania

Ronda Wimmer, PhD, MS, LAc, ATC, CSCS, SPS, LMT
CEIM Exercise Science and Sports Performance Institute
Newport Beach, California

CONTENTS

THE REVIVAL OF HOSPITAL MASSAGE

Massage in hospitals is not new. An examination of massage history reveals that ancient civilizations in India, China, Egypt, Greece, and Rome administered massage to the sick in healing halls and temples.[1] Lofty names from classical literature, invariably men, such as Homer, Hippocrates, Plato, Socrates, and Galen, appear in connection to massage and illness.[2]

By the fourth century, Christians had created houses of refuge where religious orders of both men and women tended to the sick and dying. Much of the emphasis in these early Christian shelters was on providing spiritual solace rather than physical comfort. Their purpose was to save the soul, not the body. Reference is, however, made to massage in accounts of the era.[1]

Little is known about massage during the Middle Ages, roughly designated as the fifth through the fifteenth centuries. In *The History of Massage*, Robert Calvert reports that it "was the Church that helped preserve massage within the Western world during the Middle Ages," despite its negative attitude toward the body. Touch, in the form of "laying on of hands," became part of Christian ritual and care of the sick and dying.[1]

During this period, it was church women who cared for those struck down by the plague and other epidemics, many physicians being unwilling to serve people who could not pay for their services.[3] These deaconesses were the forerunners of religious orders of sisters, such as the Sisters of Charity and Sisters of Providence, who established care facilities for the sick and the poor. Today, a number of hospitals can trace their roots to these pioneering groups of women.

The period of transition from the Middle Ages to modern times is referred to as the Renaissance. Healthcare practitioners of the day came to a new understanding of anatomy and physiology, which impacted the application of hands-on modalities. During the Renaissance, hospitals evolved from the houses of refuge and dying of early Christian times to places of rehabilitation.[4]

Guenter Risse, in his text on the history of hospitals, summarizes the eighteenth-century hospital as being focused on cure followed by teaching, research, and surgery in the nineteenth century; science in the early twentieth century; and technology in the late twentieth century.[4] Massage endured highs and lows during these periods. Some healthcare providers embraced the science and mechanization of the era, turning away from hands-on practices. Others enthusiastically prescribed it for a plethora of medical conditions.

MASSAGE AND NURSING

Massage has, at various times, been part of a physician's repertoire. The Greek physician Hippocrates is credited with saying that "the physician must be experienced in many things, but assuredly also in rubbing."[2] But for the past century and a half, hospital massage has been clearly associated with nursing. The creation of modern nursing practice is credited to Florence Nightingale, an Englishwoman who took it upon herself to nurse the wounded soldiers of the Crimean War (1854–1857). Although she does not specifically mention massage in her *Notes on Nursing*, it was part of her training program.[1]

John Kellogg, the medical director at the sanitarium in Battle Creek, Michigan, started perhaps the first training school for nurses in 1883. Massage was an important part of the nursing curriculum, and his book, *The Art of Massage*, remains a classic text. Training in hands-on modalities continued to be an integral part of nurses' training and care through the mid-1950s, after which it declined to almost nothing.[1,3]

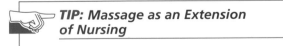

TIP: Massage as an Extension of Nursing

When presenting the idea of integrating massage into the acute care setting, one approach is to tie massage into its nursing roots. Speak to the notion that massage in hospital settings is nothing new. It is only an extension of what nurses used to do but no longer have time for.

At various times during the twentieth century, both nurses and physical therapists have administered massage. While physical therapists used massage as a treatment for various medical conditions, nurses gave massage as a comfort measure. The nightly backrub is still remembered by many older patients as a standard part of the hospital experience from the 1940s, 1950s, and even the 1960s (Fig. 1-1).

Originally, nurses were primarily caregivers. They straightened bedding, tidied patients' rooms, emptied the garbage, dusted the furniture, mopped the floor,[5] gave massage, assisted the patient with exercises, and much more. Nurses were part housekeeper, physical therapist, occupational therapist, social worker, respiratory therapist, and massage therapist. They were the ultimate holistic practitioners.

Today, nurses and physical therapists rarely include massage in their care or treatment. The modern-day nurse is in the position of case manager, leaving less time for "luxuries" such as massage. And physical therapy, like other branches of health care, has shifted toward high-tech treatments such as ultrasound and electrical stimulation.

Unfortunately, as medical care became more complex, the use of massage in hospitals and clinics was abandoned. Nurses now spend much of their time performing duties such as cardiac monitoring, passing out medications, and changing dressings. The demand on their time includes a new mountain of bureaucratic paperwork, leaving less time to spend with the patient. Even physical therapy has largely replaced human touch with ultrasound, heat lamp, or other devices. Massage therapists are the ones to re-establish healing touch in the American medical system.[6]

Daniel Eddins Andrews III, MD

A variety of factors have contributed to an atmosphere in which massage, as well as other types of personal care, was largely discontinued. Four main circumstances led to this change: (1) an increase in the patient load due to a shortage of nurses; (2) the requirement for additional documentation by governmental regulators, thereby taking time away from patients; (3) new methods of billing demanded by insurance carriers, which also increased the amount of paperwork performed by nurses; and (4) the growth of medical technology, which favored drugs and machinery over hands-on methods of care.

TECHNOLOGY AND TOUCH

At about the same time massage was left behind as a part of standard hospital care, roughly in the 1960s and 1970s, the need for massage became even greater. And that is still true today. Because of the high-tech nature of medicine, patients are cared for by a team of specialists. Despite the many advantages of being cared for by experts, there are drawbacks to having a dozen different staff members at-

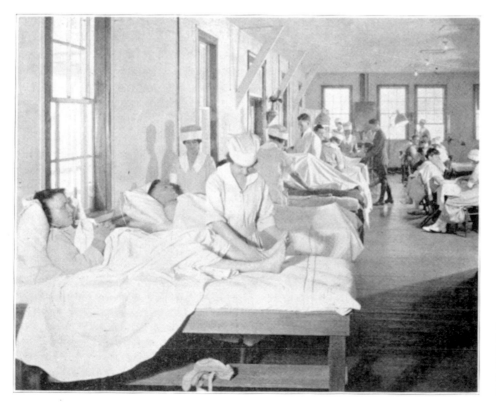

FIGURE 1-1. ■ Soldiers receive massage in medical barracks. From C. M. Sampson's Physiotherapy Technic (St. Louis, 1923). Reprinted with permission from Calvert RN. The History of Massage. Rochester, VT: Healing Arts Press, 2002.

tending to their "piece" of the puzzle. A patient's day in the hospital can consist of a steady stream of hospital staff, each treating only one specific part of the patient's health needs, leaving the patient feeling fragmented. The respiratory therapist cares for the lungs; the physical therapist sees to the legs; the nurse manages the plan of care; the pharmacist is responsible for managing pain; the nursing assistant sees to the personal care needs; the nutritionist oversees the food; the intravenous nurse attends to the catheters; the social worker cares for the psychosocial needs; and the pastoral counselor attends to the soul.

It is easy to rail against medical technology and specialization, to long for the good old days when the town doctor treated patients from childhood through adulthood. Paradoxically, however, the rise in technology, while initially leading to a lessening of hospital massage, is now partly responsible for its revival and growth. As health care has become more fragmented, the need for practitioners who can provide a sense of wholeness, such as massage therapists, is even greater. Fragmentation and wholeness, two seemingly opposite characteristics, are inextricably linked.

> *Numerous studies reflect . . . Americans' social inhibitions and cultural prohibitions when it comes to touch. Paradoxically, ongoing social and medical research demonstrates that nurturing touch is a basic human need for maintaining health and for life itself. With decreasing face-to-face opportunities for casual contact in our high-tech, low-touch society, it is no surprise that massage has been embraced as a safe structure for receiving—and giving—the human touch that we intuitively know nourishes the spirit along with the body.[7]*
>
> *Tedi Dunn, Massage Therapy Guidelines for Hospital and Home Care. 4th Ed.*

John Naisbitt foretold of this scenario in his 1984 book *Megatrends*. Advances in technology, he predicted, would be accompanied by the need for more touch. High-tech/high-touch was, in fact, one of his lead prognostications.[8] Even the bodywork profession has gone down the road of specialization, which is the natural evolution of a field as more and more knowledge and experience is gained. Although a few nurses still give some of their patients a nightly backrub and some student nurses are once again showing an interest in receiving massage training, the trend in hospitals is toward bringing in therapists who specialize in massage.

This is not to say that there isn't a place for massage or touch given by nurses, family, and friends. Each has its place in caring for patients. Helen Campbell writes eloquently of teaching family members to be massage givers (see Anecdote 13.2). And Karen Gibson, one of the field's pioneers, warns against allocating touch only to special-

ists. "We don't want to take it away from front-line practitioners, we want to supplement and encourage it."[9]

The introduction of professional bodyworkers into hospitals does, however, have advantages. Just as medical specialists are able to provide more knowledgeable care, so too are massage specialists. A bodyworker has the luxury of unhurried time with the patient that even nurses from 50 years ago did not have. Whereas a nurse may have time to rub the back or feet, a massage practitioner has time to attend to the entire person. The sense of wholeness created by this kind of attention is an important contribution to patient care.

Professional touch therapists also have a broader and deeper level of skill. Patients who previously might have been passed by as inappropriate massage candidates, such as those with congestive heart failure or low platelet levels, can now enjoy the benefits of low-impact touch modalities that only a specialist can provide. Additionally, it is the professional touch therapist who has the knowledge and time to spend teaching family how to massage their loved one.

THE NEW PIONEERS

Massage and nursing have been joined throughout human history. Therefore, it is not surprising that the pioneers in the latest chapter of hospital massage have often been nurses or others with a medical background, such as medical social worker Tedi Dunn. Along with a number of individual trailblazers, several hospitals have played a part in leading the way.

The massage program at California Pacific Medical Center in San Francisco, begun in the mid-1980s, is one of the most visible models in the new era. Dunn started the service as a voluntary activity on the 13-bed Planetree Model Hospital Unit. (Planetree is a philosophy that aims to create a healing environment in which the latest medical technology can be humanistically delivered.) Dunn and her colleague, nurse Marian Williams, were part of turning the profession in a new direction—hospital massage therapy as a specialty. Rather than massage being administered by generalists, such as nurses or physical therapists, whose duties included a laundry list of other tasks, touch therapists specially trained to work with the ill were brought into the fold. Two years after the volunteer program was initiated, paid positions were created, and a six-month internship program to train bodyworkers was added.[7]

Three others from the San Francisco Bay area—Irene Smith, Dawn Nelson, and Helen Campbell—led the way in working with the elderly, ill, and dying. Smith became known in the 1980s for teaching the massage community how to work with people who were HIV positive or had AIDS; Nelson, meanwhile, explored ways to work with another marginalized group, the elderly; and Campbell pioneered hospice and hospital massage.

BOX 1-1	*Of Special Interest*

USE OF MASSAGE IN HOSPITAL

In a survey performed by the American Hospital Association and the American Massage Therapy Association, massage was found to be the most used complementary and alternative medicine (CAM) therapy. Of the 1,007 hospitals that responded to the survey, 269 reported the use of CAM therapies, with 220 institutions using massage. Patient stress (163) and pain management (153) were two of the main reasons hospitals report using massage. Two of the patient groups commonly given massage are obstetric (121) and oncology (129). Regarding practitioners, about half of the hospitals (118) using massage therapy contract with the therapists, while 113 employ the massage providers. Only 33 of the reporting institutions bill patients' insurance for bodywork services.[10]

A number of 1980s trailblazers were found in Colorado. Among them were Barbara Carnahan and Mary Rose of the Boulder Hospice and Suzanne Wilner at the Center for Human Caring, part of the University of Colorado Health Sciences Center. Also in Colorado, Karen Gibson, a nurse massage therapist from Boulder Community Hospital in Boulder, was instrumental in moving hospital-based massage therapy forward. Building on the program developed at California Pacific, she teamed with the Boulder School of Massage to create an intern training program. Gibson's work became another model for those who followed.

Many others have been part of the pioneering effort: Sharon Piantedosi (Exeter, New Hampshire); Xerlan Geiser (Tulsa, Oklahoma); Sharon Burch (Lawrence, Kansas); Susie Ogg Cormier (Lafayette, Louisiana); Jeannie Battagin (Oakland, California); and Laura Koch (Boulder, Colorado). Koch founded the Hospital-Based Massage Network in 1995, a structure that connected and supported previously isolated hospital massage practitioners. This organization generated an exponential level of expansion that moved hospital massage to a new level. Today, hundreds of hospitals have paid employees, volunteer positions, or independent contractors giving massage to their patients (Box 1-1).

SUMMARY

There is a saying that "Everything old becomes new again." Certainly this is true of hospital massage, which has literally been around for ages. The importance of touch during illness was momentarily forgotten in the excitement of increased technology, but it has been remembered again. Today, hospital massage therapy is undergoing a transformation. What was once part of a nurse's duties is becoming a specialty unto itself, much like what occurred with physical, occupational, and respiratory therapy in the middle of the twentieth century. Massage

specialists are taking the art in a new direction. Now, instead of being part of nursing or rehabilitation services, massage has become a member of departments known by such names as Integrative Medicine, Complementary Therapies, or Holistic Health.

Historians will look back on this era as the time when the arc of the pendulum widened to include science and art, when East met West, ancient combined with modern, and technology spawned a renewal in touch. The present period, however, is only a single chapter; more evolutions will unfold. And yet, ultimately, the story will always return to the same place—the hands contain medicine. No matter what the techniques of the day are or who is designated to administer them, human touch is a vital component in caring for the sick.

REFERENCES

1. Calvert RN. The History of Massage. Rochester, VT: Healing Arts Press, 2002.
2. Beard B, Wood EC. Massage Principles and Techniques. Philadelphia, PA: W. B. Saunders, 1964.
3. Calvert RN. Pages from History: Massage in Nursing. Massage Mag 2003;103:158–160.
4. Risse GB. Mending Bodies, Saving Souls: A History of Hospitals. New York: Oxford Press, 1999.
5. Mower M. Massage Returns to Nursing. Massage Mag 1997;69:46–54.
6. Andrews DE. Guest Editorial. Massage Mag 2002;99:24.
7. Dunn T, Williams M. Massage Therapy Guidelines for Hospital and Home Care. 4th Ed. Olympia, WA: Information for People, 2000.
8. Naisbitt J. Megatrends. New York: Warner Books, 1984.
9. Gibson K. Developing a Hospital-Based Massage Therapy Program. Boulder, CO: CareBase Technologies, 1992. (out-of-print)
10. Hospitals Show Broad Use of Massage. Hands On: The Newsletter of the American Massage Therapy Association Nov/Dec 2003:7.

ADDITIONAL RESOURCES

1001 Sources to Build Your Hospital-Based Massage Program. Available through Information for People, 800-754-9790 or www.info4people.com.

Benjamin P. Rub It On, Rub It In: A Brief History of Oils and Liniments Used in Massage. Massage Ther J 2003;42(2):136–143.

Calvert RN. Pages From History: Rubbing Up vs. Rubbing Down. Massage Mag 2003;106:196–197.

Exploring Hospital-Based Massage. Available through Information for People, 800-754-9790 or www.info4people.com.

Hospital-Based Massage Network, www.HBMN.com.

Hospital-Based Massage Programs in Review. Available through Information for People, 800-754-9790 or www.info4people.com.

World of Massage Museum, www.worldofmassagemuseum.com. Located at: 811 E. Sprague Avenue, Suite E, Spokane, WA 99202.

REVIEWING THE RESEARCH

When back rubs were part of standard evening care, it was enough that they just felt good. There was no need to analyze or dissect the experience. Patients and hospital staff knew from firsthand evidence that massage was relaxing, good preparation for sleep, and mood enhancing. In today's science-oriented society, many people want the claims backed up by proof. Time and financial resources are precious; hospitals want to know which interventions provide the best outcomes at the most cost-effective rate rather than administering care based on assumption, hope, or myth.

A body of research is slowly developing that will provide guidance toward creating **evidence-based practice.** However, the surface has barely been scratched. Only two variables have had even a modicum of study, anxiety and pain, and only two patient populations, oncology and preterm infants.

The nursing profession has led the way in the study of massage for hospital patients, which is only natural since massage has historically been a part of standard nursing care. In addition, nursing has an academic infrastructure that both demands and supports research in general. Nurse researchers, because of the nature of their focus of care, will view the investigation of massage through a different lens than bodyworkers. Time and simplicity are essential to the nurse wishing to integrate massage into patient care. When readers of this book examine the research, they will notice that the massage interventions given by nurses are generally of shorter duration and consist of basic hands-on techniques such as effleurage or acupressure.

The massage profession, which is poised to enter the research arena, will take the subject in new directions, down paths that reflect its own role in health care. While a nurse must be attentive to many tasks and patients at once, leaving little opportunity to linger with a patient or step into a state of deep mindfulness, bodyworkers have the luxury of time and a single focus—the provision of skilled touch. This focus will allow them to shed light on new questions and examine such issues as the impact of mindfulness or the differences between Swedish massage and Jin Shin Jyutsu® or reflexology and Reiki. Research will help them apply the ancient art of massage to patients in the modern world.

A THERAPIST'S JOURNAL
Becoming a Researcher

I'm not a "detail" person. As a matter of fact, one of my least favorite things in life is tracking details . . . so how did I become involved in a research project tracking details? It began with my work as an LMT in the ICU of McKenzie-Willamette Hospital (a 114-bed community hospital in Springfield, Oregon). After I had done 2 years of clinical massage work for patients in units all over the hospital, the ICU Patient Care Coordinator came up with the idea of tracking the patients' response to receiving massage during PICC [peripherally inserted central catheter] placement.

We developed a tool (a Likert-scale survey) to gather data regarding the patients' perception of their anxiety and physical comfort levels, and off we went. It surprised me when I found myself focusing on the data and how to represent what it meant. We surveyed patients before and after the procedure, with and without massage. I became the person crunching the numbers and developing comparison graphs. I loved it. There it was in front of me, a clear portrait of the gift, the impact of compassionate massage.

Now I'm hooked. It's addictive in a way. It's a finite way to describe and give credibility to the power of touch, and yet each situation has mystery and variables. There is no way to tell the outcome until the data is processed, and the data has to be traceable, specific and accurate. It's all right there in the details.

—Jan Locke, LMT,
McKenzie-Willamette Hospital,
Springfield, Oregon

INCLUSION CRITERIA

To make the task of reviewing hospital-related research manageable, this chapter concentrates on people who are hospitalized. Excluded are massage studies of healthy subjects, hospice and nursing home patients, and animals; case studies; **anecdotal** reports; and dissertations on hospital massage programs.

Only studies of manual forms of massage—those in which the hands are used to manipulate tissue—are reported. Studies written in English that examine manual techniques, such as Swedish massage, acupressure, and reflexology, are the focal point. Mechanical forms of massage, such as the use of wristbands to stimulate acupressure points or pneumatic cuffs, are not included. Esoteric and energy modalities, such as Reiki or Therapeutic Touch, are often used with positive results in the hospital, but the research is still sketchy. Therefore, no attempt is made to report on these techniques at this time.

In mainstream medicine, the gold standard is the **double-blind,** controlled, **randomized** design with large numbers of subjects, an impossible yardstick for massage therapy. First, in double-blind studies, it is not known which patients are receiving the experimental protocol and which are receiving the **control** intervention. At the very least, in doing massage research, the bodywork practitioners are aware of which intervention is being administered, making it impossible to use the double-blind design. Secondly, it is difficult to obtain large numbers of subjects due to limited resources for massage research.

The aim in this review is to bring together all of the studies that have examined the effects of hospital-based massage, to paint a broad picture that is inclusive rather than exclusive. Even studies that do not have large sample sizes or that have not been randomized and controlled have a story to tell. Therefore, investigations are presented regardless of the design, sample size, or method of analysis. As massage researcher Janet Kahn states, "Research is any systematic inquiry."[1] This then is the overriding criterion for inclusion: Does the study show evidence of a consistent and methodical inspection?

The first half of the chapter groups the studies by variables, such as pain, anxiety, sleep, and **vital signs.** The second half takes the same studies and presents them in chart form by patient population, such as surgery, intensive care, **oncology,** or infants.

EXAMINING THE VARIABLES

A scouring of the hospital massage research unearthed many results that patients and healthcare providers might expect, such as the positive effect on the variables anxiety, pain, and sleep. At other times, the search produced more surprising outcomes, as in the case of vital signs. Perhaps the biggest revelation, though, was to come up nearly empty-handed on the research of certain variables, such as fatigue and depression.

Even while a noticeable number of studies exist, the unknown dwarfs the known. The effects of massage on people who are hospitalized are not fully or even partially understood. A picture is slowly emerging, but for the present, massage continues to be practiced and guided by art and instinct rather than by science.

Anxiety and pain are a good starting place for the review because they are the two most studied variables. Not surprisingly, the two have a strong interrelationship. Reduction of one reduces the other and vice versa.

ANXIETY

Massage has a high success rate in alleviating anxiety immediately following the touch session. Twenty of 2 studies showed positive results.[2–25] This finding holds true across a broad spectrum of patient populations: people with cancer,[2,3,7,12,15,21,24] those undergoing rehabilitation,[6] surgical[11,14,16,22] and psychiatric patients,[10,23] mothers in labor,[4,9] children being treated for burns,[8] and those in the intensive care unit (ICU).[5] It also is true regardless of the type of intervention. Researchers looked at a variety of massage interventions, including a 5-minute hand massage before cataract surgery, a 30-minute reflexology session on those admitted for cancer treatment, and a 20-minute **aromatherapy massage** following **cardiac** surgery.

> *Foot massage is . . . an effective way to induce deep relaxation. The simple human contact and support offered through touch is medicine in itself. But during the administration of chemotherapy, especially the first time when the person is most likely terrified, foot massage proves to be a powerful and supportive technique to reduce anxiety and lessen the common side effect of nausea. According to Ronda Fleck, MD, a radiation oncologist in Albuquerque and Santa Fe, "Massage in general helps the patient's general overall well-being and promotes healing, but I see foot reflexology during the administration of chemotherapy to be especially helpful. It makes the whole atmosphere more inviting and helps the patient to embrace their care. I have also seen cases of the patient needing less anxiety medication during chemo.*[26]
>
> —*Lonnie Howard, MA, LMT,
> Director of The Scherer Institute of Natural
> Healing, Santa Fe, New Mexico*

PAIN

Pain is one of the major stressors of hospitalization, and as it increases, so does hospital stress.[27] In the past, doctors feared that patients would become addicted or dependent on pain medications, particularly **narcotics;** this fear resulted in an underprescribing of **analgesics.** Research, however, has shown that the vast majority of patients rarely develop a dependence on these drugs.[28]

Despite a new attentiveness to pain management and more effective **pharmaceuticals,** not all pain can be managed through drugs alone. Physical discomfort is the result of a multitude of forces. The ideal pain-management program, therefore, consists of a combination of drug and nondrug interventions.

Massage consistently reduced pain in the majority of studies reviewed.[3,4,6–9,11,12,15–20,22,24,25,29–35] Eleven of 22 investigations looked at the pain of those with cancer.[3,7,12,15,20,21,24,25,29,31,34] The remaining projects were spread between surgical,[11,16,30,32,33,35] general,[6,19] maternity,[4,9] burn,[8] and heart catheterization[17,18] patients. The one population in which no improvement occurred following massage was the heart catheterization patients. This may have been a result of the baseline pain level being low to start with.

Again, the massage interventions and length of sessions varied, and yet, nearly all were successful in reducing pain. Subjects received 10-minute foot massages, 45-minute full-body sessions, 30 minutes of reflexology, and pressure to acupressure points.

Every 3 years, hospitals undergo a review by the Joint Commission on Accreditation of Healthcare Organizations (JCAHO), the accrediting body for hospitals. Pain management is an area that now receives pointed examination during the review process. JCAHO is enthusiastic about the inclusion of nonpharmacological and **complementary** interventions, particularly for pain, a fact that massage professionals could capitalize on.

TIP: Focus on Expected Outcomes

When offering massage to a patient who seems hesitant, focus on the expected outcome, such as reducing nausea or pain. For instance, when entering the room of a patient whose nurse has told you is in some pain, you might say: "Your nurse tells me you are having some pain. Sometimes a gentle foot massage will alleviate that. Would you like to give it a try?"

USE OF MEDICATIONS

Although it should be enough that massage enhances healing, improves people's hospital experience, or increases comfort, the bottom line is sometimes cost-effectiveness. Bodyworkers look eagerly for ways to prove that their discipline can be a cost saver. It is thought that massage may decrease the need for medications, especially analgesics, and, thereby, produce a cost savings. However, the evidence to support this notion cannot be implied from the present research.

The investigation into this topic is scant. Only three projects have examined the relationship between pain medications and massage,[2,16,32] the results of which were mixed. Two studies found no difference in the use of analgesics between the massage and control groups.[2,32] The other found a **trend** toward decreased use, but this trend did not reach **statistical significance.**[16]

The use of anti**emetic** drugs for chemotherapy-induced nausea was examined in a group of patients undergoing bone marrow transplantation. The massage group required significantly less nausea medication, thereby saving the hospital $750 per patient compared to the control group. Additionally, the massage group needed far less total **parenteral** nutrition (TPN), which produced another savings of $800 per patient.[36] TPN use goes hand-in-hand with emetic problems.

LENGTH OF STAY

This variable also has the potential to decrease hospital expenses in a substantial way. Again, the quantity of research is still so minimal that it is too early to make sweeping claims. However, from a review of the six studies completed to date, there is reason for cautious optimism with regard to the effects of massage and length of stay for certain acute care populations.[9,16,19,36–38]

Subject groups have included preterm infants,[37,38] postoperative patients,[16] women who have undergone bone marrow transplantation,[36] maternity patients,[9] and a group from the general hospital population.[19] All of the groups except one showed either a significant decrease or a trend toward a shorter stay.[19] The largest drop occurred with the preterm infants who received massage for 15 minutes three times a day for 10 days. In one study, these infants went home 5 days sooner than the controls.[38] In another study, they were discharged 6 days earlier. A cost analysis of the latter study showed a savings of $3,000 per infant.[37] Today, that would translate into a $10,000 savings!

The women who received massage during bone marrow transplantation went home 3 days sooner than the nonmassage group, saving the hospital $1,440 per patient.[36] Maternity patients who received massage during labor and delivery were discharged nearly a day sooner than the control group.[9] And the group that was massaged following a **hysterectomy** was discharged half a day earlier than the nonmassage group; however, this result was not statistically significant.[16]

One of the contributing factors toward length of stay for bone marrow transplant patients is the rate of **engraftment,** or how quickly the new bone marrow or stem cells begin to create **neutrophils.** Smith compared the effects of massage therapy, Therapeutic Touch, and a friendly visit on this variable. No statistically significant difference occurred.[24]

A surprising discovery was made when analyzing the benefits of our massage program. We found that on some occasions we achieved better comprehensive, multi-disciplinary care for the patient. This was accomplished by the combination of compassionate, individual attention, as well as the relaxation effect of the massage session, providing an atmosphere of comfort for the patient. Within this environment, the patient was able to state previously unexpressed needs, such as inadequate pain control, sleeplessness, financial anxieties, housing problems, nutritional problems, emotional and family stress. We were able to assist patients in these areas of their lives by the information they presented to the massage therapist, who was then able to link the patient to the appropriate resources—medical, social, psychological, nutritional—to better meet the needs of the patient as well as their families.

—Tina Ferner, LMT,
St. Vincent Mercy Medical Center,
Toledo, Ohio

NAUSEA

Nausea can be a side effect of **anesthesia**, chemotherapy, labor, or medications. Despite the creation of new antiemetic drugs, there is still a significant occurrence of nausea within the hospital population. For example, as many as 60% of cancer patients undergoing chemotherapy experience nausea and vomiting.[39] This may sound like just an annoyance, but it can cause serious complications, such as **aspiration**, dehydration, electrolyte imbalance, and disruption of a surgical site.[40]

The majority of nausea studies have investigated the effectiveness of massage with the oncology population.[2,3,31,36,41,42] The accumulative outcome of these six studies is overwhelmingly positive.

Interestingly, there is an almost complete lack of nausea research on other groups of patients using manual therapy. Dozens of acupressure projects have documented the efficacy of wristbands (also known as sea bands) for postoperative and pregnancy-related nausea.[43-49] These devices, which have a small stud in the band, generally are targeted at the P6 point and are preferable to using a practitioner because they are less labor intensive. Only one researcher compared the use of finger pressure, wristband use, and standard treatment in a group of postoperative patients. Both manually applied acupressure and the sea bands decreased nausea and vomiting over a 24-hour period compared to the nonacupressure group. However, only the finger pressure group achieved statistical significance when compared to the control.[49] In the end, cost-effectiveness is important and would probably sway the decision toward the use of

wristbands, even if manual finger pressure was more effective.

PRESSURE SORES

It would be natural to hypothesize that massage is beneficial for preventing and healing pressure sores, also known as **decubitus ulcers.** Massage and nursing education certainly teach toward this stance. A Dutch study surveyed the beliefs of hospital nurses regarding the usefulness of different methods for preventing decubitus ulcers. The application of massage and cream was believed by a majority of the nurses to be a useful intervention for those at risk for or already affected by pressure sores.[50]

However, three analyses of pressure sore–related research from nursing literature question the benefit of massage for this condition.[50-52] Consensus reports from The Netherlands and the United States recommend using moisturizers "to treat dry skin and creams during **incontinence** and to reduce friction injuries." Massage, however, is not recommended to stimulate blood flow. According to the consensus report from the U.S. Department of Health and Human Services, "the scientific evidence for using massage to stimulate the blood flow and avert pressure ulcer formation is not well established, whereas there is preliminary evidence suggesting that it may lead to deep tissue damage."[50]

The above recommendations arise from research that indicates massage does not increase blood flow and, therefore, would not speed healing or prevent skin breakdown. Most of the studies cited in the analyses showed no differences in blood flow between the massage group and the control. Insignificant effects were also found on skin temperature, a measurement that relates to circulation. In two of the studies, skin temperature actually decreased, suggesting that massage may have a deleterious effect on the skin. No significant increase in skin blood flow occurred except during the use of **tapotement,** a modality that obviously would be inappropriate to use on people who are seriously ill.

There is no clear relationship on the effect of massage and pressure sore development.[51] One study showed a positive, but statistically insignificant trend toward fewer sores in the massage group. In another, the control group had 38% fewer pressure sores than the massage group. The authors of the third project reported positive results within the massage group but had no scientific documentation.[51]

This review of research led Halfens[52] and Buss[51] to recommend that extended, robust massage should not be used for patients at risk for developing ulcers in the area of bony prominences and pressure areas. They also question the use of "soft, moderate, or standard massage." Anthony writes, "The belief held by clinicians in topical applications, physical treatments and massage in treating and preventing decubitus ulcers is in most cases misguided. With the exception of pulsed **electromagnetic** energy where evidence is accumulating in favour of this technique, no treatment seems to speed healing and most delay it."[50] The mixed data and paucity of research make it impossible to give any definitive answers about the effect of massage on decubitus ulcers. For now, touch practitioners and massage instructors should reexamine their approach to this topic.

VITAL SIGNS

Vital signs are a group of physiological assessments used to monitor a patient's status and include blood pressure, pulse, temperature, and respiration rate. Massage researchers use them as a measure of relaxation. Asked to hypothesize about the effect of massage on vital signs, a person might guess that massage decreases these variables. However, the pattern from 17 studies is inconclusive at best, but for the most part showed either no change or statistically insignificant changes.[2,5,7,8,10,11,13,14,16–18,22,30,31,53–55]

This pattern proved to be true with each of the patient populations that were studied: ICU,[5,53,55] surgical,[11,14,16,22,30] oncology,[2,7,31] premature infants,[54] children with psychiatric disorders,[10] and patients undergoing heart catheterization.[17,18] A few reductions occurred here and there, such as blood pressure, pulse, and respirations in a group of five post–**myocardial infarction** (MI) subjects;[55] the **diastolic** blood pressure of a group of bone marrow transplant recipients;[2] the **systolic** blood pressure of one of the groups of heart catheterization patients;[18] the pulse rate in burn patients undergoing **debridment;**[8] and the respiration rate in a sample of cancer patients.[7] The subjects of Grealish et al. had a reduction in heart rate following the intervention, but then so did the control group, which underwent a 10-minute quiet period.[31] Overall, respiration rate came the closest to presenting a positive outcome. Of the nine studies that examined it, five showed a decrease.[2,5,7,11,13,17,22,55]

Labyak and Metzger cite data that are useful for bodyworkers. A group of nine men who had undergone **coronary** bypass surgery were given a 10-minute back rub within 48 hours of surgery. Although the rate of breathing dropped, blood pressure and heart rate rose during the massage, leading the researchers to conclude that back massage may be too demanding on the body within the first 48 hours after surgery and therefore contraindicated for this group of patients.[55]

Two studies of heart attack (MI) patients indicate that massage can be tolerated by this particular group of cardiac patients.[53,55] A small group of men who received a 10-minute back rub post–heart attack had a positive outcome in heart rate, blood pressure, and respiration rates.[55] Another group of MI patients who received a 6-minute back massage showed no changes in **autonomic** variables.[53] Although the researchers did not find positive results, they commented on the fact that, equally important, there were no negative effects as a result of the massage. Therefore, they concluded that massage might be safe for post–heart attack patients.

👉 **TIP: Making Research Grant Connections**

Few bodyworkers have the academic credentials to be the primary investigator on a research project. This shouldn't stop them from trying to initiate a grant. Hospitals are rich with resources and people who are interested in studying health care. They employ grant writers, statisticians, and fund-raisers and have nonprofit foundations and professionals with research backgrounds and advanced degrees. If the hospital is a teaching institution, it will have connections with a nursing school, which in turn will have doctoral-level nurses who may be willing to offer guidance. The massage professional can be the driving force behind creating the grant-writing team, as well as offering his expertise on the massage protocols. A word of warning to anyone interested in the research process—be prepared to move slowly and deliberately.

CORTISOL

The measurement of **cortisol** is often used as an objective marker of stress. Menard explains in her doctoral thesis that, although high cortisol levels may be beneficial during and immediately after surgery, continued high levels may slow recovery, impair immune function, cause insulin resistance, delay wound healing, and induce sleep disturbance and depression.[16] Therefore, an intervention that decreases cortisol may enhance an individual's healing.

The studies to date show that massage does have a reducing effect on cortisol. The scientists from the Touch Research Institute measure cortisol in nearly all of their studies. This variable dropped following massage in each of their patient populations: children with psychiatric disorders[10] and adults undergoing debridement following severe burns.[8] Menard's study of postoperative patients showed a trend toward a lower cortisol level.[16] A group of people undergoing **cataract** surgery received a 5-minute hand massage before the procedure, causing a significant drop in cortisol.[14] Preterm infants have also shown a decrease in this marker.[56]

Instinctively, most conventionally trained physicians think massage is a wonderful thing. Many of them have a personal practice of receiving massage. The missing link is that they do not think of it as a medical intervention. Rather, they perceive massage as a luxury, like belonging to an athletic club or going out for a nice dinner.

Research into the use of massage as a medical intervention would move the medical practitioner to suggest and implement it more quickly for the patient. Research could also confirm whether massage is a cost-effective tool in the total care of patients. Between the change in paradigm for the practitioner and the reimbursement by third-party payers, massage would no longer be alternative, but mainstream.

—*Anne Nedrow, MD,*
Medical Director of the Women's Primary Care/Integrative Medicine Center for Women's Health, Oregon Health and Science University Portland, Oregon

SLEEP

Sleep seems to promote recovery from illness and, yet, is often lacking in an acute care setting, further contributing to the stress of hospital life. Numerous studies have shown that, despite receiving medications to promote sleep, patients in critical care units are severely sleep deprived.[57] An examination of the sleep of older people in hospitals indicates that two of the main contributors to poor sleep are pain and discomfort, both of which massage can address.[58]

Seven investigators have examined sleep and found massage to improve both its quality and quantity.[3,10,12,16,19,20,57] The cancer subjects in three different studies[3,12,20] scored higher in sleep measurements, as did a group of ICU patients,[57] children with psychiatric disorders,[10] and a generalized hospital group.[19] Menard's surgical subjects experienced a trend toward improved sleep.[16]

Swedish massage was the predominant modality used. The sessions varied in length from 6 to 45 minutes. The benefits occurred whether the session lasted 6, 20, or 40 minutes, again demonstrating that even a very short massage intervention can be effective.

DEPRESSION

Just as it is thought that a lack of sleep inhibits health recovery, so, too, may depression. And yet, it is a rarely studied symptom in the hospital population, with just a handful of investigations to date. Generally, these few studies are encouraging. Menard noted a trend toward improvement of depression following a hysterectomy.[16] In addition, a group of children diagnosed with psychiatric disorders[10] and women in labor[9] showed significant improvement in depression, as did ovarian cancer patients.[15] Two studies of bone marrow transplant patients exhibited differing results: One showed significant improvement in depression levels,[24] while the other had no significant change.[2] It is important to note, however, that these two studies can't be accurately compared because

different methodologies and measurement tools were used for each.

LESSER-STUDIED VARIABLES

A handful of variables have had minimal study. Four investigators[11,19,31,59] unanimously reported an increase in relaxation, and three others found an improvement of mood.[8,19,59] **Catecholamines** (epinephrine and norepinephrine) improved in a surgical study[14] but were unchanged in a group of preterm infants.[56] Neutrophil and **lymphocyte** levels failed to change in Kim's project.[14] Quality of life for cancer patients is improved by massage, according to two different studies.[60,61]

Fatigue is notable for a lack of investigation. Only Ahles[2] and Smith[19] included it in their studies. Both had positive results. It is surprising that, despite being a major complaint of many patients and despite massage having a reputation for increasing energy, little examination has been made of massage's effect on fatigue. When it is studied, fatigue is often included as part of a quality-of-life survey. Never has it received the focused investigation that it deserves.

The effect of a 1-minute back rub on **mixed venous oxygen saturation (SVO₂)** of intensive care patients has been investigated by Tyler[62] and Lewis.[63] While similar findings by two research teams is hardly a concrete en-

---

A THERAPIST'S JOURNAL
Grassroots Research

I have my massage students survey patients before and after each massage on four variables: pain, emotional comfort, physical comfort, and fatigue. The first year of this process, some information came to light that would have gone unnoticed without this primitive research. The first thing was that the nurses were referring mostly female patients. I hadn't realized this until I sat down the first time to average the numbers. From then on, I went out of my way to ask the nurses if their male patients could receive massage. Since then, our referrals have been well balanced between men and women.

A second piece of data that surprised me was the fatigue ranking. Patients consistently reported it higher than any of the other variables. Without those surveys, I would have guessed pain to cause the most discomfort. The data from 93 patients found that 73% perceived a decrease in their fatigue following massage. Because of the questionnaires, my students and I had a better idea of the specific good the massage was doing.

—*Gayle MacDonald, MS, LMT*

dorsement, it does warrant attention. Both projects found that a 1-minute back rub decreases SVO_2, an undesirable outcome that may indicate that a back rub causes a minor stimulus that increases heart rate and oxygen demand in many critically ill people.

Lewis also looked at the effect of positioning in relation to the back rub. Both left and right side-lying caused a drop in SVO_2, but turning to the left resulted in an even greater reduction. The stress of turning and immediately receiving massage was compared to turning and receiving the back rub after a 5-minute equilibration period. The positioning followed by a delayed back rub caused less of a drop in SVO_2. Oxygen saturation returned to clinically acceptable levels within 5 minutes of the back rub. Lewis advises that massage can be administered immediately after repositioning if the individual is **hemodynamically** stable. Unstable patients should be monitored closely and receive delayed back rub.[63,64]

EXAMINING PATIENT POPULATIONS

The purpose of this section is to summarize patient populations in chart form. The charts allow the reader to quickly access the study's basic quality by noting the sample size, use of randomization and control, and statistical analysis. While it is a handy format, much information is lost. To understand the methodological protocols, tools of measurement, statistical analyses, and results in greater detail, the full journal article must be read. Some articles can be ordered via the Internet or through interlibrary services at hospitals or medical and nursing schools.

Studies are grouped by patient populations in alphabetical order by medical specialty, such as infants, intensive care, and maternity. The order in no way reflects numbers of studies or importance. The following abbreviations are used throughout the charts:

admin—administered
avg—average
BP—blood pressure
BR—breast
CA—cancer
DBP—diastolic blood pressure
diff—difference
Dx—diagnosis
effl—effleurage
exper—experimental
gest—gestational
h—hour
hosp—hospital
HR—heart rate
ICU—intensive care unit
M—massage
med—medically
min—minutes
MTh—massage therapist

n—number
NICU—neonatal intensive care unit
nonsignif—nonsignificant
petri—petrissage
pts—patients
psych—psychological
QoL—quality of life
RR—respiration rate
SBP—systolic blood pressure
signif—significant
temp—temperature
Tx—treatment
wks—weeks
wt—weight

GENERAL HOSPITAL POPULATIONS

Several investigations grouped subjects together from a combination of medical specialties.[6,13,19,65] The wide differences in variables studied, sample sizes, and interventions make it impossible to draw any conclusions with regard to the general hospital patient. Such a patient may not exist anyway. It may only be possible to draw conclusions about specific groups of patients (Table 2-1).

INFANTS

The effects of massage on infants with medical complications, such as prematurity or exposure to HIV or cocaine, are unequivocally clear with regard to weight gain and behavioral indicators. Every study that examined weight gain showed a positive outcome,[37,38,54,65–70] which sometimes translated into a shorter length of stay (Table 2-2). Scores on behavioral assessments, such as the Brazelton Neonatal Behavioral Assessment Scale (BNBAS), also showed marked improvement.[37,38,54,67,71] The BNBAS measures clusters of criteria such as motor behavior, alertness and activity, autonomic stability, and abnormal reflexes.

Without special highlighting, several interesting items might get lost in the blur of numbers. One is a study that found that mothers who massaged their own premature infants achieved the same results as professional health caregivers in terms of weight gain.[65] Another is a study that examined the question, Is massage too demanding for the premature infant? To assess this, the oxygenation level within tissues was used as a measure. The results showed that oxygen levels stayed within a clinically acceptable range during massage.[56,71]

A final piece of information worth noting is a comment by Tiffany Field, director of the Touch Research Institute, one of the scientists responsible for many of the recent studies of premature infants. She states with regard to pressure, "... most studies that preceded ours were ineffective, most likely because they used light stroking, which was like a tickle stimulus and was aversive to the in-

TABLE 2-1 GENERAL HOSPITAL POPULATION

Author/Year	Sample	Intervention	Key Variables	Results
Smith & Stallings[19] (1996)	■ 113 hospitalized pts. (organ transplant, ortho/rehab & neuroscience unit)	■ Control—standard care ■ Exper.—30–40 min. session, up to 2 M/wk. for 2 wks. ■ Admin. By MTh	■ Pain ■ Anxiety ■ Sleep ■ Rest ■ Length of stay	■ Decreased pain & anxiety ■ Improved rest & sleep ■ No diff. in length of stay
Smith Stallings, Mariner, et al.[64] (1999)	■ 113 hospitalized pts. (organ transplant, ortho/rehab & neuroscience unit)	■ Control—standard care ■ Exper.—30–40 min session up to 2 M/wk for 2 wks.	■ Physical functioning ■ Psychological support ■ Enhanced healing	■ 98% increased relaxation ■ 93% increased sense of well-being ■ 88% positive mood change ■ 71% increased energy ■ 73% felt like a participant in Tx ■ 80% more able to move
Dunning & James[6] (2001)	■ 11 pts. w/impaired function (9 women, 2 men) ■ Age range 50–90 ■ No control	■ Each pt. received at least 3 hand or foot M ■ Essential oils lavender, bergamot, sweet orange, marjoram. 1–3% dilution	■ Pain ■ Anxiety ■ Skin condition ■ Joint flexibility	■ Signif. less pain & anxiety ■ Improved skin condition ■ No change in joint flexibility
Holland & Porkorny[13] (2001)	■ 24 rehab hosp. pts ■ Mean age 71.8 ■ Age range 52–88 ■ No control	■ Slow-stroke back M for 3 consecutive days	■ Vital signs (BP, HR, RR) ■ Psychological state	■ Decrease in SBP & DBP each day ■ Decrease in HR & RR days 1 & 3 ■ No psychological change

fants. We used deeper pressure because the infants behaved as if they preferred deeper pressure."[73]

> . . . [O]ur \bodie]s are wired to be affected by human touch from the minute we are born. I think the best scientists need to be strapped to this rocket. They need to figure out how does touch affect the newborn, the toddler, the adolescent, the adult— and the aged who are dying, often in a horrendous state of physical abandonment. . . .
>
> . . . [M]assage has a very unique role to play in our understanding of the human condition and in healing practices. I think that there is real science there, not just compassion. They are not mutually exclusive.[74]
>
> —David Eisenberg, MD,
> Director of The Center for Alternative Medicine
> Research and Professor of Medicine
> at Harvard Medical School[74]
> Cambridge, Massachusetts

INTENSIVE CARE

What is obvious when first looking at the ICU studies is that the interventions are of much shorter duration, ranging from 1 to 15 minutes, and the main focus is on physiological variables, such as heart rate, blood pressure, and respiration rate (Table 2-3). With other patient populations, these variables are used with an eye toward measuring relaxation. In the critical care arena, they often are used to measure the level of demand massage places on the body. Two studies with heart attack patients found that a short back rub had no detrimental effect.[(Searle)51,53] However, the data from another group of cardiac patients, nine men who were post–coronary bypass, showed that a 10-minute massage may be overstimulating within 48 hours of surgery.[51(Grimes)] Tyler[62] and Lewis[63] also reported SVO_2 findings that may indicate a slight level of demand on the critically ill person. As was stated earlier in the chapter, these findings suggest that the level of demand is clinically acceptable for those who are hemodynamically stable.

Positioning patients on their side may be a contributing factor on the level of demand. Right side-lying, especially when combined with a 5-minute restabilizing period before starting the massage, appeared to be the least stimulating and therefore least demanding.[63] Greater study of the relationship between massage and positioning is warranted.

MATERNITY

This population is vastly understudied. Only two investigations were found that met the inclusion criteria.[4,9] Both looked at the benefits of massage on women in labor and delivery, finding a decrease in pain and anxiety. One of

TABLE 2-2 INFANTS

Author/Year	Sample	Intervention	Key Variables	Results
Solkoff, Yaffe, Weintraub, et al. [69] (1969)	■ 10 premature infants ■ Gest. age unreported	■ 5-min., stroking daily for 10 days	■ Wt. gain ■ Activity level	■ Increased wt. gain & activity level
Solkoff & Matuszak[72] (1975)	■ 11 preterm infants ■ Gest. age 28–37 wks.	■ 7.5-min. stroking every 8 h daily for 10 days	■ Behavioral assessment	■ More rapid habituation ■ Increased alertness ■ Improved body tonus ■ More consolable
White & Lababara[70] (1976)	■ 12 preterm infants ■ <36 wks. ■ 2–11 days old	■ M during 4 consecutive h daily for 10 days	■ Wt. gain	■ Increased wt. gain ■ Increased intake of formula ■ Fewer feedings
Field, Schanberg, Scafidi, et al.[37] (1986)	■ 40 premedically stable preterm infants randomized to 2 groups ■ Avg. gest. age 31 wks. ■ All subjects in isolates	■ Control—standard care ■ M—three 15-min. sessions during 3 consecutive h for 10 week days ■ M—holding, stroking w/some pressure, 6 passive flexion/ extension movements	■ Wt. gain ■ Caloric intake ■ Brazelton Scale (BNBAS) ■ Sleep ■ Vital signs ■ Length of stay	■ 47% greater wt. gain/day ■ More active & awake ■ Higher scores on BNBAS ■ Length of stay 6 fewer days ■ Caloric intake— nonsignif. diff.
Morrow, Field, Scafidi[71] (1991)	■ 47 preterm infants randomized to 2 groups ■ 36 weeks ■ Medically stable	■ M—15-min. period during 3 consecutive h daily for 10 days	■ Comparison of transcutaneous oxygen tension during a heelstick procedure & M (O_2 tension is the level of O_2 in tissues)	■ Transcutaneous blood gas pressure higher w/M ■ O_2 tension dropped signif. during heelstick (poor outcome) ■ O_2 tension dropped much less during M (good outcome) ■ M does not appear to have medically compromising effect on O_2 tension
Scafidi & Field[68] (1993)	■ 93 preterm infants (50 massage, 43 control) ■ Mean gest. age 30 wks. ■ Mean ICU duration 15 days	■ See Field, Schanberg, Scafidi 1986	■ Wt. gain ■ Which infants would benefit most from M	■ M showed greater wt. gain ■ Infants who had experienced the following before study showed greatest benefit: 1) increased caloric intake 2) longer NICU stay 3) greatest complications
Wheeden, Scafidi, Field, et al.[54] (1990)	■ 30 med. stable preterm cocaine-exposed infants, randomized to 2 groups ■ Gest. age <37 wks.	■ See Field, Schanberg, Scafidi 1986	■ Wt. gain ■ Vital signs ■ Caloric intake ■ BNBAS	■ Postnatal complications lessened for both groups ■ M had fewer complications ■ M 28% greater wt. gain/day, better motor scores, fewer stress behaviors ■ Vital signs, except heart beat—nonsignif. diff. ■ Caloric intake— nonsignif. diff.

(continued)

TABLE 2-2 INFANTS *(Continued)*				
Author/Year	**Sample**	**Intervention**	**Key Variables**	**Results**
Scafidi, Field, Schanberg, et al.[38] (1990)	■ 40 med. stable preterm infants randomized to 2 groups, massage & control ■ Gest. age 36 wks.	■ See Field, Schanberg, Scafidi 1986	■ Wt. gain ■ Lenth of stay ■ BNBAS	■ 21% greater wt. gain/day ■ superior on BNBAS habituation cluster ■ Length of stay 5 fewer days
Acolet, Modi, Giannakoulopoulos, et al.[56] (1993)	■ 11 med. stable preterm infants—all boys ■ Gest. age 23–34 wks. ■ Mean age 29 wks. ■ No control	■ Gentle stroking to trunk & limbs using arachis oil ■ Approx. 20 min. ■ Admin. by neonatal nurse	■ Adrenaline & noradrenaline ■ Cortisol ■ Skin temp. ■ Oxygenation	■ Decreased cortisol level ■ No change in adrenaline/noradrenaline ■ Slight decrease in skin temp. ■ No change in oxygen requirement
Scafidi & Field[67] (1996)	■ 28 med. stable infants exposed to HIV randomized to 2 groups ■ Avg. gest. age 39 wks.	■ See Field, Schanberg, Scafidi 1986	■ Wt. gain ■ BNBAS	■ Signif. wt. gain ■ Improvement in most BNBAS scores, incl. stress behaviors & excitability ■ Control remained the same or declined
Ferber, Kuint Weller, et al.[65] (2002)	■ 57 healthy, preterm infants randomized to 3 groups ■ All in isolettes ■ Control (N = 19)— standard care ■ Mothers gave M (N = 21) ■ Female staff gave M (N = 17)	■ M given for 15 min. during 3 consecutive h for 10 days ■ Moderate pressure strokes to entire body except chest & stomach	■ Wt. gain ■ Caloric intake	■ Both M groups showed signif. increase in wt. gain ■ Caloric intake process more efficient ■ Mothers able to achieve same results as professionals

the projects also reported a shorter labor and hospital stay (Table 2-4).[9]

ONCOLOGY

The impact of massage on cancer's side effects and treatments has received the most scrutiny. Three common symptoms are clearly improved by massage: anxiety, pain, and nausea. Other variables have not yet been studied enough to draw any conclusions (Table 2-5).

PROCEDURAL INTERVENTIONS

Invasive or painful procedures are a common part of hospital life. Massage may eventually prove to ease the discomfort of these events, but little systematic study has been done so far. The studies categorized here are completely unrelated. Two investigations show the positive influence of massage before debridement.[8,76] Two others looked at the effects of massage given before heart catheterization.[17,18] One found no effect;[17] the other resulted in lower systolic blood pressure.[18] Parke and Kinsella determined that abdominal massage at the time of an epidural block does not quicken the onset of analgesia given to women in labor (Table 2-6).[77]

PSYCHIATRIC

A long-standing taboo against touching mentally ill patients has no doubt caused the psychiatric community to be hesitant about incorporating massage into the care of their patients. Quite naturally then, there is a lack of research in this area. The two projects reported here, one with elderly psychiatric patients and another with adolescents, found massage to be promising (Table 2-7).[10,23]

SURGERY

No clear patterns emerge from an inspection of this group of studies. Psychological variables such as anxiety are generally improved or show a trend toward improvement,[11,14,16,22] as does pain.[11,16,30,32,33,35] Nausea has received little examination except with the use of wristbands. Autonomic variables such as blood pressure and heart rate showed little difference when compared to the control groups.[11,14,16,22,30] Certainly future research will establish some benefits of massage for surgical patients, but at this time no strong statements can be made (Table 2-8).

TABLE 2-3 ICU				
Author/Year	**Sample**	**Intervention**	**Key Variables**	**Results**
Bauer Dracup[53] (1987)	■ 25 ICU pts. w/ acute myocardial infarction (18 men, 7 women) ■ Mean age 55.6 ■ No control	■ 6-min. back massage using effleurage ■ Left side-lying position ■ Given by nurse	■ Vital signs (HR & BP) ■ Electromyogram (EMG) ■ Skin temp.	■ No signif. change in HR, BP, EMG, or skin temp. ■ No detrimental hemodynamic effect from M ■ Pts. reported M felt good
Searle (from Labyak & Metzger)[55] (1987)	■ 5 males ■ Post–myocardial infarction	■ 10-min. effleurage to back	■ Systolic & diastolic BP ■ Heart rate ■ Respiration rate	■ BP dropped 6% SBP, 13.5% from baseline to 10 after M ■ HR declined 2% at 3 min. & continued to fall ■ RR dropped immed. & remained below baseline ■ No detrimental effects
Grimes (from Labyak & Metzger)[55] (1988)	■ 9 males ■ W/in 48 h postop. coronary artery bypass (CAB6) ■ Mean age 56 ■ Age range 44–75	■ 10-min. effleurage to back	■ Systolic & diastolic BP ■ Heart rate ■ Respiration rate	■ Peak rise in SBP at 3 min. (23.6%) and in DBP at 7 min. (12.9%) ■ SBP remained above baseline until 10 min. post M ■ HR rose slightly up to 3 min., then declined ■ RR declined from the start ■ M may overstimulate CAB pts. w/in 48 h postop
Tyler, Winslow, Clark, et al.[62] (1990)	■ 173 critically ill subjects (117 men, 56 women) ■ Mean age 61 ■ Age range 19–88	■ Subjects positioned supine to obtain a baseline HR and mixed venous oxygen saturation (SVO$_2$) level, then turned to side-lying for 15 min. ■ X1-min. back rub was given by RN	■ Venous oxygen saturation ■ Heart rate	■ Mean SVO$_2$ down slightly immed. after backrub, returned to baseline within 4 min. ■ Mean HR up slightly after back rub & remained higher than baseline after 4 min ■ M is slightly demanding
Dunn, Sleep, Collett[5] (1995)	■ 122 gen. intensive care pts. were randomly assigned to one of 3 groups: (N = 43) massage (N = 41) aroma therapy (N = 38) rest ■ Age range 2–92	■ M—light effl. 15–30 min. to available areas of the body ■ Aromatherapy M—same as M group using a 1% concentration of lavender in the lubricant ■ Undisturbed rest—minimum of 30 min. except for essential nursing care ■ 1–3 sessions in 5 days	■ Systolic & diastolic BP ■ HR & rhythm ■ RR ■ Anxiety ■ Mood ■ Coping ability	■ No statistically signif. differences in physiological variables ■ Aromatherapy group had signifi. improvement in mood & anxiety, although the effect was not sustained or cumulative
Lewis, Nichols, Mackey, et al.[63] (1997)	■ 57 male pts. in a surgical ICU were randomly assigned to 2 groups ■ Mean age 60.9 ■ Postop. cardiac	■ Group 1 was placed in side-lying position & immed. given a 1-min. back rub ■ Group 2 was placed in side-lying position for 5 min. before the 1-min. back rub ■ Admin. by RN ■ Subjects were randomly assigned to a right or left lateral position	■ SVO$_2$	■ Position & timing of back rub had significant effects on SVO$_2$ ■ L side-lying decreased O$_2$ saturation more than R side-lying ■ 2 consecutive interventions (position change & back rub) caused greater decrease in SVO$_2$ than delayed back rub

(continued)

TABLE 2-3 ICU *(Continued)*

Author/Year	Sample	Intervention	Key Variables	Results
Richards[57] (1998)	■ 69 male cardiac pts. randomly assigned to 3 groups ■ Age range 55–79	■ Group 1 (N = 24) received 6-min. back M from RN ■ Group 2 (N = 28) listened to 7.5-min relaxation tape at bedtime ■ 3 (N = 17) received standard nursing care ■ R side-lying	■ Sleep	■ M group experienced higher quality & quantity of sleep, slept 1 h longer than the control group ■ Nonsignif. trend toward increased sleep efficiency
Doering, Fieguth, Steuernagel, et al.[75] (1999)	■ 8 ICU pts. (3 heart trans., 3 lung trans., 2 coronary artery bypasses) ■ Mean age 53.6 ■ On mechanical ventilation	■ Vibratory M 8–10 vib./sec ■ 15 min., 7.5 min. on each side of thorax ■ Admin. by MTh ■ Supine positioning	■ Pulmonary functions ■ Cerebral blood flow velocity	■ Improvement in tidal volume & O_2 saturation (positive outcome) ■ Decrease in central venous pressure & pulmonary vessel resistance (positive outcome) ■ No change in cerebral blood flow velocity ■ No signif. change in cerebral blood flow velocity during massage ■ Increased mean tidal volume ■ Increased percutaneous oxygen saturation ■ Decreased central venous pressure ■ Decreased pulmonary vessel resistance ■ 10 min. M pulmonary resistance decreased

TABLE 2-4 MATERNITY

Author/Year	Sample	Intervention	Key Variables	Results
Field, Hernandez-Reif, Taylor, et al.[9] (1997)	■ 28 women randomly assigned to 2 groups ■ Mean age 29.7 ■ Recruited from Lamaze classes	■ Control—women & partners engaged in techniques learned in class ■ Exper.—partner gave 20-min. M beginning at 3–5 cm. dilation ■ Repeated M every h for 5 h	■ Mood ■ Stress level ■ Pain ■ Touch sensitivity ■ Length of labor ■ Length of stay ■ Anxiety	■ M group less depression, stress, labor pain, touch sensitivity, & anxiety ■ Shorter labor & hosp. stay
Chang, Wang, Chen[4] (2002)	■ 60 women, first pregnancy, randomly placed in 2 groups	■ Control—standard Tx ■ Exper.—30 min. at start of each of the 3 phases of labor ■ Abd. M, sacral pressure, shoulder/back petrissage ■ Admin. by RN researcher & partner	■ Pain ■ Anxiety	■ Increased pain & anxiety in both groups as labor progressed ■ M group signif. less pain at each stage of labor & less anxiety in early stage ■ 87% of M group reported M was helpful

TABLE 2-5 ONCOLOGY

Author/Year	Sample	Intervention	Key Variables	Results
Scott, Donahue, Mastrovito, et al.[42] (1983)	■ 10 women undergoing highly emetic chemotherapy for ovarian carcinoma ■ Age range 42–67 ■ No control (data compared to known clinical responses)	■ Pts. were coached in progressive relaxation and guided imagery techniques ■ M consisted of slow-stroke back M for 3 min.	■ Nausea ■ Vomiting	■ Shorter duration of emetic ressponse ■ Reduced frequency of vomiting ■ Decreased intensity ■ Reduced volume of emesis
Dalton, Toomey, Workman[29] (1988)	■ 16 subjects divided into 3 groups	■ Pts. were instructed to use the following interventions as needed: ■ A—progressive muscle relaxation (PMR) ■ B—PMR plus use of distraction (i.e. music) & M were demonstated ■ C—standard Tx	■ Pain	■ Groups A & B had decrease in pain ■ No difference in relief between A & B ■ Group C had highest pain levels
Weinrich & Weinrich[34] (1990)	■ 28 hosp. CA pts. (18 men, 10 women) randomized to 2 groups ■ Avg. age 61.5, range 36–78	■ Control—10 min. visit from researcher ■ Exper.—10 min. back M	■ Pain	■ Males had signif. drop in pain ■ Women no change
Ferrell-Tory & Glick[7] (1993)	■ 9 male CA pts. experiencing pain ■ Age range 23–77 ■ No control	■ 30-min. effl. to back, neck, feet	■ Pain ■ Anxiety ■ Vital signs (HR, RR, BP)	■ Signif. drop in pain & anxiety ■ HR & BP trend toward lower ■ Only RR dropped signif.
Tope, Hann, Pinkson[59] (1994)	■ 104 CA inpatients ■ No control	■ Sessions limited to 30 min. Common sites: back, shoulders, neck, feet: Effl. petri., & acupressure ■ Pts. received 2 or more M ■ Admin. by LPN/CMT	■ Mood ■ Tension ■ Comfort ■ Sense of isolation	■ 99% mentioned relaxation or release of muscle tension ■ 35% improved mood ■ 22% assistance in symptom management ■ 15% felt less isolation
Ahles, Tope, Pinkson, et al.[2] (1999)	■ 35 bone marrow transplant pts. randomized to 2 groups ■ Control (N = 18) ■ Exper. (N = 16)	■ Control group—standard care ■ Exper.—20-min. M of shoulders, head & face w/effl., petri, & acupressure ■ Up to 9 massages ■ Admin. by LPN/CMT	■ Anxiety ■ Depression ■ Fatigue ■ Nausea ■ Vital signs (HR, RR, BP) ■ Use of meds (pain, anxiety, antiemetic)	■ M group greater reduction in distress, fatigue, nausea, & anxiety early on ■ Less anxiety at mid-Tx ■ Less fatigue at predischarge ■ Lower DBP ■ No difference in med. use or overall psych. symptoms
Grealish, Lomasney, Whiteman[31] (2000)	■ 87 hosp. pts. (52 women, 35 men) ■ Served as own control ■ Primary CA sites varied ■ Age range 18–88, median age 58 ■ Control—remained in bed doing quiet activity	■ Exper.—10-min, foot M 3 consecutive evenings ■ Admin. by RN	■ Pain ■ Nausea ■ Relaxation ■ HR	■ Signif. drop in pain ■ Nausea reduced but not signif. ■ Relaxation increased signif. ■ HR dropped in both groups

(continued)

TABLE 2-5 ONCOLOGY *(Continued)*

Author/Year	Sample	Intervention	Key Variables	Results
Stephenson, Weinrich, Tavakoli[21] (2000)	■ 23 hosp. pts. with BR or lung CA ■ Served as own control ■ Median age 68.7	■ Control—no intervention ■ Exper.—10-min. reflexology session to feet ■ Admin. by a certified reflexologist	■ Anxiety ■ Pain	■ Statistically signif. decrease in anxiety ■ BR CA pts. had signif. drop in pain ■ Lung CA data could not be calculated
Hodgson[61] (2000)	■ 12 pts. randomly placed in reflexology group or placebo reflexology group	■ Placebo received gentle foot M ■ Exper. group reflexology ■ Each group got three 40-min. sessions over 5 days	■ QoL	■ All pts. reported some comfort ■ 33% of placebo had increase in QoL ■ 100% of reflexology group had increase in QoL ■ Differences between groups was statistically signif.
Dibble, Chapman, Mack, et al.[41] (2000)	■ 17 women rnadomized to 2 groups ■ _received standard Tx, _got acupressure training plus standard Tx	■ Pts. in exper. group receive acupressure training—P6 & ST 36 ■ The points were held each morning for up to 3 min. & during the day as needed during the chemo cycle (usually 21–28 days)	■ Nausea experience ■ Nausea intensity	■ Acupressure group less intensity and experience of nausea the first 10 days of the chemo cycle
Hemphill, Kemp[12] (2000)	■ 41 male CA pts. undergoing chemo	■ Control (N = 21)—20-min. verbal interaction w/nurse ■ Exper. (N = 20)—20-min. M 3x during a 1 wk. period ■ Admin. by nurse MTh	■ Pain ■ Sleep ■ Symptom distress ■ Anxiety	■ M—signif. improvement in sleep symptom distress, & pain ■ Anxiety improved in both groups
Cawthrone, Boyle[3] (2001)	■ 49 CA pts. ■ Variety of primary tumors	■ M on 2 consecutive evenings ■ Admin. by nurse MTh	■ Pain ■ Anxiety ■ Nausea ■ Sleep	■ Decrease in pain, anxiety, & nausea
Billhult Dahlberg[60] (2001)	■ 8 female CA pts. receive M for 10 consecutive days ■ Ages 54–80 ■ 75% had BR CA	■ Light stroking for 20 min. of either hand/forearm or foot/lower leg ■ Admin. to some by healthcare workers with 1-day training; others received from one of the authors	■ Qualitative experience of the essential meaning of massage in cancer care	■ M provided: - Meaningful relief from suffering - Positive relations w/ staff - Experience of being special - Feeling of greater strength - Balance between autonomy & dependence

(continued)

TABLE 2-5 ONCOLOGY (Continued)

Author/Year	Sample	Intervention	Key Variables	Results
Lively, Black, Holiday-Goodman, et al.[36] (2002)	■ 31 women with breast & ovarian CA undergoing high-dose chemo & peripheral blood stem cell transplant ■ Control N = 4 ■ Massage N = 7 ■ Average age 45.5	■ Control—standard Tx ■ Exper.—20–30-min. sessions ■ M to head with focus on SCM & cranial sacral techniques; stillpoint, frontal lift, spheno-basilar compression-decompression, temporal earl pull ■ Swedish M to leg & thigh ■ Admin. by LMT	■ Nausea/vomiting ■ Length of stay ■ TPN use ■ Cost-effectiveness	■ Decreased nausea & TPN use ■ Length of stay 3 fewer days ■ Total cost savings per pt. $2,850
Smith, Kemp, Hemphill, et al.[20] (2002)	■ 41 pts. randomly placed in a control (N = 20) or massage (N = 20) group ■ 95% males ■ Mean age 64	■ Control—nurse visit ■ Exper.—15–30-min. light eff. and petris. ■ Admin. by nurse certified in hospital-based M	■ Pain ■ Sleep ■ Symptom distress ■ Anxiety	■ Mean scores improved for all 4 variables ■ In M group: pain, sleep and symptom distress statistically signif. improvement ■ Anxiety improved in control ■ Sleep deteriorated in control
Lawvere[13] (2002)	■ 7 ovarian CA pts. hospitalized for chemo ■ Mean age 51 ■ Randomized crossover trial (pts. served as own control)	■ Control—30-min. rest ■ Exper.—30-min. Swedish ■ Admin. by MTh	■ Anxiety ■ Depression ■ Pain	■ Anxiety reduction statistically signif. ■ Pain & depression dropped insignif.
Smith, Reeder, Daniel, et al.[24] (2003)	■ 89 bone marrow transplant pts. (22 men, 60 women) ■ Randomized to 3 groups ■ Age range 18–70	■ Group 1 (N=25) 30 min. friendly visit (FV) by volunteer ■ Group 2 (N=28) 30 min. Therapeutic Touch (TT) by RN	■ Time of Engraftment ■ Complications (pain, food intake, CNS/neurological, heart, lung, liver, G1, G4, skin, circulation) ■ Pt perception of benefits	■ No diff. in engraftment rate ■ M group decrease on CNS/neurological complications only (disorientation, sleep, personality changes, convulsions, malaise, anxiety, depression, speech impairments) ■ Pt perception of benefits higher for MT v. FV ■ M & TT higher on comfort rating v. FV
Toth, Kahn, Walton, et al.[25] (2003)	■ 7 pts w/ Dx of metastic CA ■ Not randomized, convenience sample ■ Age range 52–82	■ Individualized M 10–6 min. (avg. 34 min.) ■ Pt offered M every day Pt received 1–9 massages (avg. 3.83)	■ Pain ■ Anxiety ■ Alertness level	■ Decrease in pain ■ Increase in anxiety ■ Increase in alertness level

TABLE 2-6 PROCEDURAL EFFECTS

Author/Year	Sample	Intervention	Key Variables	Results
Parke, Kinsella[77] (1996)	■ 15 women in labor (9 massage, 6 control) ■ Requested epidural analgesia	■ Control—standard care ■ Exper.—partner gave 15-min. gentle M around the umbilicus as soon as analgesia was injected	■ Effect of abdominal M on onset of epidural block & relief of pain	■ Abdominal M does not enhance the effect of the epidural ■ No signif. difference between groups
Field, Peck, Krugman, et al.[8] (1998)	■ 28 adult burn pts. randomly assigned to 2 groups ■ Avg. burn size 10% of body surface area	■ Control—standard care ■ Exper.—20-min. stroking w/ moderate pressure 1×/day for a wk. just before AM debridement	■ Anxiety ■ Behavior observation ■ Mood (depression, anger, vigor) ■ Pulse ■ Pain ■ Cortisol	■ Immed. effects: lower anxiety & cortisol level ■ Improved behavior ratings (except cooperation) ■ Pulse decrease for both groups ■ Long-term effects: lower pain rating, resting pulse, & cortisol level ■ Improved mood & behavior ratings
Hernandez-Reif, Field, Largie, et al.[76] (2001)	■ 24 children hospitalized for severe burns randomized to 2 groups	■ Control—standard dressing care ■ Exper—15 min. If prior to dressing change	■ Distress behaviors	■ M lessened distress behaviors ■ Control group had greater torso movement, crying, grimacing, & reaching out
Okvat, Oz, Ting. et al.[17] (2002)	■ 78 subjects (59 men, 19 women) randomized to 2 groups ■ Avg. age 60	■ Control—10 min. of quiet time w/ MTh ■ Exper.—10 min. of M (4 min to R side, 4 min. to L side, 1 min. to scalp) ■ Admin. before procedure by MTh	■ Feasibility of M before procedure ■ Anxiety ■ Pain ■ Vital signs (BP, HR, RR)	■ No signif. difference in pain, anxiety, or vital signs
McNamara, Burnham, Smith, et al.[18] (2003)	■ 46 subjects (34 men, 12 women) randomized to 2 groups ■ Admitted for diagnostic heart catheterization ■ Mean age 64.9 yrs	■ Contro—standard care ■ Exper.—20 min. back M (effl. & petri.) prior to procedure ■ Side-lying position	■ Vital signs (HR, BP, RR) ■ HR variability ■ Skin temp ■ Pain ■ Psychologic state	■ M decreased SBP ■ No Statistically signif. diff. beteen groups except SBP

TABLE 2-7 PSYCHIATRIC

Author/Year	Sample	Intervention	Key Variables	Results
Thomas[23] (1989)	■ 9 elderly psychiatric pts. placed in 3 groups ■ 14 nurses	■ Group 1—1-h foot M & talk ■ Group 2—1-h talk ■ Group 3—No intervention	■ Anxiety ■ Nurses' attitudes	■ Before study nurses felt M to be useless ■ After study 12 nurses felt M to be useful
Field, Morrow, Valdeon, et al.[20] (1992)	■ 72 children & adolescents (40 boys, 32 girls) ■ 36 diagnosed w/ adjustment disorder ■ 36 diagnosed w/ depression/dysthymic disorder ■ Exper. (N = 52), control (N = 20) ■ Mean age 13 ■ Age range 7–18	■ M group received 30-min. back M for 5 days ■ Admin. by psychology students trained in the M protocol ■ Control group watched relaxing video & tapes	■ Depression ■ Anxiety ■ Behavioral observations ■ Pulse ■ Cortisol ■ Nighttime sleep	■ M group decreased depression, anxiety, & cortisol level ■ Behavior was more cooperative & nighttime sleep increased ■ Pulse decreased for both groups

TABLE 2-8 SURGERY

Author/Year	Sample	Intervention	Key Variables	Results
Stevenson[22] (1994)	■ 100 post cardiac surgery pts. randomized to 4 groups	■ Group 1—standard care ■ Group 2—20-min. general conversation w/ nurse ■ Group 3—20-min. plain oil Swedish foot M ■ Group 4—20-min. foot M using neroli essential oil, 2.5% dilution ■ Performed by specially trained nurses on day 1 postsurgery	■ Vital signs (HR, RR, BP) ■ Psychological variables (anxiety, tension, calm, rest, relaxation, pain)	■ Immed. effect in groups 3 & 4 on RR only, no lasting difference ■ Groups 3 & 4 signif. better psychological results ■ Groups 4 signif. reduction in anxiety compared to group 3 at day 5
Menard[16] (1995)	■ 30 women randomized to 2 groups ■ Posthysterectomy	■ Control—standard care ■ Exper.—45-min. M beginning 1st day postsurgery continuing throughout ■ Swedish M & some acupressure ■ Admin. by MTh	■ Cortisol level ■ Systolic BP ■ Pain ■ Anxiety ■ Depression ■ Use of pain meds ■ Sleep ■ Bowel function ■ Length of stay	■ Statistical signif. not reached for most variables, but a trend toward improvement in: - Cortisol level - Systolic BP - Anxiety & depression - Pain med use (decreased) - Bowel function - Sleep - Length of stay (half day less, statistically insignif.) ■ During 4 wk. follow-up, Tx group had signif. fewer visitis to Dr.
Felhendler, Lisander[30] (1996)	■ 40 pts. undergoing knee arthroscopy were randomized to 2 groups, treatment or placebo	■ Placebo—light pressure was given to 15 non-acupoints in the same areas ■ Treatment—stimulation of 12 classic acupoints on the side contralateral to surgery w/firm pressure & a gliding movement across acupoint	■ Pain ■ HR ■ Systolic BP ■ Skin temp. ■ Blood flow	■ Tx group had lower pain scores ■ No signif. changes in autonomic variables
Nixon, Teschendorff, Finney, et al.[33] (1997)	■ 39 pts. admitted for abdominal surgery (18 men, 21 women) ■ Control (N = 20) massage (N = 19)	■ Control—standard care ■ Exper—Swedish M given to body areas of choice for minimum of 2 min., no maximum, 2x/day for 7 days ■ Performed by pt.'s nurse	■ Pain	■ Less pain over a 24 h period
Hulme, Waterman, Hillier[32] (1999)	■ 59 women who underwent laparoscopic sterilization randomized to 2 groups ■ Control (N = 30) ■ Massage (N = 29)	■ Control (N = 30) received only analgesia following surgery ■ Exper. (N = 29) received 5-min. foot M & analgesia ■ M provided by nurse researcher	■ Pain ■ Use of pain meds	■ No signif. difference in analgesia use ■ M group had less pain following surgery
Kim, Cho, Woo, et al.[14] (2001)	■ 59 pts. randomized to 2 groups ■ Mean age 57, age range 20–78	■ Control—standard care ■ Exper. hand M before surgery	■ Anxiety ■ Vital signs (BP & P) ■ Epinephrine norepinephrine, cortisol ■ Blood sugar level ■ Neutrophil & lymphocyte levels	■ Less anxiety ■ No diff. between groups in vital signs ■ Epinephrine, norepinephrine cortisol dropped in M group, increased in control ■ No diff. in blood sugar or blood cell levels

(continued)

TABLE 2-8 SURGERY *(Continued)*

Author/Year	Sample	Intervention	Key Variables	Results
Ming, Kuo, Lin, et al.[49] (2002)	■ 150 postop pts. randomized to 3 equal groups ■ Endoscopic sinus surgery under gen. anesthesia ■ Avg. age 48 ■ Age range 18–79 ■ 59% male, 41% female	■ Group 1 (control)—conversation ■ Group 2—finger acupressure to P6 & H7 for 5 min. 3x starting 1 h before surgery, last Tx 10 h postsurgery ■ Group 3—wristband acupressure	■ Nausea ■ Vomiting	■ Group 1—74% nausea, 42% vomiting w/in 24 h of surgery ■ Group 2—20% had nausea, 4% vomiting ■ Group 3—42% had nausea, 24% vomiting ■ Both acupressure groups showed improvement ■ Finger pressure had greatest improvement
Hattan, King, Griffiths[11] (2002)	■ 25 cardiac surg. pts. (20 men, 50 women) randomized to 3 groups ■ Mean age 63	■ Control (N = 7)—standard care ■ Exper. (Group 1)—guided relaxation group (N = 9) listened to 20-min. relaxation tape ■ Group 2—M group (N = 9) 20-min. foot M by MTh	■ Vital signs (HR, P, RR) ■ Psychological variables (anxiety, tension, calm, rest, relaxation, pain)	■ No diff. in vital signs between groups ■ Both exper. groups improved "calm" variable. M had greater improvement ■ Same pattern occurred w/other psychological variables, but improvement was insignif.
Taylor, Galper, Taylor, et al.[35] (2003)	■ 105 women randomized to 3 groups ■ Laparotomy for removal of possible cancerous lesions	■ Group 1 (control—standard care ■ Group 2—45-min. Swedish M ■ Group 3—20-min. sound vibration therapy ■ Interventions given postop & at same time the next 2 days	■ Sensory pain (physical component) ■ Affective pain (emotional component) ■ Distress	■ No statistically signif. difference between groups ■ M showed a trend toward less pain & distress ■ M was more effective than standard care & vibration therapy

SUMMARY

Firm conclusions are difficult to draw from many of the investigations. Sample sizes often are small, and massage methods, tools of measurement, and research protocols differ. And yet, by including all of the studies that have been systematically conducted, a broader, clearer picture of the state of massage begins to develop.

Six variables—pain, anxiety, length of stay, nausea, cortisol, and sleep—show consistent improvement from the application of massage. However, the number of studies in the length-of-stay, nausea, cortisol, and sleep groups is insufficient to boast loudly about the benefit of massage. There is reason, though, to be optimistic about future results.

The findings regarding depression, vital signs, pressure sores, and use of medications are either inconclusive and/or understudied. The vital signs results are especially weak and do not even show a trend toward efficacy.

An examination by patient population shows that conclusions can be drawn for only oncology patients and preterm infants. People with cancer clearly benefit from massage, with a reduction in pain, anxiety, and nausea. Premature babies overwhelmingly show improvement in weight gain and some behavior measurements, so much so that it is surprising that all hospitals do not have massage as standard care for these infants. Aside from these two groups, the research is either murky or insufficient.

The whole picture, however, cannot be found in numbers. In addition to listening to the data, ways must be found to listen to the patient. Many aspects of the massage experience cannot be conveyed into data—hope, for instance, or the feeling of belonging. As Cawley points out in a critique of massage methodology, massage is a subjective experience. Future studies not only must provide consistency in the intervention, but also must record qualitative data in the form of interviews to enable patients' opinions to be sought.[78]

Billhult and Dahlberg have performed such a study with cancer patients.[60] Their systematic use of interviews allowed a richer picture to emerge. Patients expressed a sense of feeling strong as a result of daily massage. They became aware that their body has possibilities. Massage gave them an experience of being important and special and contributed to the development of a positive relationship with the staff. Patients felt a new balance between dependence and autonomy. Granted, this information does not translate into cost savings or symptom management, but it speaks to the whole experience.

Massage educator Tracy Walton points out that "it is important for massage therapists to value research and to acquire basic skills in evaluating its strengths and weaknesses. It is important to become familiar with research results and use them to educate others and to shape our practice. We are health professionals—this is our duty to our clients and our professional and ethical responsibility. But, not every element of the therapeutic relationship submits itself to the rigors of scientific study. Many truths about our work remain hidden from the measurement tools of a randomized, controlled clinical trial. What happens during a massage is true—it doesn't need verification from anyone. It is often unexplainable and magical—but true, nevertheless. In fact, there are many mysterious truths about the healing power of touch, and there are many ways of knowing those truths."

The path for massage professionals wanting to work within mainstream health care is a paradoxical one. They must simultaneously strive toward science and yet never lose sight of the art, they must embrace the clinical but never at the expense of the mystery and magic, and they must maintain wholeness at the same time they are dissecting the massage experience. Much is asked of hospital massage therapists. They are called to be a bridge that connects two different worlds.

TEST YOURSELF

It doesn't take a doctoral degree, a huge grant, or expertise in statistical analysis to be a researcher. If you have a specific question, a data-collection tool, and a primitive methodology, you can systematically explore the effects of massage.

1. Make a list of five questions about the effects of massage that intrigue you. Make them very specific. This is one of the keys to a successful start. For instance: What is the effect of a 20-minute back massage on fatigue of patients hospitalized for congestive heart failure?

2. Pick one of those questions, and create a data-collection tool. For instance, a 5-point Likert Scale is easy to create and use.

1	2	3	4	5
No fatigue				High fatigue

3. How would you administer the intervention and perform the data collection?

4. Use an easy method of analysis such as mathematical averaging to see some of what the data are telling you.

REFERENCES

1. Kahn J. Research Matters. Massage Mag 2001;92:65–69.
2. Ahles TA, Tope DM, Pinkson B, et al. Massage Therapy for Patients Undergoing Autologous Bone Marrow Transplantation. J Pain Symptom Manage 1999;18(3):157–163.
3. Cawthorne L, Boyle DA. Massage As Cancer Nursing Therapeutic: Impact on Symptom Distress During Hospitalization. (Abstract of podium session, 2001 Oncology Nursing Society 26th Annual Congress, San Diego, CA.) Oncol Nurs Forum 2001;28(2):324–325.
4. Chang MY, Wang SY, Chen CH. Effects of Massage on Pain and Anxiety During: A Randomized Controlled Trial in Taiwan. J Adv Nurs 2002;38(1):68–73.
5. Dunn C, Sleep J, Collett D. Sensing an Improvement: An Experimental Study to Evaluate the Use of Aromatherapy, Massage and Periods of Rest in an Intensive Care Unit. J Adv Nurs 1995;21:34–40.
6. Dunning T, James K. Complementary Therapies in Action—Education and Outcomes. Complement Ther Nurs Midwifery 2001;7:188–195.
7. Ferrell-Torry AT, Glick OJ. The Use of Therapeutic Massage As a Nursing Intervention to Modify Anxiety and the Perception of Cancer Pain. Cancer Nurs 1993;16: 93–101.
8. Field T, Peck M, Krugman S, et al. Burn Injuries Benefit From Massage Therapy. J Burn Care Rehabil 1998; 19:241–244.
9. Field T, Hernandez-Reif M, Taylor S, et al. Labor Pain Is Reduced by Massage Therapy. J Psychosom Obstet Gynaecol 1997;18:286–291.
10. Field T, Morrow C, Valdeon C, et al. Massage Reduces Anxiety in Child and Adolescent Psychiatric Patients. J Am Acad Child Adolesc Psychiatry 1992;31(1):125–131.
11. Hattan J, King L, Griffiths P. The Impact of Foot Massage and Guided Relaxation Following Cardiac Surgery: A Randomized Controlled Trial. J Adv Nurs 2002;37(2):199–207.
12. Hemphill L, Kemp J. Implementing a Therapeutic Massage Program in a Tertiary and Ambulatory Care VA Setting. Nurs Clin North Am 2000;35(2):489–497.
13. Holland B, Porkorny ME. Slow Stroke Back Massage: Its Effect on Patients in a Rehabilitation Setting. Rehabil Nurs 2001;26(5):182–186.
14. Kim MS, Cho KS, Woo HM, et al. Effects of Hand Massage on Anxiety in Cataract Surgery Using Local Anesthesia. J Cataract Refract Surg 2001;27:884–890.
15. Lawvere S. The Effect of Massage Therapy in Ovarian Cancer Patients in Massage Therapy: The Evidence for Practice. St. Louis, MO: Mosby/Harcourt, 2002.
16. Menard M. The Effect of Therapeutic Massage on Post-Surgical Outcomes. Doctoral dissertation, University of Virginia, 1995.
17. Okvat HA, Oz MC, Ting W, et al. Massage Therapy for Patients Undergoing Cardiac Catheterization. Altern Ther Health Med 2002;8:68–75.

18. McNamara ME, Burnham DC, Smith C, et al. The Effects of Back Massage Before Diagnostic Heart Catheterization. Altern Ther Health Med 2003;9:50–57.

19. Smith MC, Stallings MA. Impact of Therapeutic Massage on Quality and Cost Indicators. Community Nurse Res 1996;229:224.

20. Smith MC, Kemp J, Hemphill L, et al. Outcomes of Therapeutic Massage for Hospitalized Cancer Patients. J Nurs Scholarsh 2002;34:257–262.

21. Stephenson NL, Weinrich SP, Tavakoli AS. The Effects of Foot Reflexology on Anxiety and Pain in Patients With Breast and Lung Cancer. Oncol Nurs Forum 2000;27:67–72.

22. Stevensen CJ. The Psychological Effects of Aromatherapy Massage Following Cardiac Surgery. Complement Ther Med 1994;2:27–35.

23. Thomas M. Fancy Footwork. Nurs Times 1989;85:42–44.

24. Smith MC, Reeder F, Daniel L, et al. Outcomes of Touch Therapies During Bone Marrow Transplant. Altern Ther Health Med 2003;9:40–48.

25. Toth M, Kahn J, Walton T, et al. Therapeutic Massage Intervention for Hospitalized Patients With Cancer. Altern Complement Ther June 2003:117–124.

26. Howard L. Integrative Approach Can Enhance Healing Capacity. Oncologistics Mag First Quarter 2003:12–14.

27. Volicer BJ, Burns MW. Preexisting Correlates of Hospital Stress. Nurs Res 1977;26:408–415.

28. Dorrepaal KL, Aaronson NK, Van Dam FS. Pain Experience and Pain Management Among Hospitalized Cancer Patients. Cancer 1989;63:593–598.

29. Dalton J, Toomey T, Workman M. Pain Relief for Cancer Patients. Cancer Nurs 1988;11:322–328.

30. Felhendler D, Lisander B. Pressure on Acupoints Decreases Postoperative Pain. Clin J Pain 1996;12:326–329.

31. Grealish L, Lomasney A, Whiteman B. Foot Massage. A Nursing Intervention to Modify the Distressing Symptoms of Pain and Nausea in Patients Hospitalized With Cancer. Cancer Nurs 2000;23:237–243.

32. Hulme J, Waterman H, Hillier VF. The Effect of Foot Massage on Patients' Perception of Care Following Laparoscopic Sterilization as Day Case Patients. J Adv Nurs 1999;30:460–468.

33. Nixon M, Teschendorff J, Finney J, et al. Expanding the Nursing Repertoire: The Effect of Massage on Post-operative Pain. Aust J Adv Nurs 1997;14:21–26.

34. Weinrich SP, Weinrich MC. The Effect of Massage on Pain in Cancer Patients. Appl Nurs Res 1990;3:140–145.

35. Taylor AG, Galper DL, Taylor P, et al. Effects of Adjunctive Swedish Massage and Vibration Therapy on Short-Term Postoperative Outcomes: A Randomized, Controlled Trial. J Altern Complement Med 2003;9:77–89.

36. Lively BT, Black CD, Holiday-Goodman M, et al. Massage Therapy for Chemotherapy-Induced Emesis in Massage Therapy: The Evidence for Practice. St. Louis, MO: Mosby/Harcourt, 2002.

37. Field TM, Schanberg SM, Scafidi F, et al. Tactile/Kinesthetic Stimulation Effects on Preterm Neonates. Pediatrics 1986;77:654–658.

38. Scafidi FA, Field TM, Schanberg SM, et al. Massage Stimulates Growth in Preterm Infants: A Replication. Infant Behav Dev 1990;13:167–188.

39. King C. Nonpharmacologic Management of Chemotherapy-Induced Nausea and Vomiting. Oncol Nurs Forum Suppl 1997;24:41–48.

40. Thompson HJ. The Management of Post-operative Nausea and Vomiting. J Adv Nurs 1999;29:1130–1136.

41. Dibble SL, Chapman J, Mack KA, et al. Acupressure for Nausea: Results of a Pilot Study. Oncol Nurs Forum 2000;27:41–47.

42. Scott D, Donahue D, Mastrovito R, et al. The Antiemetic Effect of Clinical Relaxation: Report of an Exploratory Pilot Study. J Psychosoc Oncol 1983;1:71–83.

43. Ferrara-Love R, Sekeres L, Bircher NG. Nonpharmacologic Treatment of Postoperative Nausea. J Perianesth Nurs 1996;11:378–383.

44. Lee A, Done ML. The Use of Nonpharmacologic Techniques to Prevent Postoperative Nausea and Vomiting: A Meta-analysis. Anesth Anal 1999;88:1362–1369.

45. Fan CF, Tanhui E, Joshi S, et al. Acupressure Treatment for Prevention of Postoperative Nausea and Vomiting. Anesth Analg 1997;84:821–825.

46. Stein DJ, Birnbach DJ, Danzer BI, et al. Acupressure Versus Intravenous Metoclopramide to Prevent Nausea and Vomiting During Spinal Anesthesia for Cesarean Section. Anesth Analg 1997;84:342–345.

47. Ho CM, Hseu SS, Tsai SK, et al. Effect of P-6 Acupressure on Prevention of Nausea and Vomiting After Epidural Morphine for Post-Cesarean Section Pain Relief. Acta Anaesthesiol Scand 1996;40:372–375.

48. Alkaissi A, Stalnert M, Kalman S. Effect and Placebo Effect of Acupressure (P6) on Nausea and Vomiting After Outpatient Gynaecological Surgery. Acta Anaesthesiol Scand 1999;43:270–274.

49. Ming JL, Kuo BI, Lin JG, et al. The Efficacy of Acupressure to Prevent Nausea and Vomiting in Post-Operative Patients. J Adv Nurs 2002;39:343–351.

50. Halfens R, Eggink M. Knowledge, Beliefs and Use of Nursing Methods in Preventing Pressure Sores in Dutch Hospitals. Int J Nurs Stud 1995;32:16–26.

51. Buss IC, Halfens R, Abu-Saad HH. The Effectiveness of Massage in Preventing Pressure Sores: A Literature Review. Rehabil Nurs 1997;22:229–242.

52. Anthony D. The Treatment of Decubitus Ulcers: A Century of Misinformation in the Textbooks. J Adv Nurs 1996;24:309–316.

53. Bauer WC, Dracup KA. Physiologic Effects of Back Massage in Patients With Acute Myocardial Infarction. Focus Crit Care Nurs 1987;14:42–46.

54. Wheeden A, Scafidi F, Field T, et al. Massage Effects on Cocaine-Exposed Preterm Neonates. J Dev Behav Pediatr 1990;14:318–322.

55. Labyak SE, Metzger BL. The Effects of Effleurage Backrub on the Physiological Components of Relaxation: A Meta-analysis. Nurs Res 1997;46(1):59–62.

56. Acolet D, Modi N, Giannakoulopoulos X, et al. Changes in Plasma Cortisol and Catecholamine Concentrations in Response to Massage in Preterm Infants. Arch Dis Child 1993;68:29–31.

57. Richards K. Effect of a Back Massage and Relaxation Intervention on Sleep in Critically Ill Patients. Am J Crit Care 1998;7(4):288–298.

58. Ersser S, Wiles A, Taylor H, et al. The Sleep of Older People in Hospital and Nursing Homes. J Clin Nurs 1999;8: 360–368.

59. Tope DM, Hann DM, Pinkson B. Massage Therapy: An Old Intervention Comes of Age. Qual Life Nurs Challenge 1994;3:14–18.

60. Billhult A, Dahlberg K. A Meaningful Relief From Suffering Experiences of Massage in Cancer Care. Cancer Nurs 2001;24(3):180–184.

61. Hodgson H. Does Reflexology Impact on Cancer Patients' Quality of Life? Nurs Stand 2000;14(31):33–38.

62. Tyler DO, Winslow EH, Clark AP, et al. Effects of a 1-Minute Back Rub on Mixed Venous Oxygen Saturation and Heart Rate in Critically Ill Patients. Heart Lung 1990; 19(5):562–565.

63. Lewis P, Nichols E, Mackey G, et al. The Effect of Turning and Backrub on Mixed Venous Oxygen Saturation in Critically Ill Patients. Am J Crit Care 1997;6(2):132–140.

64. Smith MC, Stallings MA, Mariner S, et al. Benefits of Massage Therapy for Hospitalized Patients: A Descriptive and Qualitative Evaluation. Altern Ther Health Med 1999;5(4): 64–71.

65. Ferber SG, Kuint J, Weller A, et al. Massage Therapy by Mothers and Trained Professionals Enhances Weight Gain in Preterm Infants. Early Hum Dev 2002;67(1–2):37–45.

66. Field TM, Scafidi FA, Schanberg S. Massage of Preterm Newborns to Improve Growth and Development. Pediatr Nurs 1987;13:385–387.

67. Scafidi F, Field T. Massage Therapy Improves Behavior in Neonates Born to HIV-Positive Mothers. J Pediatr Psychol 1996;21:889–897.

68. Scafidi FA, Field TM. Factors That Predict Which Preterm Infants Benefit Most From Massage Therapy. J Dev Behav Pediatr 1993;14(3):176–180.

69. Solkoff N, Yaffe S, Weintraub, et al. Effects of Handling on the Subsequent Development of Premature Infants. Dev Psychol 1969;1:765–768.

70. White JL, Lababara RC. The Effects of Tactile Kinesthetic Stimulation on Neonatal Development in the Premature Infant. Dev Psychol 1976;9:569–577.

71. Morrow CJ, Field TM, Scafidi FA. Differential Effects of Massage and Heelstick Procedures on Transcutaneous Oxygen Tension in Preterm Neonates. Infant Behav Dev 1991;14:397–414.

72. Solkoff N, Matuszak D. Tactile Stimulation and Behavioral Development Among Low-Birth Weight Infants. Child Psychiatry Hum Dev 1975;(1):33–37.

73. Field T. Touch Therapy. Edinburgh, Scotland: Churchill Livingstone, 2000:4.

74. Calvert RN. David Eisenberg, MD: On Massage and the Future of Health Care. Massage Mag 2002;100:84–95.

75. Doering TJ, Fieguth HG, Steuernagel B, et al. External Stimuli in the Form of Vibratory Massage After Heart or Lung Transplantation. Am J Phys Med Rehabil 1999;78(2): 108–110.

76. Hernandez-Reif M, Field T, Largie S, et al. Children's Distress During Burn Treatment Is Reduced by Massage Therapy. J Burn Care Rehabil 2001;22(2):191–195.

77. Parke TJ, Kinsella SM. The Effect of Abdominal Massage on the Onset of Epidural Blockade in Laboring Women. Anesth Analg 1996;82:887.

78. Cawley N. A Critique of the Methodology of Research Studies Evaluating Massage. Eur J Cancer Care 1997;6: 23–31.

ADDITIONAL RESOURCES

American Massage Therapy Association Foundation, www.AMTAFoundation.org.

British Libraries Allied and Complementary Medicine Database, www.bl.uk/services/information/amed.html.

Cochrane Library, www.Cochrane.org.

Cumulative Index of Nursing and Allied Health Literature, www.cinahl.com.

Field T. Touch Therapy. Edinburgh, Scotland: Churchill Livingstone, 2000.

Kahn J. "Research Matters." Massage Magazine column starting July 2001.

LookSmart's FindArticles (a magazine article search site), www.findarticles.com.

Lewith G, Jonas WB, Walach H, eds. Clinical Research in Complementary Therapies: Principles, Problems and Solutions. Edinburgh, Scotland: Churchill Livingstone, 2002.

Menard M. Making Sense of Research: A Guide for Complementary Practitioners. Toronto, Canada: Curties-Overzet, 2003.

Polit DF, Beck CT, Hungler BP. Essentials of Nursing Research. 5th Ed. Philadelphia, PA: Lippincott Williams & Wilkins, 2001.

PubMed, www.PubMed.gov.

Research Council for Complementary Medicine, www.rccm.org.uk.

Rich GJ. Massage Therapy: The Evidence for Practice. Edinburgh, Scotland: Mosby/Harcourt, 2002.

Touch Research Institute, http://Miami.edu/touch-research/home.html.

University theses, www.theses.com.

ADAPTING TO HOSPITAL CULTURE

3

Bodyworkers who enter the hospital to apply their skills, whether as employees, volunteers, students on a clinical rotation, or private contractors hired by the patient or family, will encounter an atmosphere that is much different than massage in other venues. It is more regulated, standardized, hierarchical, complicated, unpredictable, and team-oriented. Therapists will work in conjunction with a wide variety of other healthcare providers, which decreases the sense of autonomy but increases the feeling of community. Concepts that massage therapists are taught in school, such as confidentiality, Standard Precautions, liability, and scope of practice, are carried out at a more stringent level than in other massage milieus. Many factors that therapists can control in a private practice, spa, or wellness center—such as time, noise, and interruptions—are out of their control in a hospital.

Learning to function in a medical center (another term for a hospital) is analogous to traveling in a foreign land. The people in this territory speak an unfamiliar language, dress to fit their special environment, and have habits, roles, and characteristics that express their values. Like travelers who adapt to local customs, bodyworkers who embrace the ways of hospital culture will find their journey more harmonious and enriching.

Each healthcare institution has standards that reflect its uniqueness. For instance, a medical center run by a religious order will have some principles that differ from those of a hospital funded by the county government, and the environment of a teaching hospital will be unlike that of a community hospital. However, there are also practices and values shared by all hospitals. The purpose of this chapter is to outline those standards.

DRESS AND GROOMING

One way to fit in is through common dress. A practitioner may possess exquisite massage skills, and yet, if their attire and grooming deviates significantly from the institutional norm, they may never make it past the proverbial front door. While hospital clothing standards are no longer as rigid as they once were, they are still more stringent than what is often worn in the bodywork community. The following are typical norms when working in the inpatient setting. Dress in outpatient clinics, however, may be less uniform but should still appear professional.

- Name tag.
- Shoes with closed toes and heels. This is a safety regulation set down by the Occupational Safety and Health Administration (OSHA). The shoes should also be clean.
- Socks.
- Long pants or skirt that falls near the knee. (No shorts or miniskirts, even in the summer.)
- Shirt or blouse with a collar. Scrubs or lab coats are worn in some hospitals. Wearing a special-colored shirt will help the staff recognize the massage therapists more easily.
- Clothes should be clean and wrinkle free.
- Do not use scents of any kind, such as perfume, scented soaps, lotions, shampoos, or deodorants. These scents can trigger nausea.
- Maintain short-trimmed, clean nails. This is part of a professional image as well as a Standard Precaution.
- Do not wear items that dangle, such as necklaces and long earrings, and pull back long hair.
- Remove visible body piercings, except for small earrings. Many patients are older and will be more at ease if massage students and practitioners look more traditional.
- Do not chew gum!

A human resources manager recounted her experience of interviewing a group of touch practitioners for the hospital's first massage position. A number of people did not make it onto the short list because of how they were attired. They were probably fantastic bodyworkers but appeared more appropriately dressed for attending the weekend farmers' market.

First impressions matter. Dress and grooming tells an interviewer, the staff, or clinical massage instructor many things. One is that the therapist is willing to adhere to institutional policy, which is important down the road with regard to massage precautions, documentation, and Standard Precautions. It can also signal to patients that the practitioner is clean, professional, and willing to put them at ease.

HOSPITAL DYNAMICS

Bodyworkers often enter the hospital scene believing that the most difficult and challenging aspect will be in relating to people who are seriously ill. They are often anxious beforehand about the odors, tubes, machines, or incisions, fears that usually turn out to be unfounded. However, the most common angst comes not while learning to be with patients, but from two other necessities: (1) mastering the art of interacting with the doctors, nursing staff, social workers, or myriad of other staff workers and (2) settling into the rhythms and pace of the hospital itself.

Hospital life waxes and wanes unpredictably, making it difficult for touch therapists to create the restful or sacred

---

☞ TIP: Adjusting to Hospital Life

Therapists new to the hospital milieu adjust with greater ease if they are gradually introduced to the new rhythms, etiquette, odors, and medical paraphernalia. A good starting place is to spend time on the unit without patient contact. The first day, my students take a guided tour through the unit. I am careful not to expose them to too much information but to just give them small bits at a time. The focus is on such things as finding the linen room, learning how the patient assignment board works, practicing Standard Precautions, and receiving lessons in the charting system.

The next class still has no patient or nurse contact. Therapists practice doing intake with each other, learn to operate the hospital furniture in an empty room, and are given interactive tasks to perform around the unit to increase their familiarity with the area. For example, they are given several patients' names and told to find out the room number, date of birth, gender, and diagnosis and record it on the intake form. All of this is information that can be obtained without patient or nurse contact.

Usually by the third class, practitioners are somewhat accustomed to the sights, sounds, and smells of the unit and are ready to briefly interact with the nurse and give a foot massage to a patient. This has proved to be a good starting place for the first touch session. A foot massage requires minimal information from the nurse, the patient doesn't require major repositioning, and medical devices rarely interfere with this process. As therapists become more comfortable over time, they can expand the massage options to other parts of the body.

Toni Creazzo, massage intern coordinator of The Institute for Health and Healing at California Pacific Medical Center in San Francisco,

---

eases her touch therapists into hospital life by matching the new interns with interns at the end of their training cycle. The novices shadow the now-experienced therapists several times, witnessing their interactions with staff and massage sessions with patients. After the first observation period, interns write a "reflection paper" describing their experience. The group uses this as a springboard into discussion about their reactions.

The next step is to observe Creazzo at work with patients, followed by several months of her supervising their work every other week. The interns also meet weekly to debrief and explore how the experience is affecting them. In this way, the therapists have a chance to slowly become accustomed to the hospital milieu with a supportive person at their side.

---

space they desire. Nurses may need to move in and out of the room giving medications, attending to intravenous (IV) lines, or taking vital signs. Doctors' rounds, family visitors, or a consultation with the nutritionist may intrude. Ten minutes into the massage, the patient may be whisked away for an MRI (magnetic resonance imaging). Although receiving massage might seem like a high priority to the patient, massage can't always be accommodated in the way the therapist and patient would like. Not only is the bodyworker unable to control the physical environment in an acute care setting, but the patient also has minimal influence on his surroundings.

To the uninitiated, a hospital unit appears confusing and disorderly. Figuring out which of the multicolored-clad staff are nurses, doctors, students, physical therapists, or respiratory therapists is difficult. Fifty years ago, there was the doctor and the nurse, each of whom could be easily identified. In today's healthcare environment, nearly every one of the many specialists who provides direct care wears scrubs, making it difficult to know who is who. It takes time for hospital massage personnel to begin to recognize the many people and their accompanying responsibilities.

Bodyworkers new to the hospital scene often feel slighted when starting out because everyone goes about their duties with hardly an upward glance. This business-as-usual approach is taken as a snub, when it is the farthest thing from the truth. Nurses are thrilled for their patients to receive massage, but their workload is so staggering and stressful that there is no energy left over to take care of other healthcare team members.

In order to be comfortable in the hospital, massage practitioners must come to grips with at least two paradoxes. The first is that of being simultaneously sensitive to the patient and insensitive toward the standard operating procedures inherent in a large health care facility. The second paradox is how we accept hospitals for what they are, and yet strive to make them more humane places to be. No easy solutions exist for these dilemmas. The immediate answer lies in the therapist's ability to embrace opposing energies, to hold both sides at once.[1]

—*Gayle MacDonald, Medicine Hands: Massage Therapy for People With Cancer*

Bodywork practitioners should expect to take the initiative in learning each hospital's routines, especially if they are volunteering or working independently. They may have to ask where the linen is, what to do with a full urinal, or where to lock up their valuables. Whether this is the best way to orient novices, or anyone else, is questionable, but it is a reality in today's rapid-paced work life. Students will have a clinical supervisor to assist them with this orientation, and therapists employed by the hospital may have a brief training session, but hospital massage therapists will usually need to be bold about asking questions and being self-directed.

Eventually, rapport and trust will be established, and the staff will begin to recognize the massage therapist as an individual, then as a member of the healthcare team that they and the patients look forward to seeing. The bodyworker will literally be greeted with big smiles and open arms. But the transition from outsider to insider can be bumpy and long.[1]

TEAM CARE

Massage therapy, on the whole, is a solitary business. Even the practitioner who is employed by a large spa or resort, shares office space with a group of bodyworkers, or is involved with an interdisciplinary group of practitioners generally operates independently. In this model of care, the client and therapist are free to make treatment decisions on their own.

In the medical setting, people are cared for by a team. The physician or nurse practitioner is the lead decision maker, while the patient's nurse oversees the treatment plan and coordinates the various care providers, often including massage therapists. Massage is just one of many services that must all fit together into a coherent whole.

Massage may be a new concept within a hospital unit. Therefore, integration into the team won't happen immediately. The respect of and acknowledgment by other professionals must be earned. Touch practitioners can foster this by becoming familiar with the roles of other staff, staying within the bodyworker's own scope of practice, and clarifying the proper channels of decision making. They also have a responsibility to educate other staff who often don't realize the potential of massage in the acute care setting or don't understand what information a practitioner will need about a patient. It becomes the responsibility of the massage therapist to ask the right questions of team members to give a safe session. Even if the nurse is busy,

and stopping her to obtain information seems like an imposition, bodyworkers must fulfill their obligation to the patient by asking for the necessary medical data.

While touch practitioners do not have the luxury of independent action in a hospital, they have the opportunity to be part of a group from whom they can learn and seek support. They are in an atmosphere that is professionally stimulating and personally expansive. As a team member, the touch therapist learns to play a specific role and yet comes to see the broader view. This bigger picture includes the roles played by other staff members, the patient's family and medical history, and institutional and even societal needs. The bodyworker's part is an important element of a larger whole. The care given intersects and overlaps with a multitude of other forces. For the hospital practitioner, massage therapy is no longer a solitary business.

WORKING WITH THE NURSING STAFF

The majority of staff interactions will be with the nursing personnel, which include registered nurses (RNs), licensed practical nurses (LPNs), and certified nursing assistants (CNAs). Regional differences exist in the use of nursing staff. In some states, LPNs do not work in acute care settings but will be found in long-term–care facilities.

THE ROLE OF THE RN AND LPN

By and large, both RNs and LPNs provide direct patient care, coordinate other health care practitioners such as physical therapists and nutritionists, and document the patient's condition. Registered nurses, because of lengthy and in-depth training, also take on administrative responsibilities, oversee other nursing personnel such as LPNs and CNAs, and tend to patients requiring high-tech care

- To obtain pertinent patient data
- To report changes in the patient's condition
- To report medical devices that need attention
- To report a problem with an IV or piece of medical machinery
- To confer about unfamiliar skin conditions
- To obtain help with any situation that is highly technical
- To obtain assistance with linens or positioning a patient only if the CNA is unavailable

THE ROLE OF THE CNA

The CNA assists the patient with less technical tasks, such as activities of daily living (ADLs), positioning, lifting, transfers, vital signs, and basic charting. The CNA may also assist the massage therapist in the following areas:

- Providing extra bedding, sheets, towels, or pillows
- Positioning the patient

- Assisting the patient onto the commode or to the bathroom
- Changing sheets due to a bowel or bladder accident or vomiting
- Removing a urinal, bedpan, or emesis basin

HELP FROM HOUSEKEEPERS

Do not forget to cultivate a relationship with the housekeepers. They are often able to help with a variety of situations:

- Finding bedding
- Identifying staff members
- Taking care of spills on the floor, including broken glass (Do not clean up spills yourself, as body fluids may be involved.)

One way for massage therapists to more quickly establish rapport with the staff is to offer them short, seated massage sessions during spare moments (Fig. 3-1). These happen occasionally as therapists are waiting for a patient to use the commode, finish consulting with the doctor, or conclude a family visit. There is often not enough time to see another patient during the wait, and rather than letting the time go to waste, therapists can use these few minutes to offer a brief neck or shoulder massage to a staff member. This will help staff recognize the touch therapist as a

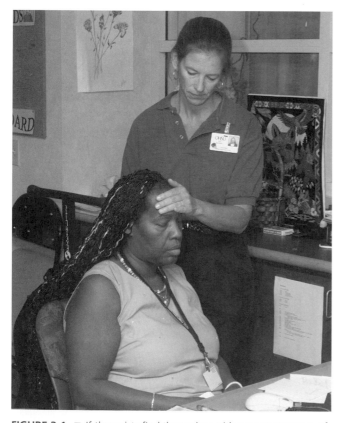

FIGURE 3-1. ■ If therapists find themselves with a spare moment, offering hospital staff a short, seated massage will help in establishing rapport. (Photo by Don Hamilton.)

person, acquaint them with the bodyworker's abilities, and trust the massage therapist with their patients.

Giving seated massage to personnel also will give the practitioner a chance to educate staff about what their discipline offers to the hospitalized patient. Many RNs are unfamiliar with the wide range of touch modalities. Initially, they may only refer a selected few patients, not realizing that there is always a way to provide skilled, comforting touch if the patient so desires. By integrating some of the comfort-oriented techniques into the seated sessions with the staff, therapists will help them quickly understand that everyone is a potential candidate for massage. In addition, comfort and relaxation is provided to a group of people who are often stressed out and overworked.

RELATING PROFESSIONALLY TO PATIENTS

At first glance, the standards of behavior expected of staff toward patients may seem as if they are meant to create distance between the two. In reality, these standards are in place for two reasons: (1) to help health caregivers establish a relationship in which the patient is free to focus on himself and (2) to create equality of care. This model of relating doesn't exclude compassion and care. In fact, it will make compassion and care all the more possible.

STURDY BOUNDARIES

Because massage creates a close bond between patient and therapist, it is imperative that bodyworkers maintain distinct emotional boundaries. Nina McIntosh points out in *The Educated Heart* that, "For [patients] to relax and drop their guard, they need the security and safety of sturdy boundaries. A safe environment is predictable, consistent, and focused on [the patients]."[2]

> *Boundaries don't create walls between client and practitioner—they help clients feel safe.*[2]
>
> —*Nina McIntosh, The Educated Heart: Professional Guidelines for Massage Therapists, Bodyworkers and Movement Teachers*

Emotional boundaries are often crossed because massage therapists are trying to meet unconscious needs of their own. The patient may bring to mind a special grandparent or brother that they miss. They may be reminded of a person with whom they have unresolved grief. Or perhaps the patient's loneliness strikes a chord deep within the practitioner.

One beginning therapist stepped over the bounds with an elderly woman who brought to mind her grandmother. Meaning only to be helpful, she visited the woman after her shift and even offered to do several tasks outside the hospital. Her own grandmother, after all, was the same age, and the therapist hoped that others were doing these things for her. While the offer to help ostensibly seemed like a kindness, in the end it became a messy tangle. The patient developed expectations the practitioner could not meet. Thus, the safe environment that allowed the patient to focus on herself was gone. The massage therapist had made the mistake of trying to fix aspects of the patient's life, forgetting that the job of professional care providers is to help patients find their own healing resources. The focus in this case had shifted from healing the patient to meeting each other's needs.

> *There is distance between ourselves and whatever or whomever we are fixing. Fixing is a form of judgement. All judgement creates distance, a disconnection, an experience of difference.[3]*
> —*Rachel Naomi Remen, MD*

On the other hand, performing an extra kindness for a patient is not always inappropriate. If practitioners do not use the task as a chance to meet their own needs and do not show favoritism, the act may be of true service. For example, Joshua had been massaging an elderly man who had been hospitalized for more than a month. The man had no family to call upon when he wished to buy the nurses a small Christmas gift. Joshua offered to do it when he did his own Christmas shopping. The two men agreed on a price range and that Joshua would bring the receipt back with any remaining money. The kindness occurred with no ulterior motive nor with any presumption that Joshua would run other errands in the future.

Sharing personal information can diminish the patient–therapist boundary, causing patients to feel a need to care for the practitioner. This takes attention away from the reason they are in the hospital: to focus on their own healing. Heidi, for instance, would always ask the massage therapist how she was feeling at the start of each session. If the therapist answered, "I'm a little tired" or "My back is sore," Heidi tried to take care of the therapist, urging her not to work too hard or too long. The therapist learned to tell Heidi that she was always "fine." Otherwise, Heidi focused on the practitioner instead of on herself.

Sometimes, however, the sharing of personal stories by the bodyworker can be supportive of the person who is ill. The prerequisite is that what is shared must support the patient's process, not the practitioner's. For example, if the massage therapist had successfully been treated for the same or a similar condition, it is often helpful to share just that much with the patient. The patient feels relief knowing that there is an unspoken understanding based on their shared experience.

Like learning to honor the rules of confidentiality, practitioners must learn how to relate to patients in a professional way. Those new to hospital work frequently make some of the following mistakes. Although these gestures appear to be the behaviors of a compassionate, caring practitioner, they cross the bounds of a professional relationship:

- Calling the patient outside of work to see how they are.*
- Calling the nurses' station to check on the patient.*
- Exchanging addresses or phone numbers.
- Giving or accepting gifts, both of which can create a sense of obligation.
- Accepting tips or other money. Tips sometimes are literally forced on a therapist. In such a case, the money could be given to a person in charge who can then return it to the patient or family member with an explanation of the hospital's policy. Some hospitals handle this situation by donating the money to the hospital foundation or buying something the entire staff can enjoy, such as cake or cookies.
- Going to the cafeteria to bring special food.
- Offering to come to the hospital on personal time to visit or give massage.
- Singling out certain patients for extra attention.
- Visiting patients at home after they are discharged, for other than professional reasons.

Sturdy boundaries benefit not only the patients but care providers as well. Hospitals are places of suffering and loss. Only with well-established boundaries can practitioners thrive in such an environment. Without them, they would be in perpetual exhaustion, overloaded by the desire to fix problems that have no solution.

*Note: The first two suggestions are aimed particularly at brand-new therapists or students. It may be permissible and even desirable for therapists to make such calls after they are more experienced with understanding boundary issues. Initially, however, such actions often are the result of misguided motivations.

EQUALITY OF CARE

Massage practitioners in private practice have the choice of refusing to work with clients if there is sufficient reason or of choosing to work with only a specific segment of the population. This is not an option when working in a public organization. Care must be given to everyone on an equal basis: men and women, rich and poor, thin and fat, grumpy and cheerful.

There are always certain people the staff love to care for. They are the cooperative, optimistic ones who make the care providers feel they are great at their jobs, who are inspirational, or who light up the room. But it is the person who is irritable and seems ungrateful that may be in even greater need of attention.

Sometimes the staff will comment on how difficult a patient is. However, when the touch therapist encounters this same person, he finds a sweet and vulnerable soul. Maintaining an open mind about each individual, no matter what other staff members have said, is important to providing equal and heartfelt care. Learning to work equally with all patients expands the therapist's comfort zone. He becomes a greater asset to himself, the hospital, and his colleagues because he is able to provide service to a wider variety of patients.

PATIENT PRIVACY AND CONFIDENTIALITY

Protecting patient privacy is a matter that is given serious attention by medical institutions. Hospital staff has always been legally and ethically obligated to keep information about a patient strictly confidential. However, in the past, some states had minimal legal protection of health information while others had strict regulations in place. The **Health Insurance Portability and Accountability Act of 1996 (HIPAA)**, which healthcare institutions gradually implemented through 2003, created national standards that ensure the privacy and security of patients' health information.

The new laws are lengthy and complicated to read in their original form. A simplified list of regulations that apply to privacy is presented in Box 3-1. Other parts of the guidelines are relevant only to personnel in billing, medical records, or administration and, therefore, are not included.

Examples of other information that must remain privileged include discussions with or conversations overheard from other healthcare workers and information told by the patient or his family. Personal information about the patient should not be discussed among the healthcare team; only that which may be relevant to the patient's treatment or psychosocial well-being should be talked about. For example, discussing such things as the patient's political beliefs, past drug use, or sexual history among the staff would be irrelevant to the patient's care and, therefore, a breach of confidentiality.

The one time a massage therapist would be ethically bound to break a patient's confidence is if the person's safety or well-being was in jeopardy. Robert, for example, was preparing to massage someone with an extremely low platelet count. Just before he entered the room, the patient had a spontaneous nosebleed, which she had packed with toilet paper. However, the blood continued flowing down her throat. The therapist asked the woman if she had notified the nurse of the bleed. "No, I will after the massage," she responded. As the reader will learn in future chapters, patients with a low platelet count have very slow coagulation time and are at risk for brain or retinal bleeds, both of which are extremely serious. Quite appropriately, Robert excused himself and left the room to report the patient's nosebleed to her nurse.

OVERVIEW OF HIPAA GUIDELINES

HIPAA's rules accomplish the following:

- Define protected health information (PHI)
- Give patients more control of their health information
- Set boundaries on the use and release of health records and require patient authorization for use or release outside those boundaries
- Establish safeguards to protect the privacy of health information
- Impose civil and criminal penalties on individuals who violate patient privacy rights
- Strike a balance when public responsibility requires disclosure of some forms of data (for example, the protection of public health)

Through HIPAA's privacy rules:

- Patients may find out how their health information may be used and what disclosures have been made.
- The release of health information is limited to the minimum reasonably needed for the purpose of the disclosure.
- Patients have the right to obtain and examine a copy of their own health records and to request corrections.
- Patients have the right to restrict the use of their health information and to request confidential communication of their health information.

The following is protected health information. PHI identifies or could be used to identify a patient or the patient's past, present, or future physical or mental health and applies to patients who are living or deceased.

- Name
- Address (or any part of the address)
- Names of relatives
- Names of employers
- E-mail or Internet protocol (IP) address
- Telephone or fax number
- Date of birth
- Social Security number
- Fingerprints or voiceprints
- Photographic images
- Any vehicle or device serial number
- Medical record number

The following types of records and activities are affected by PHI:

- Medical records, including electronic and paper
- Case histories
- Clinical reports
- Diagnostic films
- Test results
- Treatment charts and progress reports
- The oral transmission of health information[4]

If there is a need to discuss an experience outside the hospital, such as part of school clinical rounds, professional meetings, or in professional literature, omit using names or descriptions that might reveal a patient's identity, such as the diagnosis, age, date of admission, ethnicity, or name of the hospital. Rather than focusing on patients during an outside discussion, therapists should focus on their own experience.

Because of confidentiality, independent contractors, friends, and even family members wishing to give massage usually will not have access to the same medical information about a patient that a hospital massage therapist will have. For instance, if an independent contractor asks the nurse about the patient's platelet count, it probably would not be given out unless there is a physician's order for the massage and the patient has signed a release form. That data are available only to staff or official hospital volunteers.

Rules of confidentiality are very clear-cut between professional healthcare providers and patients. But when massage is being given on a more informal basis to a friend or family member, the lines can become blurred, and facts that the patient would prefer to remain private can unknowingly be passed along to others within the social circle. Giving out general information about the patient to other friends or family, such as "She's not feeling well" or "He's very upbeat," is acceptable. However, no specific facts should be given unless the patient has consented. Examples of such precise information may include that the cancer has metastasized, the patient is having trouble with his bowels, or he lost his job.

If you find yourself wanting to share information about a client outside a confidential setting (e.g., supervision group, peer group, individual supervision), ask yourself how sharing this information will benefit your client. If it doesn't benefit them, ask what need it is serving for you.

—Bob Nelson, MS, LMT, Bodywork Supervisor

It is often tempting to call family and friends to announce changes in the patient's health status, but patients must be allowed to convey the specifics of the situation in their own way and time. An extreme example of violating a friend's privacy is the woman who put an announcement in the church bulletin of her friend's upcoming surgery for breast cancer. The patient, who was sitting in church on Sunday when the notice was read out, was horrified. Of course the woman was only trying to be helpful, but she failed to understand that everyone has a unique feeling about her body and health status.

Some patients hold nothing back from friends or family. In those cases, the bodyworker might be more forthcoming about what she shares with others if the patient has given permission. If the patient's preference for sharing information is not known, then the prudent and ethical course is to withhold anything that was communicated by the ill person, even from close family members.

The following guidelines will safeguard confidential information:

- View or listen to confidential information only if necessary to fulfill responsibilities. Wanting to know

isn't a good enough reason for listening in on privileged conversations.
- Share confidential information only with those who need to know to fulfill patient care responsibilities.
- Have private discussions in private places.
- Keep confidential information such as medical records safe and secure so that others cannot see them or take them.
- Be sure that inappropriate people cannot view confidential information on the computer. Log out of the computer before leaving it unattended.
- Do not display confidential information, such as a patient's name, on appointment schedules or public sign-in sheets.

The regulations concerning privacy are explicit and seemingly simple, but mastering them requires acute vigilance. People sometimes unintentionally breach a confidence when first confronted with these new protocols. Although innocent mistakes may be made in the learning process, it is important that healthcare providers remain committed to protecting patient privacy. Everyone deserves control of the information that is made public about his or her health.

LIABILITY

Liability is an unavoidable fact of life within health care and greatly influences the attitudes and behaviors of those who work in it. When practicing in this arena, touch therapists must adopt a high level of awareness. The actions of private bodywork practitioners reflect only on themselves. Those of the hospital massage therapist impact the entire institution, which is ultimately responsible, or liable, for the care and safety of patients.

Massage therapists working in medical settings do not have the same latitude in decision making and implementing interventions as private practitioners. It is the physician or nurse practitioner who decides on the overall medical and surgical treatment plan and writes the orders to be carried out by the nursing staff, physical therapists, nutritionists, and all of the many other professional caregivers, including massage therapists. Because massage is commonly thought of as an extension of nursing, the touch practitioner often works under the direction of the patient's nurse.

Adhering to the nurse's or doctor's instruction is imperative with regard to liability. It is important to check with the appropriate staff, usually the nurse, before proceeding with anything that is outside the agreed-upon scope of practice. For example, a therapist new to hospital work thought that a patient had the beginnings of a pressure sore. Without conferring with the nurse, the therapist went ahead and treated the sore as taught in massage school. This action, however, was outside that hospital's job description for massage, which was to provide comfort-oriented touch only. Acting outside the agreed-upon job description jeopardizes the staff's trust in the massage therapist.

Even though healthcare employees are covered by the hospital's group liability insurance program, it is prudent for therapists to have a personal professional liability insurance policy. This is true whether they are volunteers, employees, or independent contractors and regardless of whether the massage is intended for relaxation or as a treatment measure. While the institution accepts major liability for patients' care, each licensed worker employed by the facility is individually liable for performing his duties in accordance with the regulations and limitations of his licensing board or governing body.

SCOPE OF PRACTICE

Massage therapists sometimes go beyond their scope of practice with private clients and offer advice on an assortment of other subjects, nutritional supplements, essential oils, and guided imagery, to name a few. When working in the hospital or other medical setting, bodyworkers must refrain from offering information or guidance that is outside their identified discipline and/or job description. There are several reasons for this. It may conflict with the treatment plan set out by the physician, endanger the patient's well-being, contradict the work of other members of the healthcare team, or go against the patient's or institution's beliefs.

The following story illustrates how a bodyworker can unintentionally drift beyond her scope of practice without meaning to. A newly licensed massage therapist had just finished working with a postpartum patient who was a first-time mother. The massage therapist was an older woman who had raised several children and was, therefore, an experienced parent. After the session was over, the practitioner pulled up a chair and discussed breastfeeding, one mother to another, offering advice along the way. To be sure, the therapist meant only to be helpful, but she also may have presented information that conflicted with what the lactation specialist had given, thereby confusing the patient and stepping on the toes of the person assigned to help mothers with breastfeeding.

When a practitioner wants to integrate complementary activities or disciplines such as aromatherapy or visualization techniques into his hospital massage practice, it is best to have the support of the nurse manager or other administrator beforehand. Depending on the hospital's culture, the approval to include new practices may be an immediate, on-the-spot OK, or it may require a number of committee meetings with final approval by a hospital governing body.

ETIQUETTE TOWARD PATIENTS, VISITORS, AND STAFF

The following courtesies toward patients, family, and staff should be observed:

- If the patient's door is shut, knock before entering. If it is partially or fully open, still knock on either the door or door frame, or in some way get permission from the patient to enter the room (Fig. 3-2).
- Until you know how the patient prefers to be addressed, approach him or her formally, using Mr. Smith or Mrs. Lopez, for example.
- If the curtain is pulled around the bed, it often means that the nurse is performing care that requires privacy, such as changing a dressing or assisting the patient with the bedpan. Most often, it is best to wait outside until the curtain has been opened.
- Only sit on the patient's bed with his or her permission. (Generally, professional caregivers do not sit on a patient's bed.)

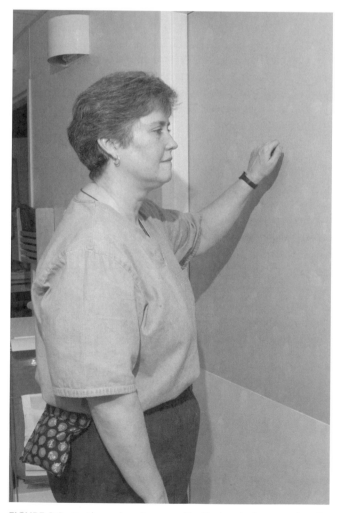

FIGURE 3-2. ■ Always knock on a patient's door before entering the room. (Photo by Richard York, Oregon Health and Science University.)

- If a doctor needs to consult with the patient partway through a massage session, ask the physician if you should step out of the room or if it is OK to continue the massage. Sometimes the doctor needs a lengthy period of privacy to discuss the situation at hand. Other matters take only a minute and can be accomplished while the therapist remains in the room.
- Nurses may need to interrupt the massage to perform tasks. As they become accustomed to having massage therapists on the unit, they will be willing to postpone nonessential responsibilities until the bodywork session is complete. The massage can often continue even through essential tasks, such as attending to IVs, giving blood products, or taking vital signs. Ask the nurse and patient if it is OK to continue the massage.
- Visits by family and friends are important. If they arrive during a massage, some visitors will wait in the hall, while others will want to be with the patient. Welcome them into the room in some way, perhaps by eye contact, a smile, or a "come on in."
- Conduct yourself with gentleness and courtesy in all parts of the hospital, such as the hallways, elevators, and cafeteria. It is impossible to know which of the people you encounter will have a parent who is dying from cancer, a spouse who has a ruptured aneurysm in the brain, or a child whose feet were just amputated because of a bacterial infection.

GENERAL HOSPITAL ETIQUETTE

Some of the following guidelines exist for hygienic reasons, some are aimed at avoiding clutter in work areas, and some are intended for both.

- Consume food and beverages in the staff lunchroom, never on the unit, at the nurses' station, or in patients' rooms. This includes use of personal water bottles.
- Store personal items in designated areas. Do not take them into patients' rooms or leave them at the nurses' station.
- Store food in designated areas.
- Change clothes in an area set aside for this purpose, such as a staff locker room.
- Do not use the patient's toilet.

SELF CARE

Giving massage in the hospital setting is often difficult for those who are trained as bodyworkers but have no other background in health care. By nature, massage therapists are sensitive, which is what makes them skillful, compas-

sionate givers of touch. Yet this strength is also a weakness in the acute care setting, where the interventions are often invasive, toxic, or hurried. Possessing extra sensitivity makes it difficult for some bodyworkers to adjust to hospital work because they feel so much of the stress, pain, and despair of patients, family, and staff.

While the joys of hospital work are immense and unimaginable, so too are the fears and questions it triggers. How do I cope with suffering? Would I respond to serious illness with grace or despair? Where should the line be drawn with high-tech health care?

In this atmosphere, self-care is vital! It may take many forms, such as attending a support or supervision group, spending time in nature, journaling, creating ritual, or limiting the number of hours worked per week. Expecting to give massage for 40 hours a week, or even 20, may be unrealistic for some. Therapists must find the limit that best serves them. So, too, they may find that caring for the self means confining their practice to certain groups of patients and not others. Some people find pediatrics too stressful because they have children of their own. Others can't work with oncology patients because it evokes painful memories of losing a loved one to cancer. Honoring those limitations is part of self-care.

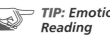

TIP: Emotional Support Through Reading

In addition to studying clinical material, those learning to work in the acute care setting find it grounding to read material that deals with the emotional aspect of the hospital experience. I require my students to read *Healing Into Life and Death* by Stephen Levine. Toni Creazzo gives her interns a choice between four books: *Kitchen Table Wisdom* by Rachel Naomi Remen, *How, Then, Shall We Live?* by Wayne Muller, *Healing Words* by Larry Dossey, or *Promise of the Soul* by Dennis Kenny. Each in their own way, these books shed light on the process of illness, teach skills in dealing with pain and grief, or inspire the bodyworker when she is feeling emotionally low. Even experienced touch practitioners benefit from constantly

Irene Smith, a San Francisco practitioner who has worked for more than 20 years with the seriously ill, offers these self-care suggestions and shares some of her own process:

There may be times when you want to seek the support of a trained professional as a guide or as someone you feel safe with while sharing your experiences or releasing emotion. Other times you may

simply need a private space to sit with your feelings and reflect inward. A safe place is as individual as each person. Sometimes a safe place for me is leaning against a tree in a quiet place in nature where I won't be disturbed and sometimes I want to be at home. Creating a safe and reflective space in the home requires some planning and some tools. Tools that I find helpful are: Kleenex, water, pillows, a blanket, a candle, aromatherapy, a musical instrument, and favorite poems. I also need a space where there is no phone and where I won't be disturbed."[5]

How touch therapists minister to their own physical and emotional needs is not important. What is essential is that they consistently and consciously set aside time and space for reflection, unwinding, and self-nurturing—walk the dog; receive regular massage; sit by the fire, in the sauna, or in the hot tub; prepare a leisurely meal; read inspirational books; rest. As Rachel Naomi Remen reminds us in *My Grandfather's Blessings*, ". . . blessing life is about filling yourself up so that your blessings overflow onto others."[6] The more touch practitioners take care of themselves, the more they can serve others.

Even a good heart can cause harm for ourselves and others if it has no rest in it.[7]

—Wayne Muller, Sabbath: Finding Rest, Renewal, and Delight in Our Busy Lives

SUMMARY

Without a doubt, the customs and conventions of medical institutions are stricter than those of the massage profession in general. The hospital setting is less flexible and requires greater standardization and accountability. There is, however, still infinite space for the massage therapist to provide skilled touch that is creative, inspired, and heartfelt.

TEST YOURSELF

Discuss the following "confidentiality" situations with classmates or colleagues. How could each be handled appropriately?

1. You discover that the patient you are massaging goes to the same church as your best friend. What information would be appropriate to divulge to your friend?

2. You are walking down the hospital hallway with a family member of a patient. The two of you are on your way to a quiet room where you can give her a seated massage. While passing the room of another patient, the family member asks you about the written instructions that are posted on the outside of that patient's door. The instructions have to do with masking, gloving, and gowning. How could you answer the question without disclosing confidential information?

3. One of the patients you have massaged has received a lot of publicity in the local news media about her medical plight. A colleague who knows that you give massage at the hospital asks if you have ever worked with this high-profile patient. What would be an appropriate response?

4. You massage a nurse who works in the hospital's oncology unit but who has been admitted to the hospital for gynecological surgery. Would it be proper to report to the oncology nurses about how their colleague is doing?

5. While you are giving a massage to a patient, he tells you that he is a prostitute who specializes in S&M. Should this information be passed on to fellow hospital massage therapists who might also be called on to work with this patient?

REFERENCES

1. MacDonald G. Medicine Hands: Massage Therapy for People With Cancer. Findhorn, Scotland: Findhorn Press, 1999.
2. McIntosh N. The Educated Heart: Professional Guidelines for Massage Therapists, Bodyworkers and Movement Teachers. Philadelphia, PA: Lippincott Williams & Wilkins, 2003.
3. Remen RN. In the Service of Life. Noetic Sciences Rev Spring 1996:24–25.
4. Oregon Health and Science University HIPAA Guidelines.
5. Smith I. Emotional Impact of Working With the Dying. San Francisco, CA: Everflowing Handbooks, 2001.
6. Remen RN. My Grandfather's Blessings. New York, NY: Riverhead Books, 2000.
7. Muller W. Sabbath: Finding Rest, Renewal, and Delight in Our Busy Lives. New York, NY: Bantam Books, 1999.

ADDITIONAL RESOURCES

Benjamin B, Sohnen-Moe C. The Ethics of Touch. Tucson, AZ: SMA Inc., 2003.
Birx E. Healing Zen: Awakening to a Life of Wholeness and Compassion While Caring for Yourself and Others. New York, NY: Viking Compass, 2002.
Bolen JS. Close to the Bone. New York, NY: Scribner, 1996.
Brasch MI. The Healing Path. New York, NY: Arkana, 1993.

Carlson R, Shield B, eds. Healers on Healing. Los Angeles, CA: Jeremy P. Tarcher, 1989.

Dass R, Gorman P. How Can I Help? Stories and Reflections on Service. New York, NY: Knopf, 1985.

Dossey L. Healing Words: The Power of Prayer and the Practice of Medicine. New York, NY: Harper Collins, 1993.

Greene E, Goodrich-Dunn B. The Psychology of the Body. Philadelphia, PA: Lippincott Williams & Wilkins, 2003.

Henderson R, Marek R. Here Is My Hope: A Book of Healing and Prayer—Inspirational Stories from the Johns Hopkins Hospital. New York, NY: Doubleday, 2001.

HIPAA guidelines, www.os.dhhs.gov/ocr/hipaa

Kenny D. Promise of the Soul: Identifying and Healing Your Spiritual Agreements. New York, NY: John Wiley and Sons, 2002.

Levine S. Healing Into Life and Death. New York, NY: Anchor Books, 1987.

Mellody P. Facing Codependence. New York: HarperCollins, 1989.

Muller W. How Then Shall We Live? New York: Bantam Books, 1996.

Remen RN. Kitchen Table Wisdom. New York: Riverhead Books, 1996.

Santorelli S. Heal Thyself: Lessons on Mindfulness in Medicine. New York, NY: Random House, 1999.

Woodman M. Bone: Dying Into Life. New York, NY: Viking Compass, 2000.

INFECTION CONTROL PRACTICES

4

The U.S. Centers for Disease Control and Prevention (CDC) estimates that each year two million Americans acquire an infection during their hospital stay.[1] Typically, **nosocomial**, or hospital-related, infections affect patients who are immunocompromised because of age, disease, or type of treatment. An aging population combined with increasingly aggressive medical interventions has created a group of people who are particularly defenseless. Additionally, with surgical care being shifted to outpatient centers, hospitals now house only the sickest patients, making acute care facilities more like a large intensive care unit (ICU). This creates further vulnerability with regard to nosocomial contagion.[2]

Hospital-related infections not only add to the patient's length of stay and cost of care but also result in many deaths and complications. The Institute for Medicine reports that these infections are responsible for 44,000 to 98,000 deaths a year in the United States.[3] In addition to patients being infected, thousands of healthcare workers acquire a disease or contagion while on the job.

The CDC and the Occupational Safety and Health Administration (OSHA) have developed protective precautions, such as handwashing and gloving, to reduce the transmission of contagious microorganisms. These protective practices are organized into two levels. The first tier, known as **Standard Precautions**, is designed for the care of all patients, regardless of their diagnosis or presumed infection status. The second tier, **Transmission-Based Precautions**, are used only when caring for specified patients known or suspected to be infected by specific **pathogens** spread through airborne or droplet transmission or by contact with dry skin or contaminated surfaces.[3]

The purpose of this chapter is to acquaint massage therapists with the protective practices they will use when working with the patient in a healthcare setting. These include handwashing, gloving, masking, and gowning. In addition, material is presented on protecting patients who are immunosuppressed, proper handling of bedding and work clothes, exposure to body fluids, and when to stay home during illness.

STANDARD PRECAUTIONS

Standard Precautions is a phrase that is just now making its way into massage vocabulary. Previously, bodyworkers were taught the term **Universal Precautions**, which refers only to bloodborne microorganisms. Standard Precautions synthesize the major features of Universal Precautions, which were designed to reduce the risk of transmission of bloodborne pathogens, and **Blood Stream Infection Precautions**, which were designed to reduce the risk of transmission of pathogens from moist body substances.[4]

These precautions apply to all patients regardless of their diagnosis or presumed infection status. All bodily fluids are treated as potentially infectious and may have their source from blood, body fluids, secretions, and excretions; broken or open skin; and mucous membranes.[4] The following are examples of body fluids, tissues, and substances that may carry pathogens:

- Amniotic fluid
- Blood
- Breast milk
- **Cerebrospinal** fluid
- Feces
- Nasal secretions
- **Pericardial** fluid
- **Peritoneal** fluid
- **Pleural** fluid
- Saliva
- Semen
- **Sputum**
- **Synovial** fluid
- Urine
- Vaginal secretions
- Vomitus
- Wound drainage

Tears and perspiration are not contagious unless they contain blood.

Those in private massage practice are sometimes casual about adhering to Standard Precautions. For example, they might think nothing of stroking over an area that is scabbed. The hospital massage therapist, on the other hand, would glove in such a situation. Paranoia is not called for when following these protocols, but serious care, attention, and diligence must be applied. It is better to be too careful than too casual.

INFECTION CONTROL TECHNIQUES

The protective practices in this chapter are presented with an eye toward ease of learning. First, each of the components—handwashing, gloving, masking, and gowning—are addressed singly. This will allow the newer practitioner a chance to master those skills one at a time. However, in real life, they are often used in combination, such as gloving and gowning. This complicates the process. Following the material on each isolated component, the precautions are taught in combinations, such as masking, gowning, and gloving.

The concept of "clean to clean, dirty to dirty" is central to the use of protective practices and garments. Once it settles into practitioners' bones, this concept will enable them to master the use of protective barriers. Readers will encounter one application of this notion in the handwashing section—turning the taps off with a paper towel. The hands, after being washed, are considered to be "clean." The taps, which have been touched by many unwashed hands, are "dirty." Therefore, the therapist is taught to touch the taps with a paper towel.

Another example will be found when learning to unglove. Practitioners will notice that the protocol for ungloving calls for them to never contact the skin, which is "clean," with the outside of the glove, which is "dirty." The clean to clean, dirty to dirty concept also will be put to use when the practitioner is removing a combination of protective barriers, such as gloves and gown. Understanding this idea is a priority.

Handwashing

The hands are the most common way to pass contagion, making handwashing the most basic Standard Precaution. All bodyworkers are required to handwash, even those who work through garments, such as Reiki practitioners or Polarity Therapists. This is necessary because contagious particles can survive in the bedding or on clothing.

Naturally, massage therapists in private practice are accustomed to washing their hands before and after working with each client. In the hospital, it is also necessary to wash after contact with surfaces in the patient's room, such as the overbed table or telephone, as well as after handling the patient's personal items, such as a razor or laptop computer.

Handwashing after such minimal contact might seem excessive until a practitioner considers the following story. A patient had a **peripherally inserted central catheter (PICC)** line removed from his arm, leaving patches of dried blood on his gown and bedding and a smaller amount on his arm. The blood had been there for hours, during which time the patient used his razor and cologne, drank from his water bottle, and ate from the tray still on the overbed table. Imagine the massage therapist entering the patient's room to ask him if he would like a massage. The patient asks the therapist to move his lunch tray and place his cologne on the bathroom shelf, all of which he has touched since the PICC line was removed.

Imagine the next scene of the above story being played out. The massage therapist enters the room of another patient, hands unwashed. Perhaps she touches that patient briefly in greeting or is asked to hand her a cup of water. Now the microorganisms from the previous patient are introduced into this next room. It is easy to understand how quickly infection can spread in a hospital.

Hospitals care for very sick people. These people have weeping skin conditions, blood around incision sites, bacterial infections that are resistant to even the most powerful antibiotics, and unknown viral infections, to name just some of the potentially contagious scenarios. Handwashing with antimicrobial soap is the first line of defense for the practitioner, for other patients, and for staff members.

Antimicrobial Soap and Water Procedure

1. Remove watch and rings and push up sleeves, if necessary.
2. Stand so that clothing does not touch the sink or get splashed.
3. Wet hands and forearms with warm water. Water that is too hot or too cold can cause skin to crack or chap, increasing the risk of infection. Keep the hands lower than the elbows with the fingers pointing down (Fig. 4-1).
4. Soap hands and forearms, working soap into a lather.
5. Wash the entire surface of the hands and forearms for 30 seconds, including the fingerstips and fingernails (Fig. 4-2). Between patients, it is necessary to wash only the hands.
6. Do not touch the sides of the sink. If your hands accidentally touch the sink, repeat the handwashing.
7. Rinse well with the fingers pointing downward. Do not shake water off the hands, as splashing spreads germs.
8. Dry thoroughly with a paper towel, then use the towel to turn off the faucet. This protects your hands from dirty faucets (Fig. 4-3).[5]

Procedure for Use of Handrubs

Until recently, American healthcare workers cleaned their hands exclusively with antimicrobial soap and wa-

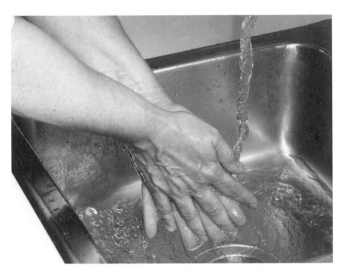

FIGURE 4-1. ■ Keep fingers pointed downward when washing hands. (Photo by Don Hamilton.)

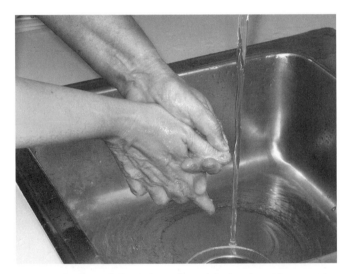

FIGURE 4-2. ■ Wash the entire surface of the hands and forearms, including fingers and fingernails. (Photo by Don Hamilton.)

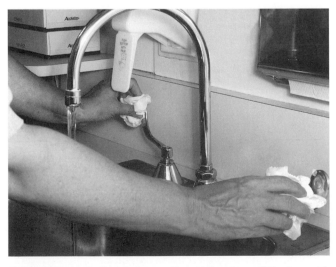

FIGURE 4-3. ■ Dry hands thoroughly and then turn off the taps with the used paper towels. (Photo by Don Hamilton.)

ter. More and more, however, bodyworkers will encounter waterless **handrubs** in the healthcare setting (Fig. 4-4). Research has shown that the use of a waterless, alcohol-based handrub is easier, faster, and more effective in disinfecting the hands. New guidelines for hand hygiene released by the CDC recommend their use because they improve adherence to hand hygiene. According to the "Hand Hygiene Guidelines Fact Sheet," these products significantly reduce the number of microorganisms on skin, are fast acting, and cause less skin irritation.[6]

Not all handrubs are equally effective. Those used in healthcare settings are more potent than commercial products sold at the grocery store. The research on these products is not as clear-cut. The information presented in this section refers to handrubs found in medical settings.

The following guidelines should be observed when using handrubs:

- Apply to the palm of one hand and rub hands together, covering all surfaces of the hands and fingers until the hands are dry. The amount of handrub needed to reduce the number of bacteria on the hands varies by product.
- Use handrubs immediately after leaving a patient's room if you have touched any surface in the room.
- Handwash with soap and water if the hands are visibly soiled (with massage lotion, for example).
- Handrubs do not eliminate the need for using gloves.[6]
- Handrubs also do not eliminate the need for handwashing with soap and water. After eating, using the toilet, or having direct contact with the patient, practitioners should wash their hands with soap and water.

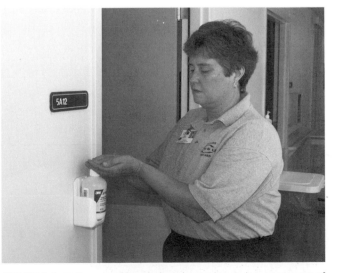

FIGURE 4-4. ■ The use of handrubs is becoming an important part of Standard Precautions in the hospital setting. (Photo by Don Hamilton.)

> ### TIP: Carrying Pouch for Personal Items
>
> Uniform supply stores sell small pouches for nurses to carry supplies in, such as scissors and tape. However, these are also handy for massage therapists to wear around their waist while at the hospital to carry waterless hand cleaner if it is not readily available at the hospital, reading glasses, pens, money, and other personal items.

Gloving

Gloves should be worn anytime there may be contact with blood, body fluids, mucous membranes, or broken skin, including the therapists'. Two types of gloves have been commonly used in hospitals: latex, a natural rubber, and vinyl, a synthetic nonlatex material. Studies have shown that vinyl gloves exhibit defects following usage more often than latex gloves. Latex, on the other hand, is banned from many hospitals because of both patient and staff allergic reactions. A third option is the nitrile glove, which, like vinyl, is synthetic. Unlike vinyl, it appears to provide comparable protection to that of latex gloves but without the allergic response to latex.[7]

Gloves used to give massage should be snug fitting so that the surface is unwrinkled. The feel of a smooth veneer will be more pleasurable to both patient and practitioner. Some lubricants, especially oils and petroleum-based lotions, will cause gloves to stretch. Not only is it difficult to massage with misshapen gloves, but the protective quality of the glove is diminished.

It is worth highlighting the point that touch practitioners must glove if the skin on their hands is not intact, including cuticle tears. This is true whether the patient's skin is broken or not. Microorganisms can be introduced to the therapist from intact patient skin via contact with areas heavily colonized with bacteria. Studies have shown that these areas include the axilla, trunk, and upper extremities,[7] all places that a bodyworker commonly comes into contact with.

Bodyworkers without prior experience in health care sometimes worry that the patient will be offended if they glove to give the massage. Because of this fear, students sometimes fail to glove in situations where they should have. Other times, massage therapists realize part way into an encounter with a patient that they should have gloved. Rather than stopping to glove, they carry on, not wanting to break the mood. A massage student participating in an obstetrics (OB) rotation did just that. While massaging the upper legs of a woman in labor, the student noticed that there was dried blood in the vicinity. However, she chose not to stop and glove. It is vital that care providers follow infection control practices regardless of any imagined judgment oth-

ers might have and regardless of whether they have to disturb the mood.

Always glove for the following situations:

- To touch any part of the patient where there is a possibility of contact with any body substances, including cuts or scabs.
- To move a urinal, bedpan, or emesis basin that has been used (Fig. 4-5). One glove is usually sufficient. Be sure to follow Step 2 under the glove "Removal" procedures when taking off just one glove.
- If the therapist has a cut, open sore, scratch, abrasion, scab, or a noncontagious rash on the hands. (Do not give bodywork sessions with any kind of contagious rash, even with gloves. Wait until the condition has cleared.) A way to determine if an area is "open" or "intact" is to wipe the area in question with alcohol. If it stings, it is "open" and should be covered with a glove. If the scratch or sore is on the end of the finger, a finger cot can be worn to protect the area.
- When any area of the patient's gown or linen is contaminated by body substances, even if the substance has dried.
- If the patient is receiving either cytoxan or thiotepa, chemotherapies used for cancer patients. There is

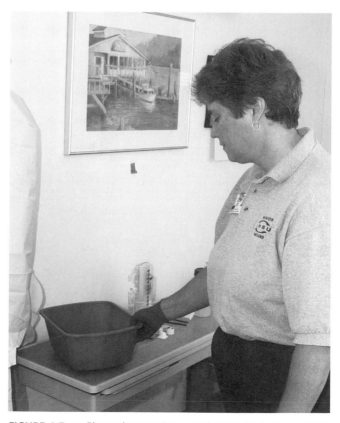

FIGURE 4-5. ■ Glove when moving a used urinal, bedpan, or emesis basin. (Photo by Don Hamilton.)

some evidence that both of these drugs eliminate through the skin.

- If steroidal cream has just been applied to the area that will be massaged.
- If the patient has **herpes** or **shingles.** Glove even when working at sites distant from the outbreak. Viral shedding can cause the condition to be present in the bedding.
- Never reuse the gloves for another patient. Also, do not use a set of gloves for more than one activity (i.e., moving a full urinal, then touching a patient).

👉 **TIP: Finger Cots**

Practitioners who frequently have cracked cuticles or cuts on the fingers and hands should carry a packet of finger cots when at the hospital. This will prevent them from having to glove just for a torn cuticle.
The use of finger cots is much more enjoyable than complete gloving.

Procedure for putting on:

1. Remove rings and bracelets to avoid puncturing or tearing the glove.
2. Wash hands and forearms.
3. Dry thoroughly. Putting gloves onto damp hands can create skin problems.
4. Put on gloves.

Removal:

1. Remove the first glove by grasping it with the gloved hand in the palm and pulling it off (Fig. 4-6). Wad this glove into the palm of the gloved hand.
2. Remove the second glove by sliding bare fingers inside the glove and pulling up (Fig. 4-7). Touch only the inside of the glove. Do not touch the outside of the glove with the ungloved hand. Remember—"clean to clean, dirty to dirty." Fold the second glove over the first dirty glove as it is removed (Fig. 4-8).
3. Place used gloves in the appropriate receptacle. Sometimes this will be inside the patient's room, for example, if the person is on **Contact Precautions.** At other times it will be outside the patient's room. Dispose of gloves after each use. When placing items into a waste container, never reach in blindly.
4. Wash hands thoroughly and dry.

If wetness is felt or anything suggests that the gloves are leaking, immediately remove them, wash thoroughly, and put on new gloves.[5]

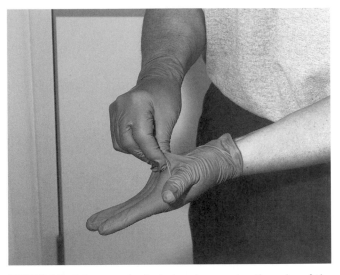

FIGURE 4-6. ■ Remove the first glove by grasping the palm of the glove and pulling. (Photo by Don Hamilton.)

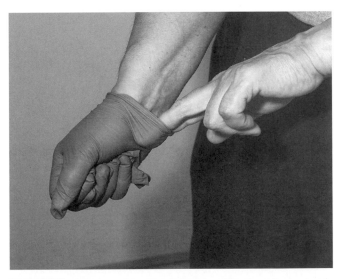

FIGURE 4-7. ■ Remove the second glove by sliding bare fingers inside the glove and pulling up. (Photo by Don Hamilton.)

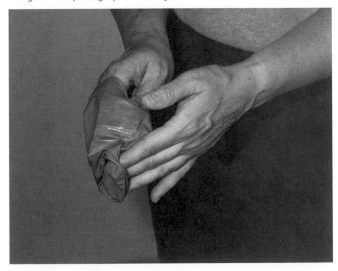

FIGURE 4-8. ■ Fold the second glove over the first as it is removed. (Photo by Don Hamilton.)

Masking

It is often necessary to mask before entering the room of a patient who is immunosuppressed or who is contagious via airborne or droplet transmission. There will be instructions on the door if this is the case. Masks should only be worn for a single usage because they become ineffective from moisture after prolonged use.

Procedure for putting on:

1. Place mask over the nose and mouth.
2. If the mask has strings that tie in the back, tie the top set first and then the bottom strings. In this way, a tight fit is created over the mouth and nose (Fig. 4-9).

Removal (reverse the process):

1. Untie the bottom strings, touching only the strings.
2. Untie the top strings, touching only the strings.
3. Place into a trash receptacle.
4. Wash and dry hands or apply handrub.

Gowning

Caregivers may need to gown for a variety of patients, such as for a patient who is immunosuppressed. This helps to protect the patient from microorganisms that may be on the clothes of those entering the room. Gowning also may be required as a protection for staff when working with those who are under Airborne Precautions, such as **tuberculosis** or Contact Precautions, such as an antibiotic-resistant bacteria.

Procedure for putting on:

1. Wash and dry hands.
2. If wearing long sleeves, roll them up above the elbows.

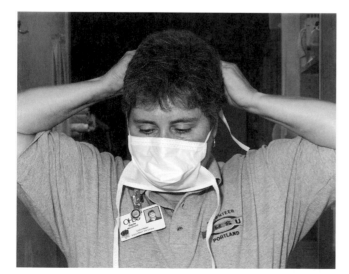

FIGURE 4-9. ■ Place the mask over the nose and mouth. Tie the top strings first so that a secure fit is formed. (Photo by Don Hamilton.)

A Therapist's Journal

Gina

One of the first patients I was assigned to at OHSU was undergoing high-dose chemotherapy. On the outside of the door were instructions requiring a 30-second handwashing and gloving before entering because of her **neutropenic** status. The nurse had referred Gina to me in hopes that massage would ease the nausea the patient was experiencing.

Before our conversation went very far, Gina felt nauseous and asked me to hand her the already-used **emesis** basin from the overbed table. When she finished, I replaced the basin, removed my gloves, placed them in the trash, washed my hands, and regloved.

Eventually the massage got under way. About 10 minutes into the session, Gina once more asked for the emesis basin. Again we patiently went through the same routine—replace the basin, unglove, wash, dry, reglove.

Twenty minutes into the session, Gina needed to use the toilet due to the significant quantities of fluids she was receiving. Although I didn't have to unglove or rewash, once again the massage came to a halt. Finally, we were then able to go another 20 minutes, this time without stopping, to the end of the massage. However, even with the many interruptions, the session of gentle touch accomplished what the nurse had hoped: Gina's nausea was gone. For a final time, I ungloved, washed, and dried.

—Gayle MacDonald, MS, LMT

---

3. Hold the gown in front of you, and let it unfold. Do not shake it. Put arms through the sleeves, and tie snugly at the back of the neck.
4. Be certain the gown overlaps in the back so that all clothing is covered.

Removal:

1. Undo waist and neck attachments. Paper gowns with Velcro attachments are common.
2. Pull down on the sleeve of the gown to start the removal process (Fig. 4-10).
3. Reach up to the shoulders and pull off the gown at the same time, folding it inward (Fig. 4-11). Roll it up into a ball.
4. Place the gown in a covered container.
5. Wash and dry hands.[5]

USING PROTECTIVE PRACTICES IN COMBINATION

Bodyworkers will observe that experienced healthcare providers perform Standard Precautions in differing pro-

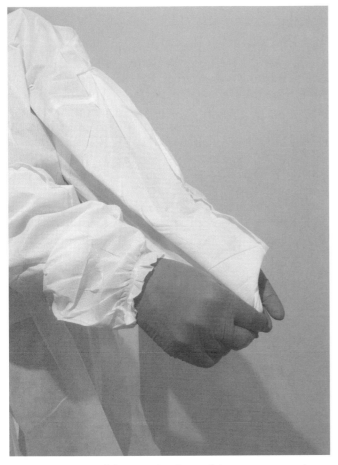

FIGURE 4-10. ■ Pull down on the sleeve of the gown to start the removal process. If gloved, grab the outside of the gown. (Photo by Richard York, Oregon Health and Science University.)

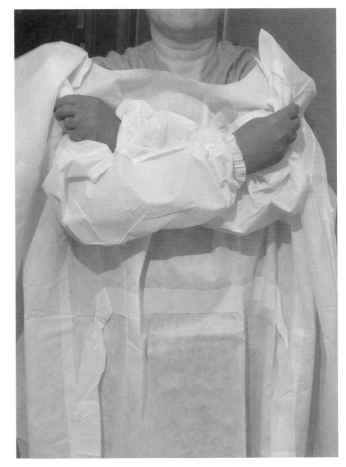

FIGURE 4-11. ■ Remove the gown by pulling off at the shoulders and folding inward. If gloved, grab the outside of the gown. Roll the gown into a ball and dispose in an appropriate container. (Photo by Richard York, Oregon Health and Science University.)

gressions. For instance, when both gloving and gowning are required, some unglove first and then ungown; others do it in the opposite order. There are differing opinions and practices about the order of performing these activities. Some staff believe that the sequence doesn't matter; others believe that a definite progression should be followed. Institutions, too, may have protocols that differ from one another. The massage therapist employed by a healthcare institution would, of course, follow the protocols required by that facility.

The sequences presented in the following section are based on ease of learning and may differ from the way in which some people put protective guidelines into practice. The important fact is that no matter the order, a safe way can be found to remove protective gear by following the "clean to clean, dirty to dirty" concept.

☞ **TIP: Infection Control Officer**

All hospitals have an infection control officer. This person can be an invaluable resource when practitioners need Standard Precautions questions answered by an expert.

Masking and Gloving

Observe the following order if it is necessary to both mask and glove.

Procedure for putting on:

1. Wash and dry hands or apply handrub.
2. Apply mask.
3. Glove.

Removal (reverse the above process):

1. Take off gloves.
2. Wash and dry hands or apply handrub.
3. Remove mask.
4. Wash and dry hands or apply handrub.

Gowning and Gloving

Procedure for putting on:

1. Wash and dry hands or apply handrub.
2. Gown.
3. Glove.

Removal:

1. Ungown. Because the gloves are still on, the practitioner must grab the outside of the sleeve to start the process. Then grab the outside of the shoulders, turning the gown inward. (Clean to clean, dirty to dirty.) See Figures 4-10 and 4-11.
2. Unglove.
3. Wash and dry hands or apply handrub.

Masking, Gowning and Gloving

Observe the following order when it is necessary to mask, gown, and glove.

Procedure for putting on:

1. Wash and dry hands or apply handrub.
2. Mask.
3. Gown.
4. Glove. (Gloving last means that the gloves have handled fewer surfaces and are cleaner than if they had been put on at the start.)

Removal:

1. Remove gown. (Only touch the outside of the gown until it is off the body.)
2. Remove gloves.
3. Wash and dry hands or apply handrub.
4. Unmask.
5. Wash and dry hands or apply handrub.

A Therapist's Journal

Standard "Overprecautions"!

Adapting my massage skills to the seriously ill was not difficult. But mastering the handwashing, gloving, gowning, and where to put the used linen of a patient with a serious infection has been a lengthy process. For me, these practices should say Standard "Overprecautions" to indicate the anxiety I have had with this part of the work. Having the chance to provide massage to hospital patients is a wonderful honor. However, this opportunity brings with it the considerable trust by and responsibility toward the patient that I will provide a compassionate, respectful, and safe massage. The patient trusts that I will follow Standard Precautions, that I will read and follow all special instructions on the door, that I will check with her nurse and read her chart, and that I will understand what having a low white count or low platelets means. Providing massage in the hospital setting carries a lot of responsibility. Although I would prefer to just focus on providing a compassionate massage, I must also follow Standard Precautions and create a balance between the two.

E.A. Dolan, LMT, Portland, Oregon

TRANSMISSION-BASED PRECAUTIONS

Transmission-Based Precautions are designed for patients who are known or suspected to be infected with highly transmissible pathogens. There are three types: Airborne, Droplet, and Contact Precautions. Just as with Standard Precautions, these practices also include handwashing, gloving, masking, and gowning, but they are carried out for different reasons.

These techniques protect staff and visitors from pathogens shed by patients and are specific to the type of disease or condition involved. Some diseases may have multiple routes of transmission and will require a combination of precautions. A sign on the patient's door, as in Figure 4-12, will specify which protocols to follow. An isolation cart containing gloves, masks, and gowns often will be positioned outside the door to these patients' rooms. Protective gear should be put on outside the room. Depending on the type of isolation, the gear will mostly likely be taken off just before leaving the room and discarded in a closed container in the room. Following are the common types of isolation and the precautions usually taken.

AIRBORNE ISOLATION

According to the CDC, airborne transmission occurs by dissemination either through the residue of small particle droplets containing pathogens that have evaporated and remain suspended in the air for long periods of time or dust particles containing the infectious agent. Pathogens carried in this manner can be dispersed widely by air currents and may be inhaled by someone in the same room or over a longer distance, depending on environmental fac-

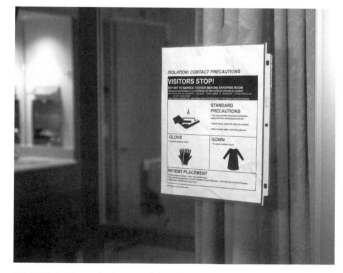

FIGURE 4-12. ■ A sign on the patient's door will indicate whether specific infection control protocols are to be followed. (Photo by Don Hamilton.)

tors. Therefore, special air handling and ventilation are required to prevent airborne transmission. Tuberculosis (TB) is an example of airborne disease in which hospitals isolate patients in rooms with negative airflow pressure, thereby keeping the TB bacteria inside the room. Measles and chicken pox are examples of other airborne diseases. Airborne Precautions involve the use of a special mask or respirator in addition to gowning and gloving.[4] However, in the case of measles or chicken pox, if the practitioner is immune to them, masking is usually unnecessary.

DROPLET ISOLATION

Droplet transmission involves contact with droplets generated during coughing, sneezing, or talking. The contagious agents do not remain suspended in the air and generally travel only a short distance, 3 feet or less, through the air. Examples of diseases that can be transmitted through this route are certain types of influenza, **meningitis**, pneumonia, **epiglottitis**, **diphtheria**, **whooping cough**, **streptococcus (group A)**, **pharyngitis**, **scarlet fever**, mumps, and **rubella**. Droplet precautions require the use of a mask when working within 3 feet of the patient.[4]

CONTACT ISOLATION

Transmission by contact can occur through direct or indirect contact. Direct contact involves transmission from one person's body to another's. Transmission by indirect contact can happen through contaminated instruments, needles, dressings, contaminated hands, surfaces in the patient's room, or gloves that are not changed between patients. The following are some conditions that warrant the use of Contact Precautions: antibiotic-resistant bacterial infections such as **VRE (vancomycin-resistant enterococcus)** and **MRSA (methicillin-resistant staphylococcus aureus)**, **enteric** infections such as certain forms of *Escherichia coli* or hepatitis A, and skin infections that are highly contagious or that may occur on dry skin, including **cutaneous diphtheria**, **herpes simplex**, **conjunctivitis**, **lice**, and **impetigo**.

Contact Precautions involve handwashing, gloving, and gowning before entering the patient's room. The protective barriers are taken off in the room and placed in a covered container before leaving. After removing the gloves and handwashing, it is important to not touch surfaces in the room that may potentially carry the pathogen, such as the overbed table or bathroom door handle.[4]

Items in the room of someone posted as a Contact Precaution should not be taken out of the room. For instance, Marta needed a chair to sit in while massaging her patient's feet. However, there was no chair in the room. The spouse of the next-door patient offered her one of theirs. Unfortunately, Marta didn't notice the Contact Precaution sign on the other patient's door. This particular patient had VRE, an antibiotic-resistant bacteria that can be communicated to other patients. Taking the chair into another patient's room potentially transfers the bacteria from one room to another. Also, avoid taking into the room items such as pens, notebooks, or lotion holsters.

PROTECTING PATIENTS DURING IMMUNOSUPPRESSION

Reverse isolation, also known as **protective isolation**, is designed to safeguard patients who are immunocompromised, such as those who have undergone organ or bone marrow transplantation or those in critical care units. Precautions may be as simple as a 30-second handwashing before entering the room, or they may entail completely masking, gowning, and gloving. In addition, living plants and fresh food and flowers often will be restricted. Protection isolation precautions vary from hospital to hospital depending on special air handling and ventilation technology. A lengthy handwashing is standard, but masking, gowning, and gloving requirements will differ. Instructions will be clearly posted on the patient's door.

LINEN HANDLING

It may be necessary to obtain additional sheets, towels, or blankets for draping, warmth, or to cover soiled areas. Linen is handled in many ways, depending on the facility. The recommended procedure is as follows:

1. Before collecting clean linen, wash and dry hands or apply a handrub.
2. Remove the necessary items from the linen closet or cart. Only take as much as is needed for each patient. Remaining linen cannot be taken into another room for use.
3. Do not let clean linen touch your clothing.
4. If any linen falls onto the floor, discard it into the soiled linen hamper, as it is considered contaminated.
5. Do not shake out linens when unfolding. This can stir up a cloud of microbes in the air, even if the linen is clean.
6. Consider any unused linen as dirty, and place it in the hamper. Do not replace it in the closet or on the cart.
7. When handling soiled linen, do not let it touch your clothes.
8. When discarding used linen in the hamper, simply place it in. Never plunge your hands and forearms down into the hamper to compact the soiled linen.

9. Do not throw used linens on the floor.
10. Wash and dry hands after handling used linen.[5]

The patient's linen or gown may become contaminated by a variety of body substances, such as urine, feces, wound drainage, or blood, requiring the therapist to glove while massaging. Ideally, linen or gowns that contain areas of contamination should be changed before starting the massage session. If this is not possible, wear gloves while massaging. A clean towel or draw sheet can be placed over the area to make for a more pleasing appearance. However, gloves should still be worn.

EXPOSURE TO BODY FLUIDS

Bodyworkers do not engage in many of the healthcare tasks that put staff at risk for encountering body fluids. They will seldom be involved with changing linens, cleaning up spills, or handling needles. With diligent adherence to Standard Precautions, touch practitioners will be safe. However, if contact occurs with body substances, immediately wash the area for 1 to 3 minutes with soap and water. If the exposure was caused by a sharp object, save the object for possible testing. Report the incident to the charge nurse or other supervisor. He or she will advise you on any further steps that should be taken.

HANDLING OF WORK CLOTHES

The purpose of the following guidelines is for the protection of the patient, the practitioner, and those who live with the practitioner.

- Always put on clean clothes just before departing for the hospital. Do not wear the same clothes to work with private practice clients or to perform other work.
- Do not smoke, and try to avoid smokers after putting on hospital clothes. Many patients are often highly sensitive to odors and can become nauseated in their presence.
- If for some reason it is necessary to bring clean clothes from home, place them in a container that is used only for that purpose. For instance, do not place hospital work clothes in a backpack or athletic bag that is also used to carry personal items such as water bottles, books, and pens.
- Change clothes in an area designated for this purpose, such as a staff locker room. Do not change in such areas as a utility room, public restroom, or staff lunch room.
- After finishing at the hospital, remove the work shirt and trousers. Do not wear them to another work site or around home. This protects those the touch therapist lives with as well as other people who receive bodywork from them.

MISCELLANEOUS PRECAUTIONS

A number of miscellaneous things are of importance with regard to infection control. This section addresses fingernail length, rings, and practices related to lotion.

FINGERNAIL LENGTH

Those who have direct patient contact must maintain short fingernails. Long fingernails are more likely to tear gloves or accidentally scratch or gouge a patient, and they provide a place for microorganisms to become trapped. This accumulated bacteria is not removed by regular handwashing, but requires vigorous brushing. The fingertips, too, are unable to be adequately cleaned when long nails are present.[8] Hospital-acquired infections have been traced back to healthcare workers with long fingernails.[9–11]

The following guidelines apply to fingernails:

- Nails should not extend more than a 1/4 inch beyond the fingertip.
- Nail decor should be within the norms of hospital culture. Also, it should not involve small objects that can come off the nail.
- Nail polish should be smooth and not chipped.
- No type of artificial nail should be worn.

RINGS

Ring wearing can create a twofold problem—protective gloves are more easily torn and skin organism counts are higher on the hands of care providers who wear rings. Research shows that the more rings a person wears, the greater the risk of contamination.[12] The guidelines about rings are very clear: Remove them while at work.

LOTION

Another component requiring attention is lotion. Many lotions provided by the hospital for patients' personal use lack good glide and therefore are not suitable for massage. The best solution is to purchase bulk quantities of lubricant specially made for massage. Therapists can then transfer what they need for a single session into a clean paper cup. This arrangement gives the therapist a good product to work with, and it prevents bacteria from being transferred from one patient's room to another's. Potentially, the latter can occur if the same lotion bottle is used for successive patients.

Several steps need to be observed to be certain the lubricant does not contribute to an infection problem:

- Ideally, massage practitioners should not take the same lotion bottle from patient to patient. If they do, the bottle should be washed with antimicrobial soap between patients.

- If therapists are unable to buy specialized massage lotion, it is then best in terms of infection control to use the single-portion bottles of lotion provided by the hospital. When the massage is over, the remaining lubricant is left with the patient.
- Use only the hospital's lotion for immunosuppressed patients or lotion specially purchased for the hospital. Lotions belonging to the therapist may have been sitting out, carried around in a backpack, or stored in a cupboard for a period of time, thereby increasing the growth of organisms in the lubricant or causing them to be rancid.
- Only set lotion bottles on tables or counters, never on the floor.
- Do not use jars that require dipping the fingers into the container unless the container will be disposed of after each patient.

TIP: Kneeling on the Floor

Therapists often kneel on the floor to achieve comfortable body mechanics when massaging certain body parts. In a hospital, that practice is especially inadvisable because of bacteria on the floor. Sitting in a chair is a more hygienic way to position one's self to massage areas of the patient's body, such as the hands and feet, that are close to the edge of the bed.

WHEN TO STAY HOME

The massage therapist who has a fever, flu, is within the first 4 days of a cold, or is infected by other communicable diseases, such as conjunctivitis or herpes, should stay at home. This is especially true when working with patients who are immunosuppressed. Also, if someone in the practitioner's family has a communicable disease, such as measles, mumps, chicken pox, shingles, hepatitis, mononucleosis, TB, or another communicable disease, confer with the unit manager or employee health nurse regarding work status.

SUMMARY

Touch therapists without prior healthcare experience often find the application of Standard Precautions to be one of the most difficult parts of learning to work in the acute care setting. It is not uncommon to have bouts of paranoia before settling into an ease and rhythm. As with any new skill, the learning period is awkward, but

eventually the use of Standard Precautions becomes second nature.

TEST YOURSELF

1. In which of the following situations should a massage therapist glove?
   A. While holding the legs of a woman in labor
   B. Airborne isolation
   C. Contact isolation
   D. If the patient has low platelet counts
   E. If the patient has herpes
   F. If the patient or practitioner has a cut that is scabbed over
   G. To move a full urinal
   H. If the patient has pneumonia
   I. If the patient is taking oral steroids
   J. If the patient is taking cytoxan

2. Massage therapist should refrain from working with patients when therapists are experiencing which of the following conditions:
   A. A runny nose and cough from hayfever
   B. Day three of a cold
   C. Conjunctivitis
   D. An open cut on the hand
   E. Herpes

3. Answer True/False to each of the following statements:
   A. If blood is not present, tears and perspiration are noncontagious body fluids.
   B. The use of handrubs is permissible to clean the hands following the administration of a massage.
   C. Fingernails should be kept short to minimize the presence of bacteria under the nails.
   D. The hands should be washed before gloving.
   E. Unused linen should be replaced onto the linen cart.

REFERENCES

1. Monitoring Hospital-Acquired Infections to Promote Patient Safety—United States, 1990–1999. MMWR Morb Mortal Wkly Rep 49(8):149 Available at www.cdc.gov/mmwr/preview/mmwrhtml/mm4908a1.htm. Accessed May 29, 2004.
2. Weinstein R. Nosocomial Infection Update. Emerg Infect Dis 1998:4(3). Available at: www.cdc.gov/ncidod/eid/vol4no3/weinstein.htm. Accessed January 4, 2003.
3. American Iatrogenic Association. www.iatrogenic.org/index.html. Accessed April 14, 2003.
4. Centers for Disease Control and Prevention (CDC), Division of Healthcare Quality Promotion. Issues in Healthcare Settings. Part II. Recommendations for Isolation Precautions in Hospitals. Updated February 18, 1997. Available at: www.cdc.gov/ncidod/hip/isolat/isopart2.htm. Accessed January 4, 2003.

5. Graves L, Mullen L, Fouts J. Nursing Assistant Training Manual. Beaverton, Oregon: Medical Express, 1992, 2002.

6. Centers for Disease Control and Prevention (CDC). Hand Hygiene Guidelines Fact Sheet. Updated October 25, 2002. Available at: www.cdc.gov/od/oc/media/pressrel/fs021025.htm. Accessed October 30, 2002.

7. Boyce JM, Pittet D. Guideline for Hand Hygiene in Health-Care Settings. MMWR Morb Mortal Wkly Rep October 25, 2002. Available at: www.cdc.gov/mmwr/preview/mmwrhtml/rr5116a1.htm. Accessed January 12, 2003.

8. McNeil SA, Foster CL, Hedderwick SA, et al. Effect of Hand Cleansing With Antimicrobial Soap or Alcohol-Based Gel on Microbial Colonization of Artificial Fingernails Worn by Health Care Workers. Clin Infect Dis 2001;32(3):367–372.

9. Parry MF, Grant B, Yukna M, et al. Candida Osteomyelitis and Diskitis After Spinal Surgery: An Outbreak Implicates Artificial Nail Use. Clin Infect Dis 2001;32(3):352–357.

10. Moolenaar RL, Crutcher JM, San Joaquin VH, et al. A Prolonged Outbreak of *Pseudomonas aeruginosa* in a Neonatal Intensive Care Unit: Did Staff Fingernails Play a Role in Disease Transmission? Infect Control Hosp Epidemiol 2000;21(2):80–85.

11. Foca M, Jakob K, Whittier S, et al. Endemic *Pseudomonas aeruginosa* Infection in a Neonatal Intensive Care Unit. N Engl J Med 2000;343(10):695–700.

12. Trick WE, Vernon MO, Hayes RA, et al. Impact of Ring Wearing on Hand Contamination and Comparison of Hand Hygiene Agents in a Hospital. Clin Infect Dis 2003;36(11):1383–1390.

ADDITIONAL RESOURCES

Occupational Safety and Health Administration, www.osha.gov.
Hand hygiene resources:
Bandolier Journal, www.jr2.ox.ac.uk/bandolier/band88/b88-8html.
University of Geneva Hospitals, Geneva, Switzerland, www.hopisafe.ch.
University of Pennsylvania, School of Medicine, www.med.upenn.edu/mcguckin/handwashing.

PRESSURE, SITE, AND POSITION—A CLINICAL FRAMEWORK

5

At first glance, the high-tech machinery, side effects from treatment, and medical devices give the impression that massaging hospital patients is a complex event. There is, however, a deceptive simplicity about giving bodywork in this setting. Once the information from the patient's chart and medical staff has been organized in the therapist's mind, the actual session is fairly uncomplicated.

In this chapter, a framework is presented that can be used for quickly and thoroughly obtaining information about the patient's condition and then organizing it to create a safe massage plan. The organizational framework centers on three specific categories: pressure considerations, site restrictions, and positioning adjustments. Most of the information about patients, such as side effects of medications, medical devices, procedures, or illness, can be placed into one of these three areas. Without a doubt, it is necessary to be knowledgeable about other parts of the patient's medical status, but the pressure, site, and position categories provide a basic structure for bringing order to the plethora of information that is given by the nurse or gathered from the medical chart.

This conceptual framework provides massage therapists with an anchor that allows them to work in any department in the hospital, from **obstetrics** to oncology to general surgery. Extensive knowledge about each medical specialty is impossible, for touch therapists as well as doctors and nurses. Bodyworkers may be thoroughly familiar with a couple of areas but have only superficial knowledge in others. With the pressure, site, and position framework as a focal point, they can move easily between areas of specialty without being completely conversant with each body of knowledge.

There is no one way to give a hospital massage. A Swedish massage therapist will administer one type of session, a Shiatsu practitioner will give another, while someone trained in Craniosacral Therapy will perform still another. The purpose of the pressure, site, and position format is to give therapists from all bodywork disciplines a common frame of reference around which they can create a safe touch session that addresses the individual needs and desires of each patient.

Many of the adjustments that patients require are self-evident. For instance, all bodyworkers are aware of the dangers of massaging too near an incision or on skin that has an open **lesion.** It is obvious that a person with breathing difficulty should not be positioned face down or a person with a blood clot should not receive circulatory modalities. In many situations, common sense is enough to guide the massage process. In other instances, it is not, and a specialized system for organizing patient information is needed.

PRESSURE CONSIDERATIONS

Pressure restrictions are the hardest group of adjustments to gauge. Massage therapists generally are taught that firm or deep pressure is necessary to release stress or knotted muscles. However, they must learn to trust that forceful bodywork is not necessary to create a profound effect. Physical symptoms such as pain, nausea, fatigue, and insomnia can be alleviated with the use of gentle touch modalities, as can emotional discomforts such as isolation, hopelessness, or anxiety.

Patients can make it difficult to hold the line on pressure because, like healthy clients, they want more firmness than the therapist is giving. This is true especially if the person has a history of receiving massage before being in the hospital. Patients have been known to plead for deeper pressure, even during times when they have dangerously low **platelet** levels or have less than 20% heart function. While it is natural to try to respect the patient's wishes, in many hospital situations, deeper pressure may cause harm to the patient or overburden body systems. Even if the patient is imploring the practitioner for more pressure, the therapist must stay within the guidelines laid out by the staff. Like physicians, touch therapists have a responsibility to "First, Do No Harm."

It must be remembered that people are in the hospital or other healthcare setting because they are acutely

TABLE 5-1 COMMON CONDITIONS REQUIRING PRESSURE ADJUSTMENTS

Systemic	Localized
Anticoagulant medication	Bone or spinal metastases
Bruises easily	Edema
Cachexia	Limb with central line
Congestive heart failure	**Lymphedema**
Deep-vein thrombosis	Lymph node removal (Hx of)
Extended bedrest	Neuropathy
Fatigue	**Osteoporosis**
Fever	Phlebitis
Neutropenia	Radiation Tx to main clusters of nodes
Preeclampsia	Skin—fragile or sensitive
Pregnancy	**Varicose veins**
Pulmonary disease	
Recent history of blood clot	
Recent surgery	
Renal dysfunction	
Risk for blood clot	
Thrombocytopenia	
Tissue fragility	

The *systemic* conditions require gentle massage or touch over the entire body. The *localized* conditions refer to just a specific area. Firmer pressure may be given to other parts of the body, depending on instructions from the health-care staff.

Some bodywork modalities can be administered with little or no modification in pressure, such as Jin Shin Jyutsu®, Reiki, Craniosacral Therapy, and Compassionate Touch®. Other techniques, such as Swedish Massage, acupressure, reflexology, Shiatsu, and trigger-point therapy, can be used by adapting the pressure to the situation. See Chapter 11 for appropriate touch-therapy modalities.

or chronically ill and require a level of care that cannot be given at home. They may have a medical condition, or side effects from treatment, that absolutely requires the use of light pressure, such as low platelets, fragile areas of skin, **neuropathy, edema,** recent surgery, bone **metastases,** or **anticoagulant** and pain medications. Nearly all patients will have some factor that necessitates decreasing the normal amount of force (Table 5-1).

The level of pressure will depend on a variety of influences: the disease, treatment, age, length of illness, blood counts, acuity of illness, and medications. Deep or even moderate pressure may place demands on a body that is too sick to tolerate them, thereby directing energy away from the healing process. Ruth Werner points out in *A Massage Therapist's Guide to Pathology* that "[m]assage therapists challenge homeostasis. We create changes in the internal environment of our clients' bodies. We influence the diameter of blood vessels and the direction of fluid flow. Massage changes the chemical balance of the body, reducing some types of hormones while increasing others, shifting neurotransmitter secretion, and altering protein levels in interstitial tissues. Our first job, before we ever touch a client, is to determine whether that person is capable of adjusting to the changes massage precipitates."[1]

TIP: Rephrasing the Request for Massage

Many hospital staff members have a stereotypical view of massage, either from their own experience or from the media. Their image is often of a vigorous experience involving strain and effort. This notion influences the staff's willingness and comfort level in referring patients for massage. Nurses sometimes dismiss patients as potential massage recipients because their platelet count is low or they are nauseated. The nurse doesn't realize that lightly applying lotion or gently resting the hands on an area is part of the practitioner's repertoire. Nor do they know what a positive effect this gentle touch could engender.

When a staff member appears hesitant about referring a patient, it is helpful to rephrase the request to create a different mental picture. A term that has worked well with many nurses is "lotioning." If the therapist knows ahead of time that extreme gentleness is required, such as for a patient with thrombocytopenia, the therapist could ask, "Would it be OK to put lotion on his feet?" This conjures up a completely different image than if the term "massage" is used. The phrase "gentle massage" also works well when trying to reframe the request.

soon learned that too much stimulation released an overload of toxins into the patient's system. I learned to go more slowly, more gently, and to work for shorter periods of time, as not to overload the person's system with too many toxins in one session.[2]

Irene Smith, Guidelines for the Massage of AIDS Patients

There are many interpretations of "gentle pressure." Someone who is a sports massage therapist will have one idea; a person who practices Craniosacral Therapy will have another. Gentle bodywork may mean just resting the hands on the body, or it may entail systematically applying lotion or using an open hand rather than thumbs to give a Shiatsu treatment. There is a broad spectrum of pressure, even gentle pressure.

Surmising the correct amount of effort and pressure is sometimes easy and straightforward. For instance, a person with a platelet level below 20,000 should be massaged *only* with the amount of pressure used to apply lotion to the skin. The patient whose legs are tight with edematous fluid because of chemotherapy or cardiac complications should also only be lightly lotioned in the lower extremities. However, the case of a 23-year-old patient with a spleen injury from a car accident is less clear-cut. A firmer pressure on some parts of his body might be well tolerated.

There is no recipe for calculating pressure. Figure 6-6 in Chapter 6 gives general guidelines for common groups of patients. To gain input, the therapist can also demonstrate various pressures on the nurse. Other tips related to pressure are listed in the Tip Box on Pressure Suggestions.

SITE RESTRICTIONS

Medical devices, skin problems, or intervention sites, to name a few, will force bodyworkers to avoid or at least be mindful of certain sites. Some areas of the body, such as an incision, a weeping skin condition, or the site of a drain, should not be touched at all. Other areas may be touched but require an adjustment to the type of touch and pressure. An excellent example is labor-stimulation points. Many bodyworkers are taught when massaging a pregnant woman not to touch these points for fear the woman will go into labor. However, lightly passing over these points as part of an **effleurage** stroke is safe. Other examples are the site of a tumor, an **epidural**, or a skin condition called **petechiae.** Kneading or stroking the site of a tumor is inappropriate, but resting the hands lightly on it is not. Care needs to be taken near an epidural, but the area can be stroked up to a few inches away from the site. Petechiae, a skin condition characterized by very small reddish-purple dots under the skin, do not need to be totally avoided. Gentle massage over the affected area is fine.

☛ **TIP: Pressure Suggestions**

- Too little pressure is better than too much.
- Place attention mainly on the skin rather than on the musculature.
- Let go of being ambitious. Do not try to fix the patient.
- Let the entire weight of the hand sink into the patient. Full-hand contact with the body will give the illusion that more pressure is being used. In addition, it is very reassuring. Sometimes in their attempt to be cautious and gentle, therapists will pull back with their hands, body, and presence. Their stroke then becomes "feathery." While a few patients enjoy this type of contact, most prefer the feel of the whole hand on their skin. Notice the full-hand contact of the practitioner in Figure 5-2.
- Position the bed so the therapist is able to stand erect rather than leaning with his weight onto the patient. Leverage is rarely needed in the hospital. Notice the therapist's body in Figures 5-2A–E.

A PATIENT'S STORY

Light-Touch Massage

I was really excited when my nurse asked me if I would like a massage from one of the hospital massage therapists. When the therapist told me she had to use light pressure, I was disappointed but decided to go ahead with it anyway. I'm so glad I did. All of the other massages I've received were sports massages. Little did I know how perfect the light touch would be while I was in the hospital to receive chemotherapy. I was able to relax deeper than I had in 20 years.

Richard U., San Francisco, California

☛ **TIP: Site Restrictions**

- Focus on what can be done, not on what can't.
- Try to give the entire body some type of attention. Areas that cannot be directly touched can be given care through the application of modalities such as Healing Touch or Therapeutic Touch.
- Be mindful of areas where body fluids might be encountered. If in doubt, glove.

A Therapist's Journal
Only a Small Part of the Body

Sometimes only a small part of the body is able to be massaged, just one arm or one tiny part of the back. A hospital massage therapist once worked with a young man who had fallen out of a window from five stories up. The patient was in a coma and had an open wound on the left hip that was stapled shut, a broken right foot, a lump on his right forearm the size of an egg, a catheter in his neck, sequential compression devices on his legs, and a broken pelvis, to name just some of his injuries. The young man's father thought it would be good to massage him, but the only part that could be stroked was a tiny bit of the left side of his back. The therapist spent half an hour on the small, uninjured part of the back, and then administered Therapeutic Touch and Reiki to the remainder of the body. The father, who had rarely left his son's side for 5 weeks, commented on how much more relaxed his son was.

Gayle MacDonald, MS, LMT

POSITIONING ADJUSTMENTS

Generally, the medical staff will allow the patient to determine which positions are comfortable. Most position adjustments involve lying prone and often are due to an incision or medical device, such as a drain, urostomy bag, or an intravenous (IV) line in the chest. Those with respiratory or cardiac conditions may need to elevate the head to ease breathing difficulties. **Orthopedic** and stroke patients require a great deal of attention to positioning to maintain alignment of the affected area. If the

patient is under a strict and continuous position restriction, a sign will be posted on the wall above the head of the bed.

Each institution should create a policy regarding patient positioning by massage therapists. Some medical conditions require specialized training to safely position patients; hip replacements and strokes are examples. Hospitals may prefer to have the nursing staff position patients who are unable to manage on their own. Other facilities may require bodyworkers to undergo instruction in how to perform **transfers** and position changes as part of their orientation to the hospital.

APPLICATION OF THE PRESSURE, SITE, AND POSITION FRAMEWORK

The following section illustrates the application of the pressure, site, and position framework using case studies from four different hospital units: **cardiology**, obstetrics, oncology, and orthopedics. The medical conditions within these case studies are dissected for pressure considerations, site restrictions, and positioning adjustments. Comprehensive information is not given for each aspect of the condition. For now, readers are given enough background about each patient so that they are able to understand the concept behind the clinical framework. Further details can be found in chapters 6 to 9, which address common signs, conditions and symptoms, medical devices, procedures, and medications.

Keep in mind the definition of massage this text is using. The typical definition is circulatory based; hospital massage, on the other hand, is comfort based. The reader will encounter medical conditions in this manual that are frequently taught in pathology classes as contraindications to bodywork (for example, fever and edema). It is

---

BOX 5-1 | *Of Special Interest*

COMMON SITE RESTRICTIONS

Avoid directly touching areas affected by:

- Bone or spinal metastases (severe)
- Communicable diseases of the skin (e.g., herpes, shingles)
- Incisions (recent)
- Intervention sites (e.g., **biopsy,** catheterization)
- Medical devices (e.g., **IV catheter,** colostomy bag, epidural)
- Monitoring devices (e.g., cardiac, **fetal**)
- Severely painful areas
- Skin conditions, weeping or painful (e.g., rash, radiation burn, fragility)

In situations where direct touch is contraindicated, there is anecdotal evidence that modalities such as Therapeutic Touch may be beneficial over the affected site. Practitioners not trained in one of these modalities can still give attention to these restricted ar-

eas by holding the hands a couple of inches above the area for several minutes.

Be mindful of the following areas. Gently resting the hands on the area or light stroking is often appropriate:

- Abdomen of a pregnant patient affected by preterm labor or other obstetrical problem
- Bone and spinal metastases
- Extremities with or at risk for deep-vein thrombosis (gentle touch is OK, but no pressure or stroking)
- Labor-stimulation points
- Painful areas
- **Phlebitis** (resting the hands on the site is OK, but no pressure or stroking)
- Skin conditions, nonweeping
- Tumors (resting the hands on the site is OK, but no pressure or stroking)
- Varicosity, mild (all strokes toward the heart)
- Varicosity, severe (massage proximal to the varices)

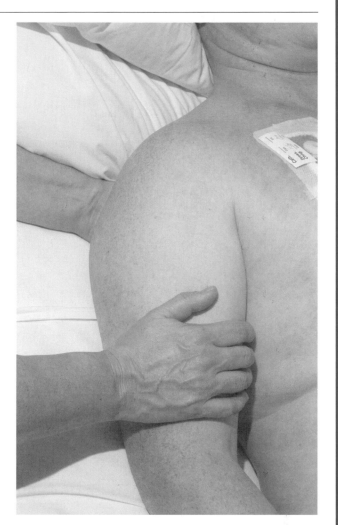

TIP: Positioning

- Therapists sometimes feel bad when asking a patient to reposition. Nurses, however, encourage the patient to make frequent position changes because it reduces the tendency of pressure sore development, improves strength, and restores confidence in the body.

- Allow patients to position themselves even though it is a slow, painful process. The therapist should assist with catheter lines or **telemetry** wires. Leave the opposite bedrail up so that the patient can use it when turning over.

- When patients need or want to remain supine, the back can be massaged by sliding the open hand under the back (Fig. 5-1). Acupressure or circular friction can then be applied by cupping the hand so that the fingertips can be directed into the muscles. Or, slide the hand just past the erector spinae group, and slightly hook the medial border with curved fingers. Slowly and gently pull the muscles away from the spine.

- A seated position on the side of the bed with support is not recommended for massaging the back of patients who tire easily.

- Patients who cannot lie prone sometimes can be positioned against the bedside table to give support while the back is massaged (see Fig. 5-2F).

FIGURE 5-1. ■ The back can be massaged from the supine position by sliding the open hand under the back. (Photo by Richard York, Oregon Health and Science University.)

| BOX 5-2 | *Of Special Interest* |

CAUSES OF COMMON POSITION RESTRICTIONS

- **Ascites**
- Breathing difficulty
- Edema
- Fractures
- Heart conditions
- Incisions
- Joint replacements
- Lymphedema
- Medical devices
- Nausea or intestinal cramping
- Pregnancy-related complications
- Tender skin (i.e., radiation burn)
- Tumors

true that rigorous bodywork would be ill-advised in those situations, but with the proper adjustments, skilled touch can be administered regardless of the severity of a person's medical condition.

The guidance given on the following pages must not be taken as the last word. It is a general framework from which to base decisions.

MR. R, A CARDIOLOGY PATIENT

Mr. R, 58 years old, had a coronary artery bypass graft (CABG) 72 hours ago. He has a **sternal** incision that is very painful and a small incision on the right leg where the saphenous vein was removed to graft onto the heart. The patient has a **peripheral IV catheter,** also known as a peripheral line, in the lower right arm, compression

TIP: Positioning Suggestions

FIGURE 5-1. ■ **Basic Positions for Receiving Massage.**

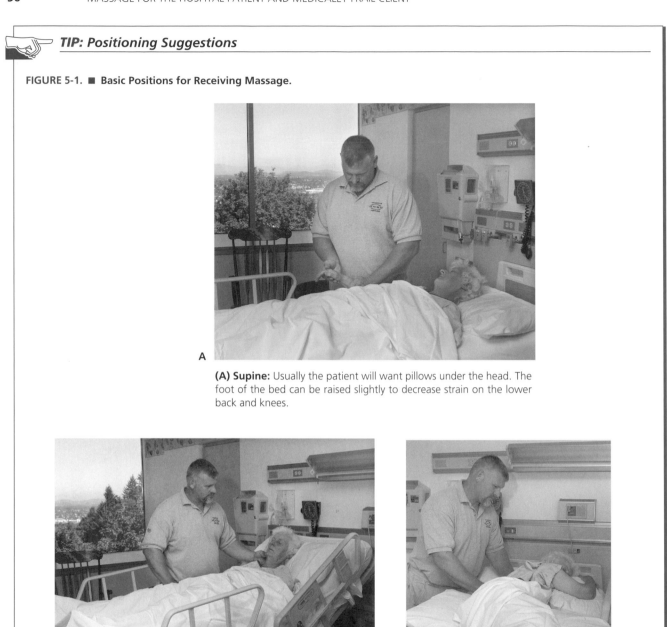

A

(A) Supine: Usually the patient will want pillows under the head. The foot of the bed can be raised slightly to decrease strain on the lower back and knees.

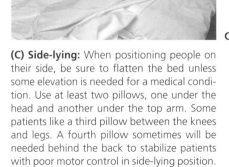

B

(B) Semireclining (also known as Fowler's position): Patients may need to be in this position to ease their breathing. Others may prefer to remain semireclining if the session is only going to include the legs, feet, shoulders, arms, and hands or if they have visitors during the massage. Be certain that the hips are at the pivot point of the bed, not the back.

C

(C) Side-lying: When positioning people on their side, be sure to flatten the bed unless some elevation is needed for a medical condition. Use at least two pillows, one under the head and another under the top arm. Some patients like a third pillow between the knees and legs. A fourth pillow sometimes will be needed behind the back to stabilize patients with poor motor control in side-lying position.

FIGURE 5-1. ■ *(continued)*

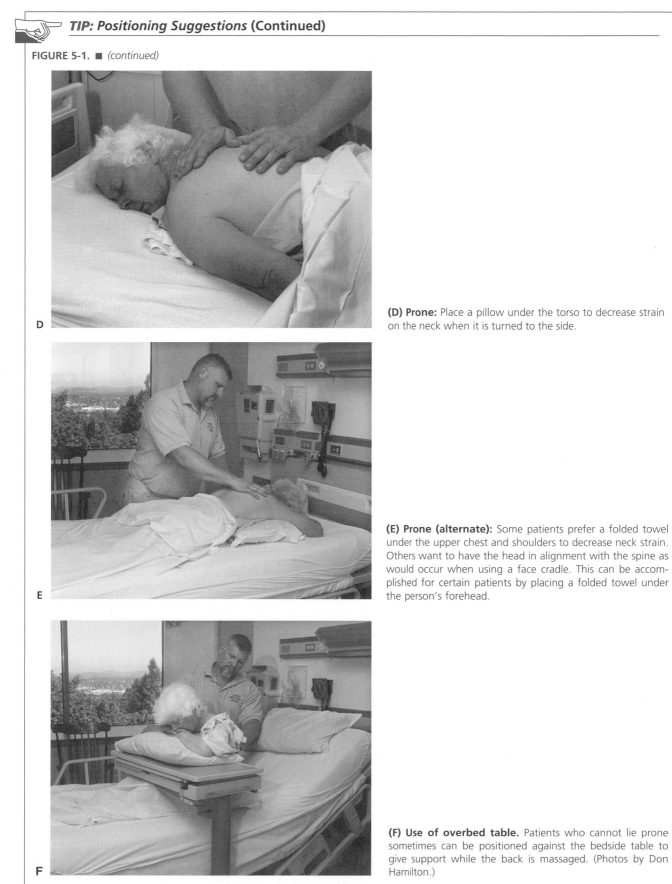

(D) Prone: Place a pillow under the torso to decrease strain on the neck when it is turned to the side.

(E) Prone (alternate): Some patients prefer a folded towel under the upper chest and shoulders to decrease neck strain. Others want to have the head in alignment with the spine as would occur when using a face cradle. This can be accomplished for certain patients by placing a folded towel under the person's forehead.

(F) Use of overbed table. Patients who cannot lie prone sometimes can be positioned against the bedside table to give support while the back is massaged. (Photos by Don Hamilton.)

hose on his legs to decrease edema and blood clots, two **electrodes** attached to the chest, and his throat is sore from the **endotracheal** tube. Mr. R smoked for 35 years, which has diminished his **pulmonary** function. He is hemodynamically stable, which means the pressures in the heart and blood pressure are stable, but he has a low-grade fever. Mr. R is on a long list of medications: aspirin to prevent a blood clot; an antibiotic; oxycodone and Vicodin for pain; Toradol, an anti-inflammatory drug also used for pain; nitroglycerin for blood pressure; Mevacor to control cholesterol; and nadolol to improve heart function. He is very fatigued. The nurses have him up twice a day for a short walk, and he takes his meals seated in a chair. Mr. R's lower back is sore from lying in bed and his shoulders hurt from being retracted to a 90° angle during surgery. Changing positions is painful, but Mr. R is interested in having a massage. His doctor has given permission for massage to the back, neck, and feet.

■ CLINICAL CONSIDERATIONS

Pressure considerations:

Mr. R's back massage should be fairly gentle for a variety of reasons:

- Inability to give accurate feedback due to pain medications.
- Low-grade fever.
- The sternal incision, which hurts at the slightest movement. Pressure on the back puts strain on the sternum.
- Fatigue.

Site restrictions:

- No circulatory massage to the legs due to the patient's increased risk for developing a **thrombus.**
- Take care around the sternum. A very light contact near the area may be OK.
- Lower right arm—peripheral IV catheter.
- Electrodes on the chest.

Positioning adjustments:

- Semireclining or right side-lying are the best positions for cardiac function.
- Side-lying may be too painful because of pressure on the sternum. Some people may tolerate short bouts.
- When the patient is in side-lying position, support his top arm to decrease pressure on the sternum.

MRS. O, AN OBSTETRICAL PATIENT

Mrs. O is 32 weeks pregnant and had been on bedrest since week 24 because of **preterm labor.** She is on magnesium sulfate ($MgSO_4$) to control the contractions, so there is a peripheral IV catheter in her right arm. She is

able to use the bathroom with help, but because the $MgSO_4$ relaxes all the muscles in the body, Mrs. O feels very lethargic. Even the muscles of her eyes are affected; she cannot see well and is easily disoriented.

Of all obstetrical patients, women hospitalized because of complications, such as preterm labor or eclampsia, require the most attention to pressure, site, and position adjustments. They are confined to bed, which further increases the risk for developing a thrombus. Therefore, only light pressure should be used on the legs. The focus should be on nurturing the mother-to-be. The safest positions are semireclining and left side-lying because they do not restrict blood flow to the uterus. And, of course, pressure to the abdomen and labor-stimulation points (see Chapter 6) should be avoided.

■ CLINICAL CONSIDERATIONS

Pressure considerations:

- Because of prolonged bedrest, the patient is at increased risk for developing a thrombus, especially in the legs. This is an indication for gentle pressure.
- As a pregnancy advances, a woman's ligaments are overstretched due to the effect of a hormone called **relaxin,** resulting in joint instability. Vigorous range-of-motion exercises are inappropriate.
- Be attentive to pressure around labor-stimulation points (see Figure 6-4).

Site restrictions:

- Stroking over the labor-stimulation points is permissible, but no pressure or concentrated attention should be paid to them.
- Peripheral IV catheter—Lower right arm.
- Abdomen—Gentle touch only, no pressure. This is partially a liability precaution.

Positioning adjustments:

- No prone.
- Left side-lying and semireclining are preferable. If the mother lies on the right side, it should be for a short period of time, perhaps 5 minutes. Start the patient on the right side, and end on the left, where she can remain indefinitely.
- When side-lying, place pillows under the head, top arm, and between the legs. Some women also like a fourth pillow or rolled towel under the belly for support.
- $MgSO_4$ can cause severe drowsiness, slowed reflexes, and flaccid paralysis. Take care when repositioning. The patient may need to move slower, may be disoriented, or may be less aware of her surroundings. Be mindful of safety. Do not leave her side with the bedrails down and the bed raised.

MS. A, A CANCER PATIENT

Ms. A, 56 years old, was diagnosed with breast cancer 3 years ago. Her treatment at that time consisted of a partial **mastectomy** on the left side, with 19 lymph nodes removed from under the arm. Four rounds of chemotherapy and 33 radiation treatments followed. Her energy now is good, but there is some lymphedema in the left arm.

The cancer has recurred in the other breast. Tomorrow morning, Ms. A will be having a mastectomy on the right side. She would like a massage in the hope that it will relieve the anxiety she feels about the upcoming surgery. The doctor has given permission for massage with no restrictions.

■ CLINICAL CONSIDERATIONS

Pressure considerations:
- In this case, the pressure adjustments are specific to a certain location. Moderate pressure is OK everywhere except in the upper-left quadrant.
- The left arm and upper-left quadrant should be massaged very gently because of lymphedema. Also, the duration to the entire quadrant should be greatly reduced. (See the Lymphedema section in Chapter 7.)

Site restriction:
- Avoid massaging into the left axillary area and inner arm. Resting the hands there is OK. This restriction is related to the lymphedema precautions.

Positioning adjustments:
- Prone—Do not allow the left arm to stay above the head for more than a couple of minutes at a time. This position can occlude the lymph flow and contribute to further swelling.
- When supine—Elevate the left arm with a pillow.
- No left side-lying due to the lymphedema.
- Side-lying on the right side is the best position for massaging the back because of lymphedema precautions.

Other:
- Study the Lymphedema section in Chapter 7. Not only should the strokes be gentle, but they should also go in the direction of lymphatic flow, which is toward the heart.

MRS. C, AN ORTHOPEDIC PATIENT

Mrs. C, 72 years old, underwent a left hip replacement 72 hours ago. The surgery and recovery went smoothly. She is on morphine for pain and anticoagulant medication due to the risk of a blood clot. Naturally, there is an incision and bruising at the left hip. A peripheral IV catheter is in the right wrist and compression hose on her legs to diminish the possibility of a thrombus. Mrs. C is beginning to be **ambulatory** but still has a **Foley catheter.** The doctor has given permission for a light back massage, but positioning is confined to the right side.

■ CLINICAL CONSIDERATIONS

Pressure considerations:
- The patient is at risk for a thrombus, necessitating light pressure to the legs.
- Because of the pain medication, the patient is unable to give accurate feedback about massage pressure.
- Avoid pressure on any part of the body that would disturb the alignment of the replaced joint.

Site restrictions:
- Left hip.
- Right wrist due to peripheral IV catheter.

Positioning adjustments:
- Supine and right side-lying are OK.
- Avoid acute flexion of the hip.
- Maintaining alignment of the newly replaced hip is essential to avoid dislocation. When the patient is lying on her side, place a pillow under her head, top arm, and especially between the entire length of her legs so that the new joint remains in neutral position. The nursing staff may want to help the patient reposition to ensure that the process is performed properly.

FURTHER APPLICATIONS

The four cases just given illustrate how the pressure, site, and position framework can be used in planning a touch session. This framework can also be applied to almost every other part of the patient's situation—medications, procedures, and as a tool to collect information. Figure 5-3 presents an example of a patient data-collection tool organized around the pressure, site, and position categories. This sample is specifically meant for obstetrical and **gynecological** patients but could be adapted for any group.

The side effects of medications can influence a massage session. Steroidal drugs, for example, are taken by many different types of patients, such as those with cancer, **rheumatoid arthritis** and **osteoarthritis,** and pulmonary diseases, and have a number of potential consequences. The three-part framework can assist the practitioner in analyzing the impact of massage on these patients. Steroids can cause easy bruising, fragile skin, osteoporosis, and edema, all of which are indications for gentle pressure. Edema also would require attention

OB/GYN Massage Patient Data Form

PART A: (Nurse)

Patient Name _____ DOB _____

Unit _____ Room _____ Nurse _____ Today's Date _____

Dx _____ Dx Procedure _____

Surgery _____ Date of Surgery _____

SENSORY IMPAIRMENT: ☐ blind   ☐ HOH   ☐ speech

PRESSURE RESTRICTIONS: Y   N

☐ DVT   ☐ phlebitis   ☐ varicose veins   ☐ long-term bedrest   ☐ easy bruising   ☐ recent surgery

SITE RESTRICTIONS: Y   N   **POSITION RESTRICTIONS:**   Y   N

_____ skin condition   _____ epidural   ☐ no walking   ☐ lay flat

_____ incision   _____ diagnostic monitor   ☐ no prone   ☐ no side-lying

_____ infection   _____ labor stim points   _____ elevate extremity or head

_____ IV site   _____ severe varicosity   _____

_____

GLOVING REQUIRED: Y   N

☐ open wound (patient or LMT)   ☐ skin condition   ☐ presence of body fluids

CHECK IF THE PATIENT HAS ANY OF THE FOLLOWING CONDITIONS:

☐ hepatitis   ☐ herpes   ☐ other contagious <u>disease</u>   ☐ allergy to lotion

other: _____

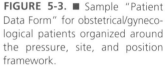

FIGURE 5-3. ■ Sample "Patient Data Form" for obstetrical/gynecological patients organized around the pressure, site, and position framework.

to positioning. In addition, steroids can cause poor wound healing, which would encourage the massage therapist to be vigilant for any sites that should be avoided.

The same analyzing process can be undertaken with regard to procedures, such as a heart catheterization. For instance, the person whose has undergone this procedure will have a site where the catheter was inserted, which the massage therapist should avoid touching. Pressure will need to be reduced due to pain and anticoagulant medications as well as the risk of bleeding into the retroperitoneal space, a side effect of the catheterization process, and because of the risk of bleeding, into the retroperitoneal space. And the patient will be required to remain supine for at least the first 4 to 6 hours, thereby affecting positioning.

Forthcoming chapters will apply the pressure, site, and position framework to medical devices, common reasons for hospital admission, and common symptoms and conditions.

SUMMARY

Like anything new, this framework, despite its simplicity, will feel a bit awkward to use at first. But in a very short time, it will become second nature. Without thinking, the massage practitioner will slot the patient's data as quickly as the doctor or nurse gives it. Touch therapists will feel confident as they expand throughout the various hospital units. Even though they may not have complete knowledge of a

specialty, the pressure, site, and position framework gives them a springboard for effective questioning strategies and critical thinking, skills that are more of an asset than the ability to memorize the details of a medical specialty.

TEST YOURSELF

Review the material presented in this chapter by answering the following questions. Use the information in the Pressure, Site, and Positioning sections if necessary. There may be more than one correct answer. Underline all correct answers.

1. Which of the following conditions indicate a high risk for a thrombus?
   A. Postpartum
   B. Postsurgical
   C. Psychiatric
   D. Osteoporosis

2. Being at high risk for a thrombus is an indication for:
   A. Reducing pressure
   B. Avoiding touch of the affected area
   C. Elevation of the head

3. Which of the following conditions require pressure restrictions?
   A. Fatigue
   B. Edema
   C. Cesarean section
   D. Congestive heart failure

4. Which of the following conditions require special positioning?
   A. Thrombocytopenia
   B. Bone metastases
   C. Neuropathy
   D. Breathing difficulty

5. Which of the following areas should not be touched directly?
   A. Weeping skin lesion
   B. Incision
   C. Edema
   D. Tumor

6. Which conditions require a reduction in the amount of pressure, either systemically or locally?
   A. Osteoporosis
   B. Fragile skin
   C. Herpes
   D. Renal failure

7. Which conditions may require attention to the patient's positioning?
   A. Pregnancy
   B. Tumor
   C. Fatigue
   D. Congestive heart failure

8. Which conditions should the bodyworker avoid direct contact with?
   A. Herpes
   B. Fever
   C. Varicose veins
   D. Neuropathy

REFERENCES

1. Werner R. A Massage Therapist's Guide to Pathology. Philadelphia, PA: Lippincott Williams & Wilkins, 2002.
2. Smith I. Guidelines for the Massage of AIDS Patients. San Francisco: Service Through Touch, 1992.

COMMON REASONS FOR HOSPITALIZATION OR MEDICAL TREATMENT

6

One of the first pieces of data to collect from the chart or the nurse is the patient's diagnosis and/or reason for receiving medical treatment. This single piece of information will enable practitioners to begin to formulate possible adjustments that must be made in the touch session. Chapter 5 outlined a framework of three categories that can assist bodyworkers in their planning: *pressure considerations, site restrictions,* and *positioning adjustments.* This chapter will continue the use of that conceptual device, applying it to some common reasons for hospitalization.

Near the end of this chapter on page 80 is a "Pressure Gauge" (see Figure 6-6), which is intended to give general guidance about the amount of force to use when massaging common groups of patients. Where pressure adjustments are indicated in the following material, it does not mean that pressure is contraindicated, but that the pressure must be modified to a varying degree. Future chapters will address in greater detail specific symptoms and side effects from medications, medical devices, and procedures.

ACQUIRED IMMUNE DEFICIENCY SYNDROME (AIDS)

AIDS is the most severe form of illness associated with the human immunodeficiency virus (HIV). HIV is fragile and does not survive outside the body for long. The virus is found in blood, semen, vaginal fluids, and mothers' milk. Although it has also been discovered in tears, sweat, and saliva, the concentration in these secretions is insufficient to cause infection. Transmission is generally through unprotected sex or needle sharing. Adherence to Standard Precautions will ensure the safety of those who come into contact with people with AIDS. In fact, the patient is at greater risk for obtaining an opportunistic infection from healthcare workers than vice versa.

Pneumocystis carinii pneumonia is the most common complication associated with AIDS. Others are **cytomegalovirus,** which can cause gastrointestinal (GI) problems, blindness, pneumonia, and infection of the adrenal glands, and **toxoplasmosis,** which can manifest with fever, headache, and **encephalitis,** causing changes in mental status. Other opportunistic infections include **cryptococcal meningitis,** which causes a number of side effects related to mental status; tuberculosis; **candida;** and herpes.

People with AIDS are also at increased risk for certain cancers. Non-Hodgkin's lymphoma and cervical cancer are seen in this patient population, but **Kaposi's sarcoma** (KS), a cancer of the cells that line certain blood vessels, is the most prevalent. It is characterized by purplish lesions on the skin, some of which may be raised and nodular, while others are flat. The lesions may or may not be painful; the pain status changes from day to day. A person with KS may feel embarrassed when having the lesions viewed or touched. Be considerate and gentle when asking permission to touch these areas.

Each complication has specific manifestations, but a general list includes fatigue, fever, easy bruising, peripheral neuropathy, shortness of breath, cachexia, oral lesions, nausea, diarrhea, and impaired mental processes. If **encephalopathy** or dementia is present, the person may have greatly reduced mental functioning, agitation, loss of balance and motor coordination, and, in the late stages, may be paralyzed and mute.

As there is not yet a cure for AIDS, patients are treated for the side effects of the disease. They may be on antibiotics for pneumonia or tuberculosis (TB), antifungal medications for candida, antiretroviral therapy to control the HIV viral load, and antidepressants.

Irene Smith, a pioneer in massage for people with AIDS, lists the following benefits of touch therapy for people with AIDS: controls pain, reduces confusion and increases orientation, encourages greater physical mobility, validates life and gives hope, reduces fear and isolation, and reinforces a more positive body image that may be lost due to debilitation and disease.[1–4]

■ CLINICAL CONSIDERATIONS

Pressure adjustments:
- Cachexia
- Easy bruising
- Fatigue
- Fever
- KS lesions

- Nausea
- Neuropathy

Sites to avoid or be mindful of:

- Bony prominences (The skin around these areas may be fragile.)
- IV catheters
- KS lesions

Positioning adjustments:

- Do not use a prone position if the patient
  - is nauseated,
  - is agitated or disoriented, or
  - has shortness of breath (SOB).
- Generally **self-limiting.** (The patient is able to set his own limits.)

Other:

The brain is a common target of the HIV virus, causing a variety of changes in mental status. See guidelines for communicating with the patient who is neurologically impaired in Box 6-1.

BOX 6-1 | *Of Special Interest*

COMMUNICATING WITH THE PERSON WHO IS NEUROLOGICALLY IMPAIRED

Any time the brain is involved in a medical condition, the patient may be easily confused, forgetful, discouraged, hostile, uncooperative, withdrawn, depressed, or emotionally unsteady. Communication often becomes difficult. The following suggestions will ease the communication process for those who have suffered a stroke, have dementia, or have brain damage[1,2]:

- If patients have had a stroke, face them on the unaffected side.
- Speak slowly, clearly, and with normal volume.
- Speak to the patient as you would any reasoning adult.
- Use short sentences.
- Ask simple questions. "Yes" and "No" questions are helpful.
- Present one idea at a time.
- Supplement speech with gestures and demonstration.
- Use the same wording consistently when asking questions or giving instructions.
- Allow the person plenty of time to speak and respond. It is difficult for patients to translate what is being said and then form a response if they feel pressured.
- Don't talk for the patient unless absolutely necessary.
- Keep distractions to a minimum. Provide a quiet environment to induce restfulness.
- Until speech returns, encourage communication through gestures, writing, or drawing if able.
- From time to time, restate what the patient has said.
- Don't act as if you understand when you don't.
- Elicit responses through statements such as, "Nod your head if you understand."
- Don't be abstract. The patient is often in a concrete frame of mind and takes everything literally. When you say you'll be back in a minute, the patient may understand it to mean "one" minute.
- Don't argue with the patient.

CANCER

For many years, **metastasis** was the dominant issue with regard to massaging people with cancer. Scientific research now has shown that the initiation and spread of cancer is the result of an accumulation of genetic mutations, some of which are **inherited,** the bulk of which are **acquired** throughout a person's lifetime. There is no evidence that increasing the circulation through mechanical means causes cancer cells to form new tumors at distant sites. If this were the case, **oncologists** would ask their patients to refrain from exercising or being active in any way. Just the opposite is true: Oncologists encourage cancer patients to remain active.

The real issues revolve around the side effects from chemotherapy, radiation, and surgery. Neuropathy, nausea, diarrhea, and fatigue are but a few. The two side effects that take center stage when working with hospitalized cancer patients are neutropenia and thrombocytopenia. It is these side effects that the doctors and nurses are most worried about in connection with massage. The neutropenic patient's immune system is compromised, leaving her vulnerable to infections. This can become a matter of life and death for some patients, not just the brief irritation of a cold or the flu. The massage therapist must take care to diligently apply Standard Precautions when working with this group.

Thrombocytopenic patients bruise easily. Sometimes they aren't even allowed to brush their teeth for fear of the gums bleeding. Massage can be given during this time, but it must be ultralight. Modalities that don't involve pressure, such as Reiki or Jin Shin Jyutsu®, are ideal. A light effleurage that basically lotions the skin also can be used. When massaging patients who bruise this easily, the practitioner should pay attention to the skin rather than the muscles.

Generally, the bodywork given to cancer patients should be gentle. Thrombocytopenia is one reason for this; fatigue is another. During cancer treatment, nearly everyone is fatigued. Deeper bodywork places a heavy burden on the systems of the body that are already working hard to deal with the disease and toxic treatments.

Radiation and lymph node removal puts many cancer patients at risk for lymphedema. Because the massage given to the medically frail is comfort oriented, the risk of a patient developing lymphedema from gentle strokes is negligible. People who have an active case of lymphedema can still have a touch session, but the safest course of action is to apply only light holds to the affected quadrant. No attempt should be made to treat the swelling unless the therapist has received extensive training in lymphatic drainage. Further information on lymphedema is given in Chapter 7.

Practitioners should glove when massaging patients who have been given thiotepa and cyclophosphamide, also known as Cytoxan, within 24 hours. There is some evidence that these two antitumor drugs eliminate through the skin. Other chemotherapies eliminate through the urine and feces; with these drugs, skin-to-skin contact poses no risk to touch therapists.

Cancer patients will be on a number of medications other than antitumor drugs. Prednisone, antibiotics, pain medication, antianxiety, and antiemetic drugs for nausea are commonly prescribed.[5]

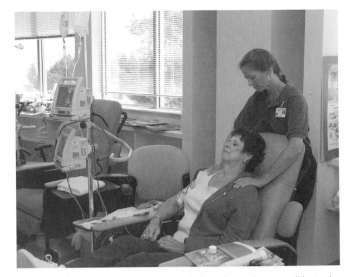

FIGURE 6-1. ■ Receiving massage during chemotherapy. (Photo by Don Hamilton.)

■ CLINICAL CONSIDERATIONS

CHEMOTHERAPY (Figure 6.1)

Pressure considerations:

- Anticoagulant medications
- Edema (usually in the legs)
- Fatigue
- Fragile skin
- Fragile veins
- Neuropathy (usually hands and feet)
- Neutropenia
- Osteoporosis (side effect from steroid use and certain chemotherapies, especially breast and reproductive system cancers, including prostate)
- Pain medications
- Skin sensitivity
- Thrombocytopenia

Site restrictions:

- Areas affected by herpes or shingles
- IV catheters
- Skin conditions (e.g., rashes, fragility)
- Tumors

Positioning adjustments:

- Central IV catheters (Some patients find it uncomfortable to lie prone.)
- Nausea (People often don't want to change positions.)

RADIATION—EXTERNAL BEAM (see Case History)

Pressure considerations:

- Bone fragility in areas with Hx of radiation
- Fatigue
- Neutropenia
- Potential skin sensitivity in the area of treatment
- Risk for lymphedema
- Thrombocytopenia

Site restrictions:

- Tumors
- The skin of the treated area may be too sensitive to touch by about the third week. Also, be aware of the area opposite the treated area. It too may be affected. Radiation burns the skin on the way out.

Positioning adjustment:

- Sensitive skin in the area of irradiation. For instance, people with breast or a head and neck cancer sometimes find it difficult to lie prone.

Other:

- The position required during radiation treatment may force the body into uncomfortable, static postures. Attention to these areas of the body may be very beneficial. For instance, during radiation for breast cancer, patients must lie with the arm on the side being positioned on the table above the head.

RADIATION—INTERNAL FORMS SUCH AS ORAL OR SEEDS

Contact during this time may be contraindicated if the patient is radioactive. Obtain guidance from the medical or nursing staff.

DISEASE-RELATED ADJUSTMENTS

Some adjustments are a result of the disease process and have nothing to do with treatment.

Pressure considerations:

- Bone or spinal metastases
- Edema or lymphedema due to obstruction by tumor
- Fatigue
- Increased risk of thrombus
- Thrombocytopenia

Site restrictions:

- Abdomen if ascites is present
- Tumor site (The area can be touched, but not pressed on.)

Positioning adjustments:

- Ascites (no prone positioning)
- Breathing difficulty due to tumors in the lungs (no prone positioning)
- Nausea
- Tumors

CARDIAC CONDITIONS

Typically, massage pathology texts advise that massage is contraindicated for many cardiac problems, such as heart attacks or congestive heart failure. However, with the broader definition of massage being used in this text, some form of bodywork is appropriate for nearly all heart patients. People with heart disease often are affected by other major health problems. Diabetes and kidney disease are two common ones. But because both of these diseases also require gentle, supportive bodywork, the massage session will not be appreciably altered by the additional conditions.

There are several factors common to many cardiac patients, each of which is an indication for gentle touch. One is the use of anticoagulants, a group of medications that prevents platelets from adhering to one another; however, anticoagulant use may also cause easy bruising if the dosage is high enough. Fatigue is another issue shared by many with heart problems that necessitates a soft approach to bodywork.

Conditions such as heart attack or congestive heart failure require the bodywork practitioner to minimize cardiac output. As has been said many times already, slow, soothing strokes or gentle touch is necessary. Because long effleurage strokes may increase venous return, smaller segmental strokes such as gentle wringing, compression, and muscle squeezing are the safest when minimizing cardiac output is necessary. A rough gauge of cardiac output can be made visually at the **jugular vein.** If there is any distension of this vessel, the pressure of the massage strokes should be decreased.

If the staff approve, therapists can massage heart patients' backs, which can especially benefit from massage. Those who have had catheterizations for such interventions as an **angiogram, stent** placement, or an **ablation,** lie supine on a hard surface for long periods of time. Heart surgery patients have sore rhomboids as a result of their arms being retracted to a 90° angle during the operation.

Psychological issues accompany serious heart disease. Major lifestyle changes often must be made, which many people resist. Other patients have to confront their own mortality or are affected by depression that is triggered by chronic pain and discomfort. Awareness of these issues is helpful for touch practitioners.[1,6–9] (Personal interview with Barbara Estes on April 12, 2003.)

Cardiac care commonly includes education activities such as guided imagery audiotapes for presurgical and postsurgical patients. Pairing massage with the tapes can be a powerful combination.

> *Bodyworkers raise people's awareness so that they get in touch with their own healing powers. . . .*
>
> Randy Cummins, Instructor, Chicago School of Massage

CONGESTIVE HEART FAILURE (CHF)

CHF is the heart's inability to pump enough oxygenated blood to meet the body's demand. The possible causes are many and varied—**hypertension,** coronary heart disease, **cardiomyopathy,** chronic lung disease, anesthesia, surgery, pregnancy, or drugs. To offset the side effects of diminished functioning, the heart rate increases, blood vessels constrict, and the heart enlarges, compensatory strategies that are themselves stressful to an already overworked heart.

The medical staff will manage the condition by reducing the heart's workload; eliminating excess fluid accumulation, which can occur in the lungs, body cavities, and extremities; and increasing cardiac output with medications. Common medications are **diuretics** to diminish excess fluid, **vasodilators** to increase the diameter of blood vessels, **beta-blockers** to slow heart contractions and control the rhythm, and antiplatelet drugs to prevent clot formation.

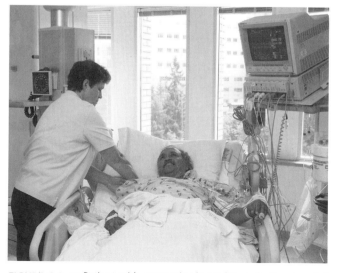

FIGURE 6-2. ■ Patient with congestive heart failure finds pain relief from massage. (Photo by Don Hamilton.)

Poor oxygenation results in SOB, fatigue, **cyanosis,** weakened immunity, anxiety, panic, and restlessness. These patients also are at increased risk for pneumonia. If they have been on prolonged bedrest, the touch therapist should be alert to the increased risk for pressure sores, thrombus, and **pulmonary embolism.**

Deep breathing is encouraged to avoid partial collapse of the lung, a condition known as **atelectasis.** Massage to the respiratory muscles can support fuller breathing. In addition, it provides rest and alleviates psychological tension, fatigue, and insomnia. CHF patients don't sleep well at night due to restlessness and anxiety, a side effect of cerebral **hypoxia.** Naturally, all bodywork should avoid placing a demand on the body (Fig. 6-2).[1,4,7–10]

■ CLINICAL CONSIDERATIONS

Pressure considerations:
- Cardiac and kidney complications
- Edema (pulmonary, extremity, and body cavities)
- Fatigue
- Psychological fragility
- Tissue fragility

Site restrictions:
- Electrodes on chest
- Oxygen-delivery device
- Pitting edema

Positioning adjustments:
- Coughing, SOB, and **dyspnea** (Avoid flat positioning; use semireclining. No prone positioning.)
- Edema (Elevate limbs. The feet should not be elevated above the heart to avoid stressing it through too much venous return.)
- Side-lying may be tolerated. (Right side may put less stress on the heart.)

Other:
- May be on water restriction.
- May need to use the bathroom frequently because of antidiuretics.
- May suffer from muscle cramps due to imbalance in electrolytes.
- Start with shortened sessions of 10 to 15 minutes.
- Observe exceptional use of Standard Precautions due to possible immunosuppression.

MYOCARDIAL INFARCTION

A **myocardial infarction** (MI) is commonly known as a heart attack. It occurs when a thrombus blocks one or more coronary arteries, depriving part of the heart muscle of oxygen. The area of the heart damaged when the oxygen supply is cut off is referred to as an **infarct.**

Treatment includes the administration of oxygen therapy and a multitude of drugs. Narcotics are given for pain; **thrombolytics** are used to dissolve the thrombus obstructing the coronary vessel; vasodilators such as nitroglycerin relax the coronary vascular system; beta-blockers are given to induce the heart to beat more slowly and with a more regular rhythm; **calcium channel blockers** decrease heart rate and blood pressure and dilate coronary vessels; and aspirin is prescribed as an anticoagulant.

An important part of cardiac nursing care is to promote restfulness, which in turn will help the heart heal by lowering cardiac workload. *The Lippincott Nursing Manual* recommends ". . . back massage to promote relaxation, decrease muscle tension, and improve skin integrity." Pain and anxiety reduction also could have been added to the above list. In addition to anxiety, a heart attack triggers a host of other psychological reactions, such as depression, grief, and lowered self-esteem. These responses can hinder healing. Anecdotal evidence indicates that massage may decrease some of these distressing feelings.[1,4,7–10] (Personal interview with Barbara Estes, LPN, LMT, on April 14, 2003.)

A number of possible complications will influence the massage session: fatigue and shortness of breath caused by decreased oxygenation, edema, and risk of bleeding due to thrombolytic drugs. Reducing the heart's workload is important. This can be accomplished through the use of gentle pressure and positioning the patient in specific ways.

■ CLINICAL CONSIDERATIONS

Pressure considerations:
- Edema
- Fatigue
- Inability to give accurate feedback due to pain medication.
- Light massage to the legs is often OK with doctor or nurse approval.
- The need to minimize cardiac output. Maintain awareness of heart rate and distension of the jugular vein.
- Risk of bruising due to thrombolytic and anticoagulant medications.

Site restrictions:
- Electrodes on chest
- IV catheters

Positioning adjustments:
- Some patients will be able to lie in any position.
- Elevate head if patient has SOB.
- Right side-lying puts less strain on the heart.
- Patient should rise slowly from a supine position.
- When rising from the bed to a seated position, the patient should sit with his feet on the floor to minimize **orthostatic hypotension.**

OPEN-HEART SURGERY

Open-heart surgery is commonly performed to replace a valve, repair the aorta or a congenital heart defect, or graft new blood vessels onto the heart. This last surgery is called a coronary artery bypass graft (CABG). Following surgery, the patient will be on oxygen and a number of medications—aspirin to decrease the chance of a blood clot, pain medication, drugs to regulate the heart's rhythm, and **antihypertensive** drugs such as beta-blockers, calcium channel blockers, and vasodilators.

Many of the complications are similar to those of other heart conditions. (Refer back to the MI section.) Patients are at risk for renal and cardiac insufficiency, decreased oxygenation, breathing difficulties, **coagulation** problems, thrombus, **hypotension**, fever, edema, hepatitis, and anxiety. In addition, the person who has been through open-heart surgery will have significant sternal pain due to the **sternotomy** and leg pain if blood vessels were removed to provide new coronary vessel grafts. They will have additional medical devices, a chest drain, an endotracheal tube, sequential compression devices on the legs to maintain circulation, a Foley catheter in the bladder, and possibly a **Swan-Ganz catheter** in the neck to monitor pressures in the heart.[1,4,7–10]

The sternal pain will be one of the major influences on any massage session. The prone position is not possible, and many patients will be unable even to lie on their side because of the pressure it places on the sternum. The neck, upper shoulders, arms, hands, and feet will be the areas most easily accessed.

■ CLINICAL CONSIDERATIONS

Pressure considerations:
- Coagulation problems
- Edema
- Fatigue
- Fever
- Pain medications
- Risk for thrombus
- Sternotomy

Site restrictions:
- Electrodes on chest
- IV catheters
- Leg incision
- Mindfulness of the legs due to increased risk of a thrombus
- Sternal incision

Positioning adjustments:
- No prone.
- May tolerate short bouts of right side-lying.
- Elevate head if there are breathing difficulties.
- Elevate lower extremities if edematous.

CHOLECYSTITIS

Cholecystitis is inflammation of the gall bladder and is most often caused by gall stone obstruction. The stones are a byproduct of cholesterol that has supersaturated the bile. Commonly, there will be pain in the upper right quadrant that radiates to the right scapula or shoulder. Nausea, vomiting, and a low-grade fever also may be present. Treatments involve removal of the gall bladder, oral medications to decrease the size of or dissolve the cholesterol stones, infusion of an agent directly into the gall bladder via a catheter, or the use of laser or hydraulic shock waves to break up stones in the common bile duct. Patients are given pain medication and antibiotics.[1]

A THERAPIST'S JOURNAL

Cardiac Nursing and Massage

Being an experienced cardiac nurse and massage therapist allows me opportunities to touch patients in ways that benefit us both. I remember a patient who recently had open-heart surgery, a multicoronary bypass graft. This patient, a 60-year-old man, was having difficulty coordinating his breathing exercises because of incisional pain. I commented to the cardiac surgeon that I felt the patient could use some skilled touch and gentle shiatsu massage, to which he readily gave his blessing. I explained to the patient that what I was going to do would hopefully bring pain relief and deep breathing, both of which are important in the recovery process of open-heart patients.

Twenty minutes prior to starting, I premedicated him with hydrocodone/acetaminophen tablets. I began the session by laying my hands near the incision in his chest, encouraging him to imagine a place that was emotionally comforting. In just a few minutes, his breathing pattern slowed. He truly relaxed and was able to take the slow, deep breaths he had been taught. As I applied extremely light pressure on his rib cage, we practiced deep breathing in a 1-2-3 in-and-out manner. After about 20 minutes, I left the room and allowed him to rest. The next morning, I was greeted by the surgeon, who was totally amazed at the difference in the patient, who had a great night's sleep and was breathing markedly better.

Barbara Estes, LPN, LMT,

Providence Medical Center,

Portland, OR

■ **CLINICAL CONSIDERATIONS**

Pressure considerations:
- Fatigue
- Fever
- Nausea
- Pain medications

Site restrictions:
- Abdomen
- Incision
- IV catheters

Positioning adjustments:
- Incision (Side-lying is usually OK.)
- No prone positioning if nausea or abdominal discomfort is present.

CHRONIC OBSTRUCTIVE PULMONARY DISEASE (COPD)

Three conditions commonly cause COPD: **asthma, chronic bronchitis,** and **emphysema.** All three disorders cause airways to narrow, preventing the lungs from performing efficiently. Airflow into and out of the lungs requires more time, slowing the exchange of oxygen and carbon dioxide. The end result is labored breathing, also known as dyspnea. Over a period of time, poor lung functioning causes the heart to overwork, the potential consequence being right-sided heart failure. Management of the disease is through medications such as bronchodilators, **corticosteroids,** cough suppressants, and decongestants.

Emphysema not only creates narrowing in the airways, but also causes the alveoli to lose their natural elasticity, become overstretched, and rupture. The person with this disease is then only able to partially exhale. Development of an excessively enlarged chest is a characteristic byproduct.

People with COPD are prone to serious respiratory diseases such as pneumonia, acute bronchitis, and influenza. Diminished air exchange also results in fatigue, a weakened immune system, and tissue fragility and cyanosis in the extremities. Tissues injure more easily and heal more slowly, with a lesser quality of repair. Constant breathing difficulty and fatigue makes the patient irritable, apprehensive, anxious, depressed, and powerless. During an episode of respiratory insufficiency, these patients may be sleepy, restless, aggressive, panic-stricken, or confused.[1,3,11,12]

Gentle massage that does not tax the body benefits these patients in many ways. Narrowed airways force the respiratory muscles to overwork. Therefore, attention to the neck and thoracic area will be welcome. During times of anxiety and hopelessness, touch can soothe tension and give the person a sense of control. In addition, massage can play a part in developing relaxation skills, an impor-

tant component in learning to live with a chronic respiratory problem.

■ **CLINICAL CONSIDERATIONS**

Pressure considerations:
- Cardiac and kidney complications
- Easy bruising (if on regular steroid or bronchodilator medication)
- Edema
- Fatigue
- Psychological fragility
- Tissue fragility

Site restrictions:
- Areas of fragile tissue
- Oxygen-delivery device

Positioning adjustments:
- Elevate head to ease breathing.
- Encourage the patient to move slowly when repositioning due to possible dizziness or disorientation.
- Repositioning may cause fatigue and dyspnea.
- Most likely unable to lie flat in either supine or prone position due to dyspnea and coughing.
- Side-lying may be tolerated. (Right side may put less demand on the heart.)

Other:
- Become familiar with the side effects of steroidal, pain, and cough-suppressant medications.
- Practice good Standard Precautions because of the patient's general immunosuppression and increased risk of contracting a respiratory infection.
- Be mindful of pulmonary irritants such as perfumes or oils.
- Avoid overfatigue, which contributes to further respiratory distress.

DIABETES

If this chapter were organized by frequency of diseases rather than alphabetically, diabetes would be at the start of the chapter. Massage therapists will encounter this health situation more often than any other, especially within the hospitalized or medically fragile population. Diabetes can be the result of a variety of influences—pregnancy, medications, certain infections, heredity, or diseases, such as cancer or hyperthyroidism. Long-term diabetes damages blood vessels and nerves. Nerve damage leads mainly to **peripheral neuropathy.** Deterioration of the larger blood vessels increases people's risk for heart disease, hypertension, stroke, and **aneurysm,** while small blood vessel damage causes kidney and eye problems. **Atherosclerosis** develops at a more aggressive rate. Not only is plaque laid down on the inside of blood vessels, but it can be deposited throughout the body. Poor circulation also gives rise to

---

A PATIENT'S STORY

It's Never Too Late to Try Something New

I was in the hospital overnight because of a kidney problem. To my amazement, a foot massage was offered to me by a student massage therapist. I was hesitant and only agreed to try it because my daughter wanted me to. I'm 75 years old and have never had a massage. Plus, I was uncomfortable about having my feet massaged because the big toe on my right foot was removed 3 weeks previously, a side effect of diabetes. The student said that she could just massage my hands and the unaffected foot. So, I gave it a try. I liked it so much that I even let the masseuse touch the foot that had had the amputation. I had no idea it could feel so good! It's never too late to try new things.

Dottie R., Portland, OR

---

edema in the limbs, as well as diminished wound healing and fragile skin. In the advanced stages of diabetes, the connective tissues can be very fragile and easily injured. **Ulcerations** and **gangrene** are a possibility and can eventually lead to amputation, most often in the extremities.

For the most part, diabetes is managed with insulin and **hypoglycemic** drugs on an outpatient basis. If a patient has been hospitalized, it is because she is experiencing a severe episode of destabilization. Secondary complications, such as renal disease or gangrene, are the other common reasons a person with diabetes is hospitalized.

The medical history of a person who has had the disease for a long time can be complicated and may require a number of massage adjustments. Diabetes is characterized by periods of instability. Massage should not be demanding on the body and thereby contributing to a disruption of the **homeostatic** equilibrium. In his book, *Massage Therapy and Medications*, Randall Persad warns against increasing the metabolic demands on the body or the workload of the heart for those with advanced diabetes. Shorter sessions, perhaps 20 minutes, are advisable at the beginning to gauge the person's response to the massage.[11] Noninvasive modalities may be best during periods of severe instability. (See Chapter 11 for a list of these techniques.)

Patients with diabetes are more susceptible to infection, and once they have an infection, it is slow to resolve. Practitioners need to practice exceptional Standard Precautions, especially near areas of fragile skin or open lesions. Good handwashing is a must.

The tissue in areas that have received repeated insulin injections tends to become fibrotic. It may have poor color and sensation. Like a scar, it can cause tugging on nearby structures, reduce range of motion, and create edema distal to the area. Massage or stretching to these sites should be performed with care.[1,3,11,12]

■ CLINICAL CONSIDERATIONS

Pressure considerations:
- Cardiovascular and renal disease
- Destabilization
- Easy bruising
- Edema
- Fatigue
- Fragile connective tissue
- Fragile skin
- Inaccurate feedback about depth of pressure
- Old injection sites
- Peripheral neuropathy

Site restrictions:
- Fragile skin
- Old injection sites
- Slow-healing wounds
- Ulcerations

Positioning adjustments:
- Cardiac complications (e.g., breathing difficulty)
- Edema
- Ulcerations

Other:
- Become knowledgeable about cardiovascular complications, kidney disease, and stroke.

GASTROINTESTINAL (GI) BLEEDING

Bleeding in the GI tract can be a side effect of various prescription drugs, alcohol use, a tumor, ulcerative **colitis,** a bacterial infection, stress due to trauma or surgery, **diverticulitis,** or an ulcer. Common symptoms that accompany a GI bleed are fatigue, weakness, shortness of breath, diarrhea and abdominal cramping, dizziness, increased heart rate and decreased blood pressure, and dehydration and **electrolyte** imbalance. Patients may be given vasopressin, a drug to slow the bleeding, and a **histamine** blocker to interfere with the acid-secreting action of histamine. Massage precautions are fairly common sense.[1,12]

■ CLINICAL CONSIDERATIONS

Pressure considerations:
- Coagulation problems
- Fatigue and weakness
- Nausea

Site restrictions:
- Abdomen
- IV catheters
- **Nasogastric** tube

Positioning adjustments:
- Elevate head if short of breath (no prone positioning).
- Reposition slowly if the patient is dizzy or affected by low blood pressure.

- May not want to reposition if the patient is affected by nausea, diarrhea, or abdominal cramping.
- Right side-lying will place the least strain on the heart.

👉 **TIP: Ask Questions!**

One purpose of this book is to give touch therapists enough information to intelligently ask questions and then to systematically categorize the answers. There is no way in these few pages to convey everything practitioners need to know. They must ask, ask, ask. Ask nurses, ask physical therapists, ask social workers, ask nutritionists, ask respiratory therapists, ask questions of everyone. All hospital employees learn from those around them. Knowledge from books is only the beginning. And remember—there are no stupid questions!

HEPATITIS

Hepatitis, inflammation of the liver, is most often caused by a viral infection of the liver. Seven types of hepatitis virus are known, but three types, A, B, and C, cause 90% of the cases. Type A is transmitted most commonly through the fecal-oral route. Types B and C are primarily transmitted via blood but also can be transmitted through semen and vaginal secretions. The symptoms for each type are similar and include fatigue, fever, headache, nausea, vomiting, and jaundice. Hepatitis B and C also may display skin disruptions, light sensitivity, edematous areas of skin, **myalgias,** arthritis, and **vasculitis.**

The majority of hospitalized hepatitis patients are affected by types B (HBV) or C (HCV). GI problems, fatigue, and fever are the main reasons for hospitalization. In addition, they might be impacted by **coagulopathy** due to impaired liver function. In severe cases, encephalopathy can occur, causing altered thought processes and personality changes in which the person alternates between excitability and lethargy.

HBV and HCV are not transmitted by casual contact but generally through unprotected sex or needle sharing. In the healthcare setting, workers contract hepatitis through inadvertent needle sticks. Since bodyworkers do not engage in such tasks, there is a negligible chance of them coming into contact with the virus. By following Standard Precautions, massage therapists can safely massage patients with hepatitis.[1,3]

■ CLINICAL CONSIDERATIONS

Pressure considerations:
- Areas of edema
- Easy bruising caused by coagulopathy

- Fatigue
- Fever
- GI problems
- Myalgia

Site restrictions:
- IV catheters
- Skin disruptions
- Use only noncirculatory modalities on the abdomen.

Positioning adjustments:
- Self-limiting for many patients.
- May desire minimal movement if nauseated.
- May prefer left side-lying if upper right quadrant is tender.

KIDNEY FAILURE

The onset of renal failure can be acute, triggered by shock, severe bleeding, burns, decreased cardiac output, or **nephrotoxic** drugs or substances such as antibiotics, nonsteroidal anti-inflammatory drugs (NSAIDs), or solvents. It also can be a chronic condition in which the kidneys progressively lose function. As with CHF or COPD, renal failure is part of a multiple-system deterioration.

The complications are similar to CHF and COPD—electrolyte imbalance, blood pressure problems, fluid retention or dehydration, increased potential for infection, shortness of breath, fatigue, and rapid heartbeat, for example. In addition, the skin of renal patients is dry and more susceptible to breakdown due to itching and poor skin integrity from edema. The mental status of some patients in kidney failure can be highly impaired because of high levels of toxicity.[1]

Massage adjustments are comparable to those of the CHF and COPD patient. Refer to those sections for guidance. Comforting, undemanding modalities are advisable during periods of severe failure.

KIDNEY STONES

Kidney stones, the common name for **nephrolithiasis,** are formed from the crystallization of substances such as calcium, uric acid, and the amino acid cystine, which are excreted in the urine. Most stones pass out of the body spontaneously. Those that lodge in the kidneys or other part of the urinary tract cause an obstruction that can lead to edema, a secondary infection, and sometimes kidney damage. The pain caused by this condition is legendary and will manifest in the area where the stone is lodged. Other symptoms such as chills, fever, nausea, vomiting, diarrhea, and abdominal discomfort also are common.

One form of treatment used to disintegrate the crystallized formations is the use of high-energy shock waves directed at the stones from outside the patient. Larger stones are broken apart by hydraulic shock waves or a laser beam administered through a **nephroscope** that is inserted into the kidney or ureter. Another method of treatment is the placement of a catheter into the kidney; a solvent is then infused through the catheter into the stone. Surgery is performed only in a small fraction of cases.

The treatment process can induce a variety of complications that will affect a massage session. **Sepsis** can result from the dissemination of infected stone particles or bacteria that has occurred from obstruction. Abdominal distension, nausea, vomiting, and diarrhea are common. Shock-wave treatment can result in a **hematoma** from bleeding around the kidneys. Patients usually will be on large doses of pain medication.[1]

Despite the painful nature of this condition and the use of invasive therapies to correct it, massage can be given and may greatly relieve the physical discomfort and emotional stress associated with kidney stones.

■ CLINICAL CONSIDERATIONS

Pressure considerations:
- GI discomfort
- Pain medications
- Sepsis
- Tenderness in lower back

Site restrictions:
- Abdomen
- Lower back due to side effects from treatment
- IV catheters

Positioning adjustments:
- No prone if nauseated. The patient may prefer minimal movement.
- Side-lying is OK if the patient is comfortable.

OBSTETRICS

Obstetrics (OB) is one of the medical specialties most affected by the litigious nature of Americans. People expect healthy babies and are more likely to sue when things go wrong. Obstetricians have left the field in droves because of exorbitant malpractice insurance premiums. The result is an increased cautiousness. Massage therapists must factor this into their work, especially with women hospitalized because of a high-risk pregnancy.

There are a handful of precautions that must be observed when massaging all pregnant patients regardless of whether they are healthy or have a high-risk condition. During pregnancy, a woman is at increased risk for devel-

oping a thrombus because the body increases its clotting capacity to ensure that she does not bleed a dangerous amount during delivery. Therefore, massage to the legs should be superficial and never deep. This includes during the **postpartum** period.

As a pregnancy advances, a woman's ligaments are overstretched due to the effect of a hormone called relaxin, resulting in joint instability. This is especially true of the sacroiliac joint. Vigorous bodywork that mobilizes the joints is inappropriate.

Attention to positioning is important for these patients. Because the weight of the uterus can put pressure on the aorta and inferior vena cava, it is best to limit right side-lying to avoid decreasing the blood supply to the mother and baby. Left side-lying allows for maximum maternal heart function and fetal oxygenation. When supine, the patient should be in semireclining position, also referred to as Fowler's position. When the patient is lying flat, the weight of the uterus rests against the inferior vena cava, which can result in low maternal blood pressure and decreased circulation to both the mother and baby, a condition known as **supine hypotensive syndrome.**

HIGH-RISK PREGNANCY

A number of complications can force hospitalization during pregnancy. If contractions start too early in the pregnancy, referred to as preterm labor, a woman may be hospitalized on bedrest until the contractions are stopped or the fetus reaches a viable age. Hypertensive disorders; **placenta previa,** a condition in which the placenta implants in the lower part of the uterus; and **abruptio placentae,** the premature separation of the placenta from the uterus, can all require hospitalization.

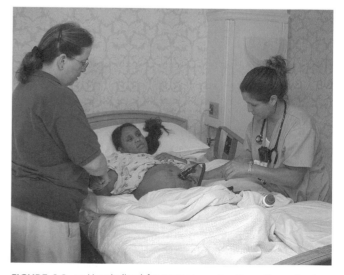

FIGURE 6-3. ■ Hospitalized for preterm contractions, the patient relaxes during a massage. The nurse is performing an ultrasound check on the baby. (Photo by Don Hamilton.)

A high-risk pregnancy places even greater demands on the prospective mother's heart, lungs, vascular and lymphatic systems, kidneys, and liver than a healthy pregnancy. This is an indication for extra gentle, nurturing, supportive massage. In addition, the mother is anxious about the health of her unborn baby and is not inclined toward any activity that would pose a threat to the pregnancy, such as vigorous massage.[1,13] However, if she has been on bedrest for a prolonged period of time, the patient's back will be sore, and she will be bored, restless, and feel sluggish from inactivity. Some careful bodywork will be welcomed (Fig. 6-3).

> *. . . [Some] anecdotal evidence indicates that deep, bone-to-bone pressure to the uterus and ovary zones can readily initiate labor or kick-start languid labor contractions. Obviously, then, any ischemic compression or pressure to the center of the medial or lateral calcaneus is contraindicated during pregnancy until after the due date. Unfortunately, many practitioners and books written by non-reflexologists mistakenly misconstrue this precaution as a total contraindication to touching the heels or the feet of pregnant women. Only bone-to-bone pressure to these exact reflexes will create these negative prenatal effects.[13]*
>
> Carole Osborne-Sheets,
> Pre- and Perinatal Massage Therapy

■ CLINICAL CONSIDERATIONS

Pressure considerations:

- Abdomen (only gentle holds)
- Edema

LABOR-STIMULATION POINTS

In Chinese medicine, pressure on certain points can stimulate uterine contractions, which is helpful for a woman whose pregnancy has gone full-term. However, pressure should not be applied to these areas if the woman is hospitalized because of preterm complications. This is a moot point anyway, because deep, or even moderate, pressure should not be administered to the legs of pregnant patients due to the increased risk for blood clots. Light effleurage strokes that pass over these points can be used safely.

POINTS WITH GREATEST POTENCY:

- Liver 3—In the webbing between the big toe and second toe.
- Kidney 3—Between the Achilles tendon and inner ankle bone.
- Spleen 6—Four patient fingers up from the top of the inner ankle bone. Press against the tibia.

POINTS WITH LESSER POTENCY:

- Gall Bladder 21—On top of the trapezius halfway between the nape of the neck and the acromial process.
- Large Intestine 4—Between the webbing of the thumb and index finger.
- Urinary Bladder 31–34—One each is located in the sacral grooves.

The same guidelines apply to the reflex zones of the uterus and ovaries. The uterine reflex zone is located on the inside of the heel, and the ovarian zone is on the outside of the heel.

- Labor-stimulation points (Figure 6-4A and B, Box 6-2). It is, however, OK to gently pass over these points when lotioning the feet and legs.
- Legs (Only apply lotion or rest the hands on the legs because of the increased risk for blood clots.)
- Preeclampsia
- Varicosities

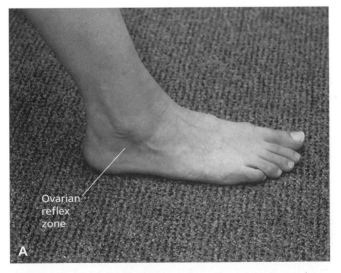
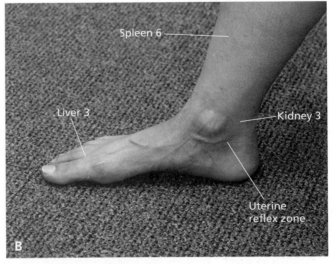

FIGURE 6-4. ■ Labor-stimulation points. The most potent points are found in the feet and lower leg. (A) Labor-stimulation zone to the lateral side of the foot. (B) Labor-stimulation points to the medial side of the foot and leg. (Photos by Don Hamilton.)

- As a pregnancy advances, a woman's ligaments are overstretched due to the effect of a hormone called relaxin, resulting in joint instability, especially the sacroiliac (SI) joint. Vigorous bodywork that mobilizes the joints is inappropriate.

Site restrictions:
- Abdomen (gentle touch only)
- Fetal monitor
- IV catheters
- Labor-stimulation points (Only gently massage over the points; no focused bodywork, no matter how gentle, should be applied to the points.)
- Severe varicosity (Massage only proximal to the site.)

Positioning adjustments:
- No prone positioning.
- Limit right side-lying because it may decrease the blood supply to the mother and baby. The weight of the uterus can put pressure on the aorta and inferior vena cava.
- Left side-lying allows for maximum maternal heart function and fetal oxygenation.
- Offer to place a pillow or towel under the belly for support when the woman is side-lying. Some mothers find this comfortable; others do not.
- When supine, the patient should be in a semireclining position, also referred to as Fowler's position.
- Take care when helping reposition a patient who is on magnesium sulfate. She may be disoriented or weak.

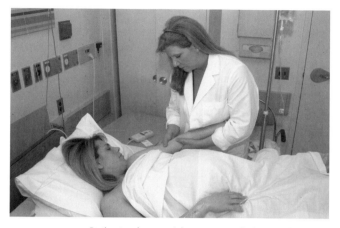

FIGURE 6-5. ■ Patient relaxes with massage during early labor. (Reprinted by permission of Stonybrook University Hospital Medical Photography Department. Photo by Jeanne Neville.)

LABOR AND DELIVERY

More than any other patient population, women in labor and new mothers can receive bodywork that is more vigorous than the normal patient. These patients are not sick; they are experiencing a natural event. Unfortunately, this event has become overly medicalized.

The use of epidurals in obstetrics has never been more popular. Once the device has been placed, the mother-to-be and the nurse are usually under the impression that no other pain management is necessary or useful. An epidural, however, only diminishes the pain sensations. Many laboring women are still uncomfortable and anxious, feelings that massage can address. It can help stimulate labor, allow the patient to rest, and decrease pain.

During early labor (1 to 3 cm dilation), full-body massage that includes long strokes down the back, legs, and arms will feel good (Fig. 6-5). (Practitioners need to glove if they are in contact with the lower back or legs or if the bedding is soiled with body fluids.) The light, downward direction of the strokes encourages a sense of openness and outwardness. Therapists can also perform firm circles to the sacrum with the palm of the hand, apply acupressure along the spine, and pay special attention to the labor-stimulation points. It is during labor that these points are most potent. Contrary to popular belief, they are not particularly affective when administered to the woman not yet in labor. (Personal interview with Carole Osborne-Sheets on November 21, 2003.)

Giving massage during active labor (4 to 7 cm dilation) demands flexibility and focused concentration on the part of the therapist. While there are fewer precautions to implement than with a medically fragile patients, the needs and emotions of women preparing to deliver a baby change frequently, making it an intense experience for everyone in the room. One moment the laboring woman may be enjoying the sensations of massage, while in the next it becomes intolerable. During contractions, she may not want any touch or just "still" touch.

Women aren't always sure what they want in the midst of labor. The touch therapist may have to lead them by saying, "I am going to rub your feet for two contractions. You tell me how it feels." Communicate in shorter phrases rather than long sentences. This will allow the laboring woman to stay connected to that deep, primal place that birthing can lead to. During labor, the cortex shuts off, allowing the lower brain to take over. (Personal interview with Carol Gray on March 17, 2001.)

If she is tolerating massage between contractions, effleurage to the inner thighs will help relieve fatigue and trembling of the legs. If the legs cramp, extend and stretch them after contractions. Pressure to the sacrum and massage to the buttocks feels good to some women during this phase of labor; to other women, simple massage to the feet, shoulders, jaw, and scalp may be more relaxing.

Depending on the wishes of the patient and the hospital staff, the massage therapist may or may not be allowed to stay in the room during the transitional phase (8 to 10 cm dilation) and delivery. If the bodyworker is able to remain, her role will be to provide reassurance to the laboring woman, to encourage breathing, to help her assume whatever position is comfortable, to hold her hand, or to support the legs.

The massage literature contains a wealth of material on pregnancy massage that the reader is encouraged to study. These books list many ideas to ease the discomfort related to labor, such as the use of birthing balls, certain positions, or walking. The hospital massage therapist usually is not free to suggest the use of these directly to the patient; instructions for positioning and walking must come from the nurse. A massage therapist acting in the role of **doula** or a massage therapist who has a long-standing rapport with the labor and delivery staff may be more influential in this area.

There is also an array of relaxation skills that can be helpful during labor. However, often the hospital massage therapist is meeting the mother-to-be for the first time and has not had a chance to develop a rapport with her. New skills such as focusing or breathing techniques are difficult, although not impossible, to learn in the middle of such an intense experience.[1,13–15]

■ CLINICAL CONSIDERATIONS

Pressure considerations:
- Generally self-limiting in the upper body.
- Apply superficial pressure to the legs.
- Preferences may change from one minute to the next during labor.

Site restrictions:
- Epidural site (Gentle massage within a few inches of the site is OK.)
- Fetal monitor

Positioning adjustments:
- Self-limiting
- When the patient is side-lying, support with a pillow under the abdomen may feel good.

POSTPARTUM

Following delivery, women who give birth vaginally can be massaged with few precautions in the upper body. Their muscles are sore and fatigued from the exertion of delivery and respond well to firm bodywork. Most are not inclined to lie prone, but the nurse usually leaves the decision to the patient. Attention to the neck, shoulders, arms, and hands will be welcomed. The pelvic bones and attachments will be unstable; therefore, deep compression that displaces the musculature or mobilizing techniques to the area should be avoided. Also, the legs should only be given gentle attention, as a thrombus is still a possibility. Patients who have had an epidural may have a headache. Massage to the head and neck are effective in relieving the discomfort.

Those who deliver by cesarean section require the same protocols as any surgical patient. Attention must be given to an increased risk for a thrombus, especially in the legs. Because of incisional pain, positioning is more difficult; the new mother may prefer to remain supine. She will be on pain medication and unable to give accurate feedback regarding pressure.

■ CLINICAL CONSIDERATIONS

VAGINAL DELIVERY

Pressure considerations:
- Generally self-limiting unless specific conditions, such as varicose veins, warrant decreased pressure.
- Firm pressure to the neck, shoulders, arms, and hands feels particularly good.
- Avoid firm pressure to the legs because of the continued risk of a thrombus.

Site restriction:
- Epidural site (Gentle massage within a few inches of the site is OK.)

Positioning adjustments:
- Self-limiting

CESAREAN DELIVERY

Pressure considerations:
- Extremely light pressure to the legs
- Moderate pressure to the arms, neck, and back is generally OK.
- Pain medications

Site restrictions:
- Abdominal incision site
- Epidural site (Gentle massage within a few inches of the site is OK.)
- IV catheters

Positioning adjustments:
- No prone positioning.
- Side-lying is OK if the patient desires.
- The patient may prefer minimal movement due to incisional discomfort.

All pregnant women are capable of receiving some kind of touch. Those who experience loving touch in the form of massage during their pregnancies are better able to provide it to their infants. Each new life then becomes an opportunity to break the cycle of touch deprivation.

Carol Gray, home-birth midwife and LMT

ORTHOPEDICS

The massage therapist who works with orthopedic patients will encounter a world of medical hardware such as pins, screws, rods, plates, and apparatus used to stabilize the body, such as slings, halos, and traction devices. The types of patients vary. There are those having elective surgery for joint replacements, most often knee and hip; elderly people, especially women, who have broken their hip in a fall; and victims of trauma, often due to motor vehicle accidents.

Positioning is a primary concern with orthopedic patients. If the hospital staff allow patients to make position changes in the bed, maintaining skeletal alignment is imperative. For instance, the person who has had a hip replacement eventually will be able to assume a side-lying position on the unaffected hip, but it is important to place a pillow between the entire length of the legs so that neutral alignment is preserved, thereby placing no stress on the newly replaced joint. The person who has had a knee replacement can have the knees bolstered while receiving massage in supine position. Afterward, however, the knee should be repositioned so that it is flat and does not remain in flexion. Following back surgery, spinal alignment is important. Positions or movements that cause the spine to torque or twist should be avoided.

Bruising is a common occurrence with orthopedic patients. It can happen near the surgical site or be the result of falling or colliding. Once the discoloration has become yellow-green, gentle massage can be administered in the bruised area if the patient is agreeable. Elderly orthopedic patients are likely to have osteoporosis. Be mindful of this when massaging the noninjured parts of the body. Many of these patients will be on high levels of pain medication, which inhibits their ability to provide feedback to the massage therapist. Additionally, they may be on anticoagulants, another indication for gentle massage because of the possibility of easy bruising.

When using lubricants near orthotics, be cautious. The skin in splinted areas is best kept dry. Also, some lubricants can soften plaster cast materials.[1] (Personal interview with Lisa Walters, OT, LMT, on March 14, 2003.)

Despite the medical equipment that must be worked around and the many precautions, systematic touch is very beneficial for this group. It promotes circulation in the affected areas, provides pain relief, and can assist the work of the rehabilitation staff who are working to increase range of motion, rebuild strength, and control edema. Massage practitioners, however, should provide only touch therapy unless they have been given approval by the physical therapy staff to integrate range-of-motion or other movement exercise into the massage session.

■ CLINICAL CONSIDERATIONS

FRACTURE OR TRAUMA

Pressure considerations:
- Edema often occurs in the affected limb.
- Pain medications
- The patient may be on anticoagulants because of the risk for a thrombus.
- Veins of the lower extremities and pelvis are highly susceptible to a thrombus after a fracture in the lower regions.

Site restrictions:
- The involved area may be affected by muscle spasm, which is the body's attempt to stabilize the area. Massage in the vicinity of the surgical site should be very gentle and in no way destabilizing.
- During the drying period, 1 to 3 days, a cast should not be subjected to wetness or soiling. Also, to prevent the buildup of heat, a fresh cast should not be covered with a blanket.
- Avoid getting lotion on the cast.
- Take notice of the skin around the edge of the cast for signs of irritation.
- Be aware of the potential for pressure sores around boney prominences.
- Be aware of signs that circulation is being cut off by the cast. These are a cold, numb, or tingling sensation in the area, or blue or pale fingernails or toenails in the affected extremity.
- It may be all right to reach under the cast of certain patients and massage the accessible skin.

Positioning considerations:
- Elevate the fractured limb above the level of the heart.
- Frequent repositioning is beneficial for preventing pressure sores.
- Ensure that bedding and clothing are wrinkle-free. This helps prevent irritation to the skin for those people who are severely immobilized.
- Avoid resting the cast on hard surfaces or sharp edges that may dent or flatten the cast, which then may cause pressure sores.

Other:
- Anxiety and depression can occur if a significant part of the patient's body is casted. The person is subjected to immobility in a confining space, dependence on others, and loss of control. Massage may take the edge off these emotions.
- The decrease in activity combined with pain medications may cause constipation. If the foot or hand is accessible, attention to the bowel reflex zones may be beneficial.
- Patients' breathing also will be diminished due to decreased activity, which can contribute to pneumonia. Encourage some deep breathing during the

massage session to facilitate lung expansion and movement of respiratory secretions.

HIP OR KNEE REPLACEMENT

Pressure considerations:

- Avoid pressure on any part of the body that would disturb the alignment of the replaced joint.
- Decrease pressure to the legs because of anticoagulant medications and the increased risk for a thrombus.
- Pain medications

Site restrictions:

- Affected joint
- IV catheter

Positioning adjustments:

- Supine and side-lying on the unaffected side are OK.
- Avoid acute flexion, adduction, and internal rotation of the hip following a hip replacement.
- Maintain alignment of the new hip to avoid dislocation. When the patient is side-lying, place a pillow under the head, top arm, and especially between the entire length of the legs so that the new joint remains in a neutral position. The nursing staff may want to help the patient reposition to ensure that the process is performed properly.
- Following knee replacement, avoid leaving the knee in flexion after the massage. Elevate the leg on pillows to control swelling.

PNEUMONIA

Pneumonia isn't just a single disease but can be one of more than 50 different diseases, each of which inflames the lungs. Bacteria, viruses, or inhalation of irritants such as chemicals or vomitus can be the cause. The various pneumonias are divided into three main categories: community acquired, which are triggered by microorganisms found in the community, such as pneumococci or influenza; hospital-acquired; and aspiration pneumonia, caused by aspirating foreign matter. Pneumonia is often secondary to another condition, such as immunosuppression, COPD, or cardiac failure.[1,12]

■ CLINICAL CONSIDERATIONS

Pressure considerations:

- During the most acute phase, especially when the patient is **febrile** and fatigued, bodywork should consist of very light stroking and/or holding techniques.
- Pressure can be a slight bit firmer after the acute phase.

Site restrictions:

- Oxygen-delivery device
- IV catheters

A THERAPIST'S JOURNAL
A Great Relief

As she came out of anesthesia following a hip replacement, the patient, a 58-year-old woman with advanced young-onset Parkinson's disease, had painful muscle spasms in much of her body. Although the spasms had subsided somewhat, she still had significant generalized rigidity and pain at the surgical site. In addition, the patient reported increasing abdominal discomfort from not yet having a bowel movement.

I started with massage to the shoulders, back, upper extremities, and non-surgical leg. Work on the affected extremity consisted of massage to the foot followed by gentle strokes up the leg toward the surgical site. Near and at the surgery site, modest pressure was used, but with no articulation of the hip joint and only slight movement of the muscles and soft tissue. I ended by massaging the abdomen for five minutes using broad circles over the area, vibration over the small intestine, and focused tracing of the colon.

The patient reported being comfortable throughout the 30-minute session, with increased relaxation and reduced pain. I noted some decrease in muscular rigidity. In a follow-up, the patient reported that 45 minutes after the massage she had a bowel movement, which provided great relief. She was so delighted with the massage that she arranged for a practitioner to come to the nursing home four times a week throughout the two-week rehabilitation period.

Lee Daniel Erman, NCTMB
(copyright © Lee Daniel Erman),
Stanford Hospital and Clinics—
Inpatient Massage Therapy Program of the
Office of Community and Patient Relations

Positioning adjustments:

- Change of position is good to prevent pooling of secretions in lungs.
- Due to cough or dyspnea, the patient will need to maintain an upright position.

Other:

- Deep breathing is good.
- If the patient is hypoxic, his mental status may be altered.

SEPSIS

Sepsis occurs as a result of an infection entering the bloodstream. The body's response is to kill off the unwanted bacteria, but in the die-off process, toxins are released that can cause shock. Pulmonary failure, diminished kidney function, or multiple-system organ failure can occur. Only lotioning or other undemanding techniques are appropriate during the acute phase. Slightly more pressure may be tolerable and beneficial when the person has stabilized. Massage for the septic patient will be similar to that for the person suffering from kidney failure or CHF. See those sections for massage guidance.[1]

STROKE

Stroke is the common term for a **cerebrovascular accident** (CVA), the cause of which is disruption of the blood supply to the brain. A CVA can be the result of partial or complete blockage of a cerebral blood vessel by a blood clot, decreased blood flow to an area of the brain, or bleeding in or around the brain.

The side effects of a stroke are dependent on where in the brain the occluded vessel is located. Usually weakness or partial paralysis, also known as **hemiparesis,** will occur on one side of the body. The affected side may have spasticity, diminished awareness of touch and proprioception, and lack of discrimination of size, shape, and texture. Mental processes may be affected and can manifest as changes in memory, judgment, concentration, and confusion. Impaired speech and vision, as well as incontinence, are also common. Following the stroke, patients are at risk for deep-vein thrombosis, aspiration pneumonia, joint contractures, edema, fatigue, and depression and other emotional states, such as hostility, uncooperativeness, and discouragement.

Strokes may be treated with thrombolytic drugs to dissolve the blood clot and anticoagulants to prevent formation of additional clots. Diuretics are given to reduce cerebral edema, and calcium channel blockers are given to reduce blood pressure and prevent spasm of the vessels in the brain. After the acute phase is over, medications may also be administered to reduce spastic paralysis.

Rehabilitation is a central piece of treatment. Physical therapy helps to reestablish range of motion, build strength, and regain motor control. Occupational therapy teaches the patient how to move and perform **activities of daily living** (ADLs). Massage therapists should work in conjunction with the rehabilitation experts.

Special attention to positioning is necessary when caring for these patients. Because of a lack of motor control and strength, the person who has suffered a stroke is unable to hold certain positions and requires special devices or supportive items to maintain body alignment and prevent contractures. The nursing staff will use footboards, night casts, splints, or braces to accomplish this.

Attention to position is also important to relieve the pressure of body parts pressing against the bed or another body part. For instance, when the patient is in

A THERAPIST'S JOURNAL
"Yes, reflexology!"

When I first told my dad that I had wanted to become a massage therapist, he was not happy. His dream was for me to get a degree in accounting or business. However, as I was completing the massage therapy training, my dad was diagnosed with severe cirrhosis of the liver and placed on the transplant list. His illness gave me many opportunities to utilize my training.

While going through massage school, I also worked for his computer company as an office manager. Most of the time, it was just him and me in the office. Many days he would just lay on the couch while I worked. After work, I also cared for him before going home to be with my own family.

Much of our massage time was spent working with his feet and hands, using essential oils, giving reflexology and Reiki, or whatever other technique I might be learning. At first I was afraid to touch him, fearing it would hurt him or make him feel worse. As time went on, I became more and more comfortable. In this time together, we would talk about our lives. We had been through many struggles over the years, and during massage we were able to find peace over them.

The first time he had to go to the hospital, I felt so helpless. Even with all of the training I had already received, I wasn't sure what I could do to comfort him. I went home one night and prayed for something that would help. There in front of me was an ad for the Clinical Aromatherapy course with the M technique. I signed up immediately.

As time passed, my Dad's feelings about me being a massage therapist changed dramatically. He would thank me all the time and let me know that he didn't know what he would do without me. It brought us so much closer. Massage was a way that we could connect in a special way, and I felt there was something I could do for him.

I was in my second module of the aromatherapy course when he went into the hospital for the last time. The paramedics were called to transport him because he was in so much pain and his abdomen was full of ascites. Unbeknownst to us, Dad was septic. It looked as though he would survive the systemic infection, but then pneumonia took over and his body didn't have enough strength left to fight it off.

I was more confident about comforting him with touch during his final hospitalization. During that time, he was struggling so much against the IV lines that he had to be placed in restraints. I asked the nurse if I could massage his hands and feet using essential oils. She agreed that it might *calm him down. My father was also hallucinating because of the toxins that had accumulated in his system and didn't really know where he was. But, as the nurse let him know that I would be giving him a massage as I had done so many times before, he actually said "Yes, reflexology!" It amazed me that he would know this.*

The nurse left the room, and it was just dad and me. I took off the restraints and began to apply the M technique to his feet. He relaxed for the first time that day. In that short moment, I had such a connection with him. This was the moment that all the massage training was for. It lasted for only a few minutes because the nurse returned to attend to him, but that moment seemed like an hour.

When the nurse left, I did a little more massage and then just sat next to him, surrounding him and me with a bubble of loving energy. For at least 20 minutes, he was able to rest peacefully without the restraints. On the fifth and last day of hospitalization, we knew that he would not survive. A dear friend of ours, who is also in massage therapy training, came in. What a blessing for Dad and me. She and I both held one of his arms, gently massaging him and sending loving energy. She then gently massaged my shoulders and back, which I needed desperately.

During his final day, we were able to move Dad to the hospice home. The family gathered around him. I continued just to hold and touch him at times. The hospice staff let us know that hearing is the last sense to go, so we talked of good times together, sharing the happy and dear experiences we had with our dad, grandfather, brother, friend. His last hour was a peaceful one, free from the struggle and pain he had endured for so long.

As I cope with grief, I am blessed to have a dear friend who is a massage therapist. I think of her as an angel sent from heaven to walk with me at this time. She holds that sacred space for me to experience whatever is needed. As her hands massage my body, I once again feel the places that had become numb from heartache. I will get through this difficult time, and when I do, I will be able to walk with others in greater understanding.

Kim Howell, Phoenix, Arizona

side-lying position, a pillow must be placed between the knees and ankles to avoid the discomfort of one bony prominence pressing against another. While the normal hospital patient could move her knee if it became uncomfortable, the person who is severely weakened or paralyzed cannot.

Positioning is the major adjustment for the massage therapist. If the patient wishes to have her back massaged, situate her on the unaffected side with pillows placed under the head, between the knees and ankles, under the top

arm, and behind the back. A pillow may be necessary behind the back to maintain the side-lying position.

Shoulder pain can occur in the affected side of a partially paralyzed person. To prevent it, the paralyzed arm should not be allowed to dangle unsupported. Also, because the shoulder joint is unstable due to lack of muscular control, do not position the person by pulling on the affected arm or shoulder.[1] (Personal interview with Lisa Walters on March 14, 2003.)

Massage can support the return to health of stroke patients by increasing circulation, diminishing joint contractures, and providing sensory stimulation, which in turn improves motor use. The unaffected side also can benefit from attention to muscles that are overused. Patients who receive massage before seeing the rehabilitation staff are often more alert for these therapies.

■ CLINICAL CONSIDERATIONS

Pressure considerations:
- Easy bruising due to thrombolytic or anticoagulant medications
- Edema
- Fatigue
- Poor proprioceptive and touch awareness
- Risk of further thrombus
- Unstable joints on the affected side

Site restrictions:
- IV catheters
- Joints on the affected side, particularly the shoulder area

Positioning adjustments:
- Supine and side-lying on the unaffected side are best.
- Do not pull on the affected arm or shoulder when assisting the patient into position.
- When the patient is side-lying:
  - Use pillows under the head, between the knees, under the top arm, and against the back.
  - Position the affected limbs to avoid pressure on bony areas, such as the elbows, ankles, and knees.
- When the patient is in a seated position, elevate the affected arm and hand to prevent edema.
- Barring other factors, such as breathing difficulties, return the bed to a flat position after the massage to prevent hip flexion contracture.

Other:
- Avoid doing things for patients that they can do themselves.
- When the massage session is over, return the bedside table, telephone, and TV remote to the unaffected side.

Pressure Gauge

Level Four • Self-limiting barring other factors	**4**	Labor Postpartum—vaginal delivery (upper body) Healthy preoperative
Level Three • Nurturing yet firm pressure • No forceful depth • No attempt to be ambitious • Skin does not remain reddened	**3**	Neuropathy (mild) Fatigue (minimal) Osteoporosis (low risk of fracture) Myocardial infarction (recovery period)
Level Two • Light contact with superficial muscles • Heavy lotioning • No depth • Places no demand on the body	**2**	Bone metastases (moderate risk of fracture) Cachexia (boney prominences visible) CHF COPD Extended bedrest Fatigue Fever (low grade, noncontagious) Nausea Neuropathy (moderate pain) Neutropenia (ANC>500) Osteoporosis (low risk of fracture) Postoperative (upper body) Pregnancy (legs of all women) Renal failure Thrombocytopenia (<50,000) Tissue fragility Varices (discolored veins)
Level One • Lotioning • No pressure • Energy techniques • Places no demand on the body	**1**	Bone metastases (moderate risk of fracture) Bruises very easily Cachexia (boney prominences visible) Edema Fatigue (severe) Fever (<100, noncontagious) Fragile skin and tissue (severe) KS lesions (closed, intact) Lymphedema or risk of it Neuropathy (severe) Neutropenia (ANC<500) Osteoporosis (severe risk of fracture) Postoperative (legs) Thrombocytopenia (<20,000) Varices (veins that are bulging, ropey, twisted)

The "Pressure Gauge" is meant only as a general guideline. The circumstances of individual patients may allow or require slight variations in the amount of pressure used. However, it can't be overemphasized that too little pressure is better than too much.

FIGURE 6-6. ■ Pressure Gauge. No matter how medically fragile a person is, he or she can receive some type of skilled touch if the therapist adapts the pressure.

SURGERY

Surgery is an injurious event to the body, as well as to the entire being. Systematic touch can be instrumental in piecing together the whole person and in releasing the trauma. When receiving massage, whether it is after a gynecological surgery, a coronary bypass, or the removal of a tumor, postsurgical patients require some common adjustments. An increased risk of blood clots is one of the primary considerations. When blood vessels are injured, as they are during an incision, platelets adhere to one another to form a plug that staunches the flow of blood.

These cells can clump together in the body and come to rest on the interior of blood vessel walls, forming a thrombus. Heavy massage could dislodge this accumulation of platelets, thereby creating a pulmonary embolism. Patients who have had surgery to an area with an abundant supply of blood vessels are at greater risk for a blood clot. The abdomen and chest cavity are good examples, as opposed to the tonsils or hands.

There are a variety of ideas about how to approach the lower extremities, which are the most frequent site of a thrombus following surgery. Some hospitals forgo massage to the legs during recovery from surgery and focus on the hands, arms, neck, and shoulders. Others approve of the use of light effleurage or noncirculatory modalities. Still others lightly massage only the feet. Each hospital should examine this issue and create its own protocol.

Even when hospital-wide guidelines have been established, individual nurses may have their own inclinations regarding this matter. This is especially true for nurses who took their training during the time when it was advised that the legs of hospital patients should never be massaged. Because massage therapists are usually accountable to the patient's nurse, the nurse's preferences must be honored.

The recovery room is an excellent place to begin administering systematic touch. For some patients, it can ameliorate pain, decrease anxiety, and provide faster recovery from anesthesia. Nausea is a common side effect of anesthesia. General massage or specific attention to the acupressure nausea points has been shown to be helpful.

After patients have returned to the room, application of a noncirculatory modality such as Reiki or Jin Shin Jyutsu® is very soothing. During this time, they will be on pain medication and unable to give coherent or detailed feedback. Anticoagulants may make patients susceptible to bruising. Repositioning usually is not possible or advisable. Of course the incision site cannot yet be massaged, but patients report decreased incisional pain from the application of an off-the-body modality such as Therapeutic Touch over the surgical site.

Medical devices may present the bodyworker with many areas that must be avoided. Surgical patients often have sequential compression devices on their legs, a Foley catheter inserted into the bladder, an IV catheter in at least one wrist, and possibly a drain at the surgical site. This group of patients may more often necessitate gloving due to the drainage of body fluids, which not only will be around the treated area but also may seep into the gown and bedding. Staying alert to this is important. If in doubt about whether to glove, err on the side of caution and glove.

■ CLINICAL CONSIDERATIONS

Pressure considerations:
- Anticoagulant medications
- Fatigue
- Increased risk of a thrombus (no circulatory massage to the legs, but light massage to the feet is usually OK)
- Pain medications
- The psychological need to be pieced together

Site restrictions:
- Abdomen if Foley catheter is in place
- Incision
- Medical devices (e.g., drains, epidural, colostomy)

Positioning adjustments:
- Generally no prone postioning due to:
  - incision,

- medical devices,
- nausea, or
- pain.
- Side-lying may be tolerated, especially on the untreated side.
- The patient may not want to reposition due to pain or disorientation.

A THERAPIST'S JOURNAL
Massaging the Surgeon

The previous day the patient, a 40-year-old surgeon, had the tip of her left thumb surgically reattached after cutting it off in a power-tool accident. She requested massage to alleviate the pain and soreness in her left shoulder and neck, which she attributed to the position during surgery and the overall stress of the situation. When asked, she also indicated that her hand and thumb were quite painful, but she assumed that massage couldn't do anything for that.

I first repositioned her, adjusting the bed and pillows so that her spine was straighter and her hand was elevated in a way that reduced the strain on the arm and shoulder. These adjustments produced some immediate relief. I began with moderate massage on the neck, back, shoulder, and upper arm on the uninjured side. Focused work on palpably tight rhomboids, levator scapula, and trapezius was given and then brief generalized massage to the feet, legs, lower back, and hips. During this time I encouraged her to breathe slowly, deeply, and gently and to notice in detail the sensations in her body. The patient indicated that the massage felt good.

Finally turning my attention to her left arm, I instructed the patient to indicate immediately if she felt any discomfort. As I worked slowly down from the left shoulder towards the left hand, the tight muscles in her arm released their tension. Eventually, I was able to massage down to the left hand, starting with the fingers and then carefully to the thumb itself. The surgeon expressed surprise and pleasure that massage could be performed right up to the surgical site. At the end of the session, she had considerably less pain, an overall increase in well-being, and greater circulation and increased "naturalness" to the thumb. According to the patient, the 45-minute massage had substantially helped in the recovery and healing process.

Lee Daniel Erman, NCTMB
(copyright © Lee Daniel Erman),
Stanford Hospital and Clinics—
Inpatient Massage Therapy Program of the
Office of Community and Patient Relations

Mrs. James

Mrs. James, 62 years old, was admitted to the hospital for a third reoccurrence of non-Hodgkin's lymphoma. She and her husband had tried for more than a year to control the tumors with alternative therapies. The event that finally brought her to the hospital was a tumor in her back pressing on the spinal cord; it had become impossible for Mrs. James to walk.

Radiation was started immediately and given every day for 2 weeks. A peripherally inserted central catheter (PICC) line was placed in the upper right arm to allow for the administration of Rituxan along with a steroid called Decadron. The treatments were very fatiguing but effective. The tumors shrank from the size of grapefruits to golf balls within a week. The growth in the back no longer impinged on the spinal cord, and Mrs. James slowly regained movement in her legs.

At one point, the patient's bowels became impacted, despite the use of stool softeners. The bladder stopped functioning, requiring a Foley catheter. This probably was a side effect of radiation and the spinal impingement. On day 10, Mrs. James's right arm swelled, which the nurse suspected to be the result of a blood clot related to the PICC line. Ultrasound confirmed this, and the PICC line was pulled. Anticoagulants were given to prevent further clot development, and the arm was hot-packed.

Mrs. James has one more radiation treatment and will then be discharged. She is still unable to walk or even support herself because of severe neuropathy of the feet. Chemotherapy will continue on an outpatient basis every 3 weeks for 4 months.

The first day, the massage therapist stopped in to see if the patient would like a massage. Mrs. James was too exhausted and did not want to be touched. However, her husband quickly accepted the offer of a 10-minute chair massage. Interestingly, the longer the husband was massaged, the more alert his wife became. By the time the therapist finished the short, seated massage, the patient was sitting up in bed with her glasses on and a bright expression on her face.

The next time the massage therapist stopped in, a week later, Mrs. James's energy had increased, and she felt more in the mood for a touch-therapy session. Because of the blood clot in the right arm, the nurse requested that no massage be given to that arm, as well as the shoulder and upper back on that side. Besides the right arm and shoulder, the other site restrictions were her feet due to discomfort from neuropathy and the area along each side of the spine that had been treated for the impinging tumor. Because of fatigue and extended bedrest, the body was massaged gently. The swelling in the arm prevented Mrs. James from positioning on the right side, and prone wasn't an option. The decision was made to stay supine. The therapist lotioned the legs and left arm, followed by work to the left side of the neck and upper shoulders. Massage to the face and scalp finished the session.

URINARY TRACT INFECTION (UTI)

Urinary tract infections are caused by the presence of pathogenic bacteria in the urinary tract. People might be hospitalized because of a UTI, or it may develop secondary to another condition, such as an indwelling urinary catheter or as a result of treatment for kidney stones. Common symptoms are the frequent and urgent need to urinate, pain or discomfort just above the pubic bone, abdominal tenderness, fever, nausea, and vomiting. Elderly patients with a UTI may also undergo a change in their mental status. The condition is treated with antibiotics.[1]

The massage plan for patients diagnosed with only a UTI is straightforward. Massage for individuals in whom the UTI is secondary to other factors will be more complex and require the therapist to study other sections of this book.

■ CLINICAL CONSIDERATIONS

Pressure considerations:
- Fatigue
- Fever
- Nausea and vomiting

Site restrictions:
- Abdomen
- IV catheters

Positioning adjustment:
- No prone due to abdominal discomfort and nausea

SUMMARY

This text can only provide a thumbnail sketch of each medical condition. Pathology texts, medical dictionaries, and nursing manuals are needed to more deeply study diseases and their treatments. This book cannot replace those texts but is a complement to them.

One of the main purposes of *Massage for the Hospital Patient and Medically Frail Client* is the creation of an intellectual infrastructure that will lead new and experienced therapists to develop critical thinking skills. The ability to ask the right questions and to connect the dots between knowledge and practice is more desirable than memorization of a vast quantity of information. The pressure, site, and position framework combined with the knowledge of some basic concepts is the skeleton around which intake skills and questioning strategies can be built. Touch therapists who can combine critical thinking with the practice of Standard Precautions, develop the ability to perform gentle massage, relate to patients, and act in concert with the other healthcare professionals will be on their way to mastering massage in the medical setting.

TEST YOURSELF

Practice what you've learned so far by reading the following case histories. On another sheet of paper, make three columns: pressure, site, and position. List the conditions from each history that apply to each category.

1. Mr. Williams is 68 years old and was admitted to the hospital with diabetic-related side effects. A scratch on his left foot developed into a serious infection after he waded in dirty water. Despite heavy doses of antibiotics, the infection could not be controlled, which is not uncommon with diabetes. The doctor was in favor of amputating the foot and the entire lower leg, but Mr. Williams insisted on a more conservative approach, removal of only half the foot.

   The procedure was performed 2 days ago. The surgical site requires elevation and is dressed with a compression bandage. There is some seepage in the area. The right foot is affected by neuropathy. The patient has a Foley catheter in the bladder and a urine-collection bag attached to the side of the bed. Pain medication, insulin, and antibiotics are being given through an IV catheter inserted in his left wrist.

   Other long-term side effects from diabetes include poor eyesight, causing Mr. Williams to be very dependent on his wife; 3 years ago he had coronary bypass surgery; and his skin is fragile.

2. Mrs. Jennings, a 48-year-old massage therapist, had her gall bladder removed laparoscopically 6 hours prior. The organ was removed in hopes of ameliorating nausea she suffered when eating, particularly fatty foods. Normally, the patient would have been discharged to recover at home, but she became very nauseated, vomiting every 45 minutes for the past 3 hours. Mrs. Jennings was given antiemetic medication, which was helping. Pain was addressed with Percocet. Additionally, she was on naproxen for arthritis. Although nothing was being given through the IV catheter, the device was still in place at her left wrist. There was a small amount of bleeding around the tiny incisions made in her abdomen. The nurse, knowing that Mrs. Jennings was a massage therapist, asked if the patient would like the hospital's bodywork practitioner to give her some massage.

REFERENCES

1. Nettina S. The Lippincott Manual of Nursing Practice. Philadelphia, PA: Lippincott Williams & Wilkins, 2001.
2. Smith I. Guidelines for the Massage of AIDS Patients. San Francisco: Everflowing, 1992.
3. Werner R. A Massage Therapist's Guide to Pathology. Philadelphia, PA: Lippincott Williams & Wilkins, 2002.
4. Nursing 2003 Drug Handbook. 23rd ed. Philadelphia, PA: Springhouse Lippincott Williams & Wilkins, 2003.
5. MacDonald G. Medicine Hands: Massage Therapy for People With Cancer. Findhorn, Scotland: Findhorn Press, 1999.
6. Osborn K. Creating Spirit Through Structure and Energy. December/January 2004 Massage Bodywork: 28–33.
7. Bauer WC, Dracup KA. Physiologic Effects of Back Massage in Patients With Acute Myocardial Infarction. Focus Crit Care Nurs 1987;14:42–46.
8. Labyak SE, Metzger BL. The Effects of Effleurage Backrub on the Physiological Components of Relaxation: A Meta-Analysis. Nurs Res 1997;46(1):59–62.
9. Tyler DO, Winslow EH, Clark AP, et al. Effects of a 1-Minute Back Rub on Mixed Venous Oxygen Saturation and Heart Rate in Critically Ill Patients. Heart Lung 1990; 19(5):562–565.
10. Lewis P, Nichols E, Mackey G, et al. The Effect of Turning and Backrub on Mixed Venous Oxygen Saturation in Critically Ill Patients. Am J Crit Care 1997;6(2): 132–140.
11. Persad R. Massage Therapy and Medications. Toronto, ON: Curties-Overzet Publications, 2001.
12. Mayo Clinic Family Healthbook. New York, NY: William Morrow and Company, 1990.
13. Osborne-Sheets C. Pre- and Perinatal Massage Therapy: A Comprehensive Practitioners' Guide to Pregnancy, Labor, Postpartum. San Diego, CA: Body Therapy Associates, 1998.
14. Stillerman E. Mother Massage. New York, NY: Dell Publishing, 1992.
15. Waters B. Massage During Pregnancy. Mesilla, NM: BluwatersPress, 1998.

ADDITIONAL RESOURCES

American Cancer Society, www.cancer.org or 800-227-2345.
American Diabetes Association, www.diabetes.org.

American Heart Association, www.americanheart.org.

American Liver Foundation, www.liverfoundation.org or 800-465-4837.

American Lung Association, www.lungusa.org.

American Stroke Association, www.strokeassociation.org or 888-478-7653.

Leukemia and Lymphoma Society, www.leukemia-lymphoma.org or 800-955-4572.

National Kidney Foundation, www.kidney.org.

Nelson D. From the Heart Through the Hands. Findhorn, Scotland: Findhorn Press, 2001.

Project Inform (HIV information), 800-822-7422.

Smith I. Christmas With Chuck (video about massaging a man with AIDS). Available through Information for People, 800-754-9790.

Stillerman E. Mother Massage. Massage Mag 2000;87:82–95.

Stillerman E. Partner Labor-Support Massage. Massage Mag 2000;88:144–154.

Stillerman E. Postpartum Massage. Massage Mag 2001;89:146–155.

Warren J. Labor and Massage. Massage Ther J 2002;40(4):92–101.

WebMDHealth (Web site that offers a multitude of information on a wide variety of diseases and organizations), http://my.webmd.com.

Yates J. A Physician's Guide to Therapeutic Massage: Its Physiological Effects and Treatment Applications. 2nd ed. Vancouver, BC, 1999. Available through the Massage Therapists Association of British Columbia, www.massagetherapy.bc.ca.

COMMON CONDITIONS AND SYMPTOMS

7

The purpose of this chapter is to present more detailed information about conditions that are common to a variety of diseases, such as edema, fatigue, and bruising. While a symptom may appear the same in all patients, the underlying cause can be very different, and, therefore, require individual adjustments in the massage session. For example, a touch practitioner could encounter edema in five patients. With one patient, it may be a byproduct of congestive heart failure (CHF); with another, pregnancy may be the cause. Prednisone use, extended bedrest, a blood clot, and many other situations can also cause edema. In four of the above scenarios, light massage could be safely given; in the fifth, any type of stroking motion would be contraindicated. By becoming more familiar with various symptoms, bodywork practitioners will have a deeper understanding of the massage precautions.

BRUISING AND BLEEDING

People bruise easily for a variety of reasons. Diabetics bruise easily because their disease causes blood vessels to become fragile. Poor oxygenation, such as occurs with CHF or chronic obstructive pulmonary disease (COPD), can cause tissues to become fragile and therefore more susceptible to trauma. Advanced age also can cause patients to bruise more easily as a result of fragile tissues.

A bruise can be painful and unsightly, which is sufficient reason for massage therapists to take care when working with those whose tissues are fragile. However, bruising can also occur because of a platelet disorder, which potentially has more serious implications. **Platelets** are the component of the blood that causes clotting. When the numbers of platelets are insufficient, bruising occurs easily and clotting time is slow. More dangerous than bruising, however, is the risk for bleeding.

The lack of platelets is referred to as thrombocytopenia. A normal platelet count is between 150,000 and 450,000 per cubic millimeter of blood, expressed as 150–450. (The zeros are dropped off to make the numbers more manageable.) Thrombocytopenia is defined as a platelet count of less than 100,000.[1]

A number of medications, most notably the anticoagulants—such as aspirin, heparin, and Coumadin—and antitumor drugs, cause physiological changes that affect the platelet count. Specific diseases cause the platelet level to be low due to decreased production. Leukemias, multiple myeloma, and some lymphomas are examples, as well as liver diseases. **HELLP syndrome,** a severe complication of pregnancy-induced hypertension, causes low platelets.[2] Platelets can also be destroyed as a result of an infection such as *Escherichia coli*, trauma to the body, or drugs. Liver disease, too, is often accompanied by coagulopathies.

While a platelet count of 100,000 is below the norm and technically qualifies as thrombocytopenia, it is not a dangerous level. Unless there are other influencing factors, patients can be given the usual bodywork that most any hospitalized person receives. However, when levels drop to 50,000, usually expressed by healthcare staff as 50, special attention must be paid to the amount of pressure. It should not exceed anything more than just the superficial layer of musculature.

A platelet count of below 20,000, or 20, will necessitate ultralight touch, focusing just on the skin. Lotion with good glide should be used to avoid any drag or friction on the skin. The reason for these precautions is that a count below 20 puts the patient in danger of bleeding, the most serious of which are brain and retinal bleeds. Without sufficient platelets, any bleeding, whether internal or external, no matter how miniscule, is difficult to stop. Occasionally, the platelet level is so low that patients aren't allowed to brush their teeth for fear of causing the gums to bleed. The group of patients that is most at risk for this level of thrombocytopenia is those who receive high-dose chemotherapy, such as bone marrow and stem transplant patients. Platelet counts below 10 are not unusual in this group. (See Chapter 13 for more information specific to bone marrow and stem cell transplantation.)

Applying lotion in a systematic way with a very gentle effleurage stroke is safe, as are techniques that do not employ pressure or stroking, such as cranialsacral therapies or Polarity Therapy. However, patients with seriously low platelets often will be hesitant to accept touch therapies, as will their doctors and nurses for fear the touch will be too heavy and cause bleeding. Most hospital staff are unfamiliar with the broad range of bodywork modalities. Their knowledge may come from the experience of receiving massage as a healthy person or from information seen in the popular media where massage is given in a more vigorous manner. The touch practitioner can help by using such phrases as "gentle massage" or "light touch" and briefly demonstrating on the doctor's or nurse's back. (Be certain to ask permission from the doctor or nurse before reaching out to demonstrate on his or her back.) Referring to the massage as "lotioning" is also a helpful way to word it and truly describes what will occur with these patients.

■ CLINICAL CONSIDERATIONS

Pressure considerations:
- Easy bruising or risk for bleeding is an indication for light pressure, generally at Level 1 or 2 as indicated by the Pressure Gauge (see Figure 6-6).
- When massaging thrombocytopenic patients, use a lotion with good glide to avoid friction to the tissues.

Site restrictions:
- Areas with hematomas

Positioning adjustments:
- Usually self-limiting

CONSTIPATION

Readers might be surprised at how serious and painful constipation can be. Patients are sometimes admitted to the hospital solely for this reason. Narcotics are the chief culprit due to a slowing of peristaltic activity in the colon, but other drugs, such as chemotherapies, also contribute. Decreased activity and fluid intake additionally play a part.

Constipation can range from mild to impacted, the latter requiring medical intervention. Massage is not usually effective in those situations. In mild to moderate cases, various touch modalities, such as Polarity Therapy, Swedish massage, and attention to the points on the foot that reflex to the elimination system, have been known to be beneficial. If the patient can't tolerate direct touch to the abdomen, indirect techniques such as reflexology may be helpful.

■ CLINICAL CONSIDERATIONS

Pressure considerations:
- Patients are usually in such discomfort because of the constipation that it creates a sense of pain that envelops the entire body. Even if constipation is

their only complaint, they will probably require gentle force over the whole body.

Site restrictions:
- Most likely, the person will be unable to tolerate touch to the abdomen.

Positioning adjustments:
- Frequently, the patient is too uncomfortable to change positions or be in any other position except supine.
- Supine is the most comfortable position. Prone and side-lying are rarely possible.

EDEMA

Edema is the accumulation of fluid between cells and can be the result of many different factors. It can be part of a disease process, such as heart or renal failure, or an obstruction, such as a blood clot or tumor. Certain medications, inflammation, or an electrolyte imbalance can be the cause. Pregnancy, too, nearly always is accompanied by swelling in the extremities, as is extended bedrest.

Edematous tissues are not only puffy, but fragile. The skin integrity may be poor due to being overstretched, thereby increasing the chance of a pressure sore or skin breakdown. People with edema often have reduced blood flow, which further aids in skin breakdown.[2]

Werner states, "Most edemas contraindicate circulatory massage,"[3] which is certainly sound advice when massaging a person whose major organ systems are easily overloaded. However, since massage with hospital patients and medically frail clients is focused on comfort-oriented, noncirculatory bodywork, many people with edema can receive some type of touch therapy, including light lotioning to the legs. Patients with swelling due to pregnancy, lack of ambulation, and fluid retention due to medications, such as steroids or antitumor drugs, can safely receive gentle effleurage to the legs. So, too, can most people with renal or heart insufficiency. The key is to not place an extra demand on these systems, which can be accomplished with nonforceful pressure and shortening the length of the session.

It is still appropriate to caution against any type of massage stroke gentle or otherwise, to areas that are edematous due to local infection or a blood clot. Swelling due to obstructions, such as a tumor, would also preclude the use of any type of touch that moves fluid. However, many hospital massage therapists have safely substituted techniques, such as Reiki, that do not use pressure or stroking.

The guidelines listed below are intended for use with patients with edema. Later on in this chapter, the phenomenon of lymphedema is discussed. With a few exceptions, the guidelines are similar. However, the two types of edema have very different causes and outcomes and call for separate discussion.

■ CLINICAL CONSIDERATIONS

Pressure considerations:

■ Edematous tissues are fragile. Use only the amount of pressure required for lotioning.

■ The skin in the swollen area may also have poor integrity if the edema is a chronic condition.

■ Reduced pressure may be necessary to prevent overloading major organ systems.

■ A limb with edema due to a blood clot should not be massaged with any stroking motions. Resting the hands gently on the limb is the only allowable touch.

Site restrictions:

■ Limbs with obstruction or infection-related edema should be avoided. Resting the hands on the limb or energy modalities may be substituted with staff approval.

■ A limb with edema due to a blood clot should be avoided.

Positioning adjustments:

■ Elevate affected limbs.

■ Be mindful of placing the person in a side-lying position on an edematous limb, as it may be uncomfortable. Additionally, the weight of the body may create an occlusion, especially in the upper body.

Other:

■ When using a light effleurage or light rhythmical compressions with the palm, stroke only toward the heart (Fig. 7-1 A–C).

■ Begin massaging the most proximal section of the limb (the upper arm or thigh, Fig. 7–1A), then move down to the next section (the forearm or lower leg, Fig. 7–1B), and then do the hand or foot (Fig. 7–1C). Strokes applied to the hand or foot should also go in the direction of the heart. Massaging in this sequence allows the area "upstream" to empty, thereby creating space for the fluid that will drain from the lower regions.

■ Give attention to the joints, as fluid pools there.

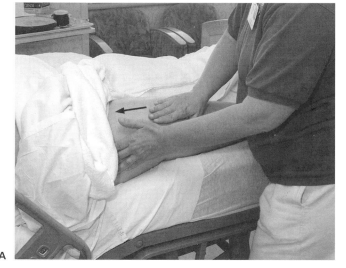

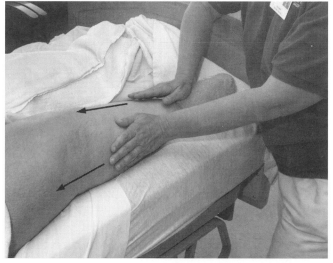

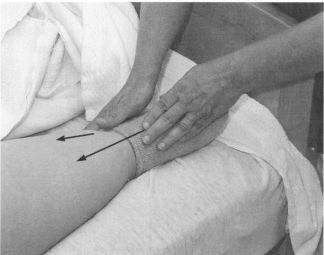

A   B   C

FIGURE 7-1. ■ Massaging the edematous limb. Stroke only toward the heart. Do not bring the stroke back toward the feet or hands. Hand-over-hand stroking gives the feeling of continuous contact. (A) Begin by massaging the most proximal section of the limb (the upper arm or thigh). (B) Move next to the middle section of the limb (forearm or lower leg). (C) Ending with the foot or hand, still performing strokes toward the heart. Long integrative strokes from the distal to proximal end of the limb will give the feeling of wholeness. (Photos by Don Hamilton.)

FATIGUE

As with many other conditions, fatigue is a multifaceted state. It may be due to a low red blood cell count, as occurs with anemia or chemotherapy. Poor oxygenation, a result of COPD or CHF, can leave people feeling tired. Many medications, such as cancer therapies, anticonvulsants, and certain heart medications, can contribute to fatigue. There is also a psychological component brought on by fear, loss of control, or hopelessness. Even if all of the above factors were absent, being confined to bed decreases circulation, thereby creating a sense of lethargy.

There is no evidence yet that massage has a positive effect on fatigue. Patients, however, consistently report feeling more energy following a bodywork session. Not surprisingly, massage should not place a demand on the body if the patient reports fatigue. Nearly always, there is multiple organ involvement for these patients.

■ CLINICAL CONSIDERATIONS

Pressure considerations:
- Administer light pressure so as to not place a demand on the body.

Positioning adjustments:
- Severely fatigued patients may tolerate only minimal repositioning.

Other:
- During severe episodes of fatigue, sessions may need to be shortened.

FEVER

Fever is taught in pathology classes as a strong contraindication to massage, which then is incorrectly translated to mean "Do Not Touch." However, it is now apparent to the reader that some form of touch therapy can nearly always be performed no matter how severe a person's medical condition. The only time a bodyworker should avoid contact with a febrile patient is when the fever is caused by a condition that could be communicated to the practitioner.

Fever is an immune response against temperature-sensitive organisms such as bacteria and viruses. In the hospital setting, fever could be due to the disease the patient was admitted with; it could have been introduced via a catheter or during surgery; a low white blood cell count from cancer chemotherapy could be the reason; or the fever could be a reaction to a blood transfusion or medication.

The body is hard at work during a febrile episode. To speed up the distribution of white blood cells, the heart rate increases about 10 beats per minute per degree of body heat. Cell wall permeability is increased, which allows for faster chemical reactions and therefore faster

recovery for damaged tissues. Immune activity is stimulated, particularly T cells, B cells, and antibodies.[1,2]

Systematic touch that does not place a demand on the body is generally permissible when a patient has a fever. Light lotioning strokes or resting the hands on the body is well received in this circumstance. Gentle, compassionate touch will sometimes temporarily lower an elevated body temperature, giving the patient a momentary respite from the discomfort of a fever.

■ CLINICAL CONSIDERATIONS

Pressure considerations:
- Avoid any kind of bodywork that places a demand on the body.

Positioning adjustments:
- The patient usually feels unwell and may not want to reposition.

IMMUNOSUPPRESSION

Severe immune suppression most often occurs because of the person's disease or drug regimen. For example, leukemia, **aplastic anemia**, AIDS, and **non-Hodgkin's**

A THERAPIST'S JOURNAL

Laura: 2 Hours of Relief

Laura had received high-dose chemotherapy 2 weeks previously for breast cancer. She had been discharged from the hospital and then readmitted with a fever, presumably triggered by neutropenia. Laura and I had worked together on previous occasions. Despite the fever, the nurses approved of another gentle touch session. This time, the two of us decided that Reiki would be the best modality to use. The fever had not abated the entire week, despite the administration of medications for it, and Laura was feeling very tired and unwell.

Even through the sheets, the heat from her body was evident as soon as I laid my hands onto her. As the session progressed, Laura's body seemed to be cooling. I was sure it was my imagination. In my wildest dreams I never expected gentle touch to lower body temperature. We stopped after half an hour, with Laura feeling better than she had in a week.

Out of curiosity, I asked the CNA to take Laura's temperature again. When it was taken just before the session, her temperature was 103.2°F. Following the session, it was 98.6°F. Granted, it did not remain there for more than a couple of hours. But those 2 hours of relief were important to Laura. They reminded her that healing was possible.

Gayle MacDonald, MS, LMT

lymphoma are diseases that reduce immune function. This is because the level of either white blood cells or lymphocytes is lowered or the white blood cells or lymphocytes do not function normally. Medications, too, can suppress the white blood cells. At the top of the list are corticosteroids, with prednisone being the most common. Another group of pharmaceuticals that depress the immune system are antitumor drugs. For most people, immune function also declines with age. However, the decline is not as extreme as that caused by disease or certain drugs.

Two terms associated with lowered immunity are **leukopenia**, which is a decreased level of all white blood cells, and **neutropenia**, low levels of neutrophils, a specific white blood cell. The neutrophil count is especially important for cancer patients, as it is "the single most important predisposing factor to infection."[1] The importance of infection cannot be overstated. It is the most common cause of death for those with cancer.

Patients who have had high-dose chemotherapy, such as precedes bone marrow or stem cell transplantation, experience the most severe immunosuppression. The normal level of white blood cells is between 4,500 and 10,000 leukocytes per cubic millimeter. However, those numbers are most often denoted as 4.5–10. All of the zeros are dropped off to make the numbers more manageable.

High-dose chemotherapy causes the white blood cell count to drop as low as 0.1. During this time, patients are at an extremely high risk of infection from microorganisms that are benign to a healthy person. To the person with neutropenia, they can be lethal. Even fresh food and flowers are not allowed because of the bacteria and fungi on them. Generally, the white count starts increasing a week or so after the transplant, but it takes months, and for some people even years, before the low end of the normal range is achieved.

The immune systems of people who go through organ transplantation, such as kidney, liver, or heart, are purposely suppressed with drugs such as cyclosporine and prednisone to prevent rejection of the new organ. The level of suppression, usually 50% of normal, is far less than that of bone marrow or stem cell transplant patients, but it is kept low for the remainder of their lives.[1,2]

Infection has already been listed as a complication of a deficient immune system. Other complications are increased risk of malignancies, fungal infections, malaise, fatigue, and fever. While fever is commonly taught as a contraindication to massage, lotioning the body or applying techniques such as Reiki or Therapeutic Touch are safe in this circumstance.

■ CLINICAL CONSIDERATIONS

Pressure considerations:
- The person who is severely immunosuppressed generally does not feel well and often has a fever. The pressure should be very light so as to not be demanding on the body.

Site restrictions:
- It is important to avoid skin that is not intact because of the risk for infection. Open areas become a portal of entry for infectious organisms.
- Be mindful of a fungal infection on the feet. Gloves should be worn if a fungal infection is present.

Positioning adjustments:
- Fatigue may influence the willingness to reposition.

Other:
- Handwashing is extremely important with these patients. It is the number one most important action for preventing patient infection. Always perform the handwashing immediately before touching the patient and after the room has been set up.
- Therapists who are sick, or feel on the verge of being sick, should not work with immunocompromised patients until the illness is no longer contagious. It may even be wise to avoid this group until the major symptoms of the illness have passed. During immunosuppression, patients often are fearful of being around anyone who is coughing or blowing their nose, even if the period of communicability is over.
- Massage is helpful during this time because people often feel socially isolated due to the fear of infection.

INFLAMMATION

Hospital patients exhibit a wide variety of inflammations. Surgical, trauma, and wound sites often have some degree of inflammation. Intravenous (IV) catheters and the medications given through them can create inflammation. Phlebitis, the inflammation of a vein, and **cellulitis**, an acute infection of the skin and subcutaneous tissue, are common inflammatory conditions encountered in hospitals. Cellulitis develops most often in the presence of damaged skin or poor circulation.

Inflammation can be a local phenomenon, or it can spread systemically. Cellulitis, dermatitis, and sprains, for instance, are examples of local inflammations, while influenza and meningitis are systemic diseases. Viruses and bacteria can trigger the inflammatory process both locally and systemically.

The symptoms of a local inflammation are redness, swelling, and pain. Loss of function, itching, the formation of blood clots, and pus are other signs. Some inflammatory conditions, such as phlebitis and lymphangitis, also may present with a red streak that runs proximal from the site of inflammation.[4] Systemic inflammation is characterized by fever and fatigue.

■ CLINICAL CONSIDERATIONS

Pressure considerations:

- Anti-inflammatory medications make it difficult for the patient to give accurate feedback.
- If the inflammatory event is accompanied by fever, no demanding bodywork should be performed. The body needs its resources for healing. See the section on "Fever" in this chapter.
- Even if the inflammation is due to local infection, it is safest to give gentle massage to the entire body.

Site restrictions:

- Avoid contact with areas of local inflammation related to infection.
- Avoid massage strokes in areas affected by musculoskeletal injury. Resting the hands on the area is permissible if it is comfortable for the patient.

Positioning adjustments:

- Positioning will vary depending on the situation.
- An inflamed wound may preclude certain positions.
- Inflammation that triggers swelling may require elevation.
- Fatigue due to systemic inflammation may affect the patient's willingness to reposition.

LYMPHEDEMA AND ITS ASSOCIATED RISK

Lymphedema is a condition that seldom receives significant attention in basic massage training. This book offers a chance, albeit a minimal one, to shine a light on the relationship between massage and this condition. Nearly all bodyworkers, whether they specialize in massage for those with medical conditions, work in a spa, or have a private practice, will encounter people with a history of cancer treatment. Although lymphedema can be caused by congenital influences, surgery, or be the result of trauma, cancer treatment is one of the most common causes. If lymph nodes from the superficial clusters in the neck, axilla, or groin are removed or irradiated, which is the case for many, many cancer patients, those people are at risk for lymphedema.

One of the keys to safe practice with these clients is understanding the way in which the superficial lymphatic fluid drains. In people whose lymphatic system is intact, lymph converges in the body toward two main groups of nodes, the axillary and inguinal. As shown in Figure 7-2, two main watersheds divide the body into quadrants. If some of the nodes in a quadrant have been removed and/or damaged by radiation therapy, the capacity of the

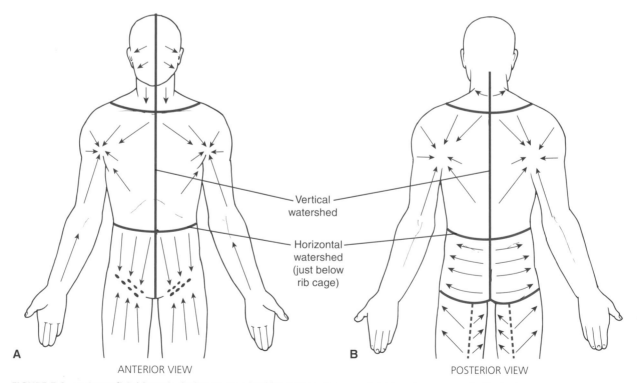

A   ANTERIOR VIEW   B   POSTERIOR VIEW

Vertical watershed

Horizontal watershed (just below rib cage)

FIGURE 7-2. ■ **Superficial lymph drainage.** In a healthy patient, the superficial lymph converges in the body toward two main groups of nodes, the axillary and inguinal. Two watersheds divide the body into quadrants. A third watershed just above the clavicles is the destination point for the lymph from the head and neck.

lymphatic system is lessened in that area. The combination of surgical removal and radiotherapy further increases the possibility of lymphedema occurring.

A third watershed is present just above the clavicles. It drains lymph from the neck and head. Removal of nodes from the main clusters in the neck, or radiation to this area, can create lymphedema in the neck or head.

The lymphatic system has been likened to a sewage treatment plant with the lymph nodes acting as the filtering system for plasma protein molecules, fats, cellular debris, and bacteria and viruses. If the lymph nodes have been removed or damaged by radiation, the "sewage" contained in that part of the lymphatic system goes unfiltered or is poorly filtered. Movement through the system also occurs more slowly, creating a backup into the affected quadrant. This backup of excess fluid and protein is lymphedema. Joachim Zuther, an expert in Manual Lymphatic Drainage, refers to lymphedema as "protein-rich edema."[4] Unfiltered protein is one of the problematic aspects of lymphedema that sets lymphedema apart from "edema." Left unfiltered, excess protein causes tissues to thicken and become fibrotic. Lymph then stagnates, providing a medium for bacterial growth, and in turn increases the risk of infection.

Many massage therapists are unaware that overly vigorous massage can trigger lymphedema or exacerbate an existing case of it. Deep, or even moderate, bodywork can cause hyperemia, which is characterized by reddening of the skin. The affected quadrant of a person whose lymphatic capacity has been diminished cannot always handle the greater fluid volume created by hyperemia. Vigorous massage can also initiate the inflammatory process, which triggers the release of histamines. Histamines cause fluid to migrate to the area, further burdening a compromised lymphatic system.[4]

Therefore, people with lymphedema or even those who are at risk for it should not have bodywork to the affected quadrant that causes hyperemia. For instance, a patient who has had nodes removed from both sides of the inguinal area and/or radiation treatment to the pelvis, such as would occur for uterine or prostate cancer, is at risk in both of the lower quadrants and should receive only light bodywork below the rib cage. Someone who has had nodes removed and/or radiation to the axilla, as happens with breast cancer treatment, is at risk in the arm and trunk on the treated side. He or she should have only light massage to the entire treated side above the rib cage. (The rib cage is the watershed that divides the upper quadrants from the lower quadrants.)

Lymphedema is a serious condition. There is no cure for it, only constant monitoring and management. Not only are people at increased risk for infection in the affected limb, their body image, as well as activities of daily living, can be affected. The excess fluid creates heaviness in the limb, which can cause discomfort, joint pain, loss of mobility, and postural problems. Once a person has had an occurrence of lymphedema, future episodes may happen more easily and take longer to vanish. Even if people at risk for lymphedema have never had an incidence, they remain vulnerable indefinitely. The literature recounts many stories of people whose lymphedema did not occur until years after treatment.

Trauma to a compromised lymphatic system can induce lymphedema. For some individuals the trauma is an airline trip; for others it is an infection, having blood pressure taken on the at-risk arm, carrying buckets of rocks, or receiving a flu shot in the affected limb. Massage involving deep pressure has been the trauma that initiated an episode for some, especially those treated on an outpatient basis or in a practitioner's private practice.

Mary had completed her breast cancer treatment 5 years prior and had never had an incidence of swelling on the treated side. One day while in the breast cancer center following a mammogram, she discouragingly showed her now swollen arm to a nurse massage therapist. The nurse quizzed Mary in an effort to trace the cause of the swelling. It surfaced during the questioning that the patient had received a deep-tissue massage the day before. Although she had been given a number of massages since finishing treatment, this was the first deep-tissue session. And, while Mary reported that the bodywork felt comfortable and pleasant in the moment, the nurse suspected that it was the cause of the swelling.

☞ **TIP: Intake and Lymph Nodes**

I instruct all of my massage students to ask clients if they have had lymph nodes removed or irradiated. That question should be part of a standard massage intake, even a 5-minute neck-and-shoulder massage at a health fair. Any bodywork that causes the skin to redden can potentially cause lymphedema.

We had an unfortunate occurrence at our hospital that drives home the point. The incident happened to a nursing assistant (a CNA) after receiving a seated massage. She had been treated for breast cancer several years prior, including lymph node removal and radiation therapy. Following a short chair massage, the CNA was ill the next day and had swelling in the affected arm. While the swelling eventually dissipated on its own, it was more than a year and a half before the CNA would consider another massage.

Bodywork given to people in poor health is usually so gentle that lymphedema or the risk of triggering it does not play an important factor when planning the massage session. It is those who are being treated on an outpatient basis, such as in the radiation oncology department or clients who finished their treatment years ago, that present the most complicated scenario for massage practitioners. They tend to be more energetic and want more vigorous massage. Unfortunately, there is no way to know which of the individual patients who are at risk for lymphedema will develop an occurrence of it. Many go their entire life without an incidence, others have a constant level of residual fluid in the affected limb, others wax and wane, and some teeter unknowingly on the brink of lymphedema until a certain confluence of events overloads the lymphatic system. For one breast cancer patient, it was the strain of moving from one house to another, followed by an out-of-town guest for a week, which caused her to become "run-down," and then the final straw—moving buckets of rocks while landscaping the new front yard. These events increased the burden on the patient's lymphatic system, a system that could no longer handle such an overload.

The statistics regarding lymphedema occurrence vary widely. Breast cancer patients are most commonly affected. The range for them has been reported to be as few as 5% of those treated for breast cancer to as high as 40%.[5,6] However, the lymph nodes of many other cancer patients are either surgically removed or irradiated, also putting them at risk. The person treated for a head and neck cancer may have the nodes in the neck dissected or irradiated. The axillary nodes of a lung cancer patient or the inguinal nodes of a colon or ovarian cancer patient may be affected by treatment. It is vital to ask all people with a history of cancer treatment if they have had lymph nodes removed or treated with radiotherapy.

Massaging the person with lymphedema or at risk for it can be complex. The rehabilitation services department of many hospitals has practitioners such as physical and occupational therapists who are extensively trained to work with those who have lymphedema. They are excellent resources and can help develop institutional guidelines for the massage of patients with or at risk for lymphedema. The "Clinical Considerations" listed in this section can also be of help in creating guidelines.

The management of lymphedema is a complex situation and requires a great deal of training. Only practitioners with lengthy, supervised training, such as occurs with Manual Lymphatic Drainage or Lymph Drainage Therapy, should attempt to reroute excess, accumulated lymph. Touch practitioners without training in lymphedema management should refer clients to a specialist. When massage clients are under medical care for lymphedema, confer with their lymphatic practitioner about adjustments that need to be made in the massage session. Often times, lymphedema specialists prefer that their patients wait until the swelling is under control before they receive massage, or they may request that the patient receive no massage in the affected quadrant.

It is impossible to present more than a thumbnail sketch in this text. Therapists are encouraged to further study this topic and become adequately trained so that they can perform relaxation massage safely. The adjustments listed below are intended to give therapists basic guidance in the administration of comfort-oriented bodywork to people at risk for lymphedema. Those wishing to be part of a client's lymphedema management team need considerable training.

■ CLINICAL CONSIDERATIONS

Pressure considerations:

- If the person is at risk for lymphedema, use a level of pressure on the affected quadrant that does not cause hyperemia. Controlled fascial release techniques that do not redden the skin are permissible, as is gentle trigger-point therapy.
- Do not perform exaggerated stretches or twists.
- If the patient has lymphedema, only rest the hands on the affected quadrant until guidance has been received by the patient's lymphedema specialist. The remainder of the body can be massaged with adjustments relative to the patient's general health.

Site restrictions:

- Massage the untreated side first. If it is a patient's first massage, be gentle even with the untreated side to gain his trust.
- Stroke only toward the heart on the treated limb as was shown in the "Edema Protocol" in Figures 7-1 A–C. This is the direction that lymph is trying to flow—toward the heart.
- Massage segments of the limb sequentially using a proximal-to-distal order. For instance, begin with the shoulder, then the upper arm, the forearm, and the hand. End with long strokes that connect the entire limb. Refer back to Figures 7-1 A–C in the "Edema Protocol."
- Limit the amount of time to no more than a few minutes in the affected quadrant. This will ensure that the area is not overworked. Even gentle work can overburden the lymphatic system by moving too much lymph. Remember, the quadrant is more than just the limb!
- Do not aim strokes at areas of nodal involvement (Fig. 7-3 A and B).
- Keep strokes lateral on the affected upper arm or leg (see Fig. 7-3 A and B).
- If the affected quadrant is in the upper body, massage the back with strokes that move down past the rib cage (Fig. 7-3C). The rib cage is the demarcation line between the upper and lower quadrants. The opposite is true if the lower quadrants are affected. Extending the strokes up past the rib cage, with the patient's permission, would be helpful because the lymph nodes in the upper body are undamaged.

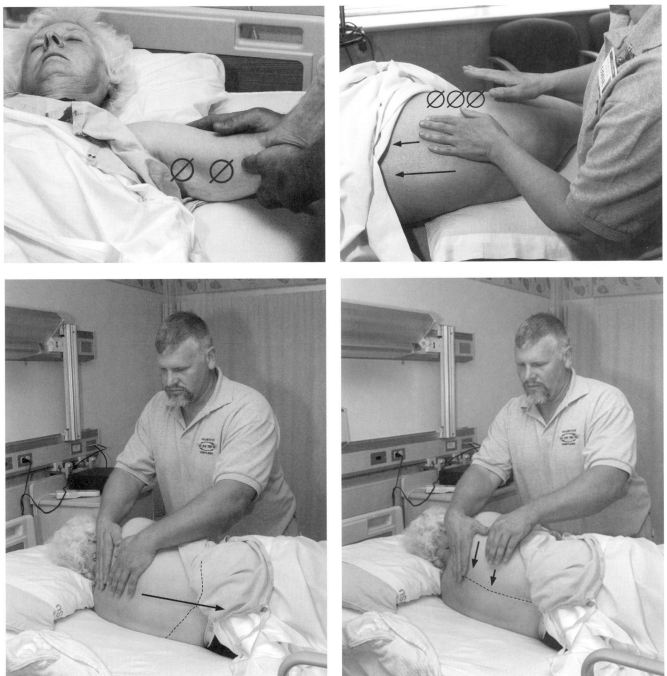

FIGURE 7-3. ■ Massaging the person at risk for lymphedema. (A) The therapist is demonstrating two things: 1) Do not aim strokes at areas of nodal involvement, in this case, the inside of the arm. 2) Keep strokes lateral on the affected limb. (B) The therapist demonstrates lateral strokes on a lower limb at risk for lymphedema. The strokes should follow the side of the leg, avoiding the top and inner part of the leg. (C) If the affected quadrant is in the upper body, massage the back with strokes that move down past the rib cage. A dotted line marks the horizontal watershed of this patient. (D) Strokes that travel "lateral to medial" on the back of the affected are also safe for the patient at risk for lymphedema in the upper extremities. (Photos by Don Hamilton.)

- With patients at risk for lymphedema in the upper quadrants, strokes that travel "lateral to medial" on the back are best (Fig. 7-3D).

Positioning adjustments:
- Do not allow an affected arm to hang off the massage table or be occluded by the position in a massage chair.
- Do not position the patient side-lying on an arm with lymphedema.

Other:
- Educate clients and patients beforehand so that they understand why light pressure is being used. Most people will not fuss about the lighter pressure if they understand the reasoning.
- The person at risk for lymphedema can still have firm pressure in the nontreated quadrants, assuming that their general health is sufficient. When told this, most people accept the limitations on the affected side. For instance, someone treated for breast cancer can have deeper massage below the rib cage (i.e., to the gluteals, hamstrings, or quadratus lumborum). Someone treated in the lower quadrants can have firm pressure in the shoulders, scapula, and around the thoracic spine.

NAUSEA

A quiet session of bodywork can help diminish nausea, which often is a side effect of cancer treatment, anesthesia, labor, or medications. Patients who have received bodywork while in the hospital know that the style of touch is noninvasive and are more likely to want this gentle touching. Those who have not had bodywork will often decline, thinking that any extra stimulation or interaction will add to their discomfort. For some patients who don't feel well, being touched seems too much to bear. As always, the decision must be left to the patient.

Nauseated patients may have an emesis basin by their side and may even need to stop during the session to use it. If it is necessary to move the basin at any time, glove the hand that will be in contact with the basin. After removing the glove, wash your hands before resuming with the patient.

☞ **TIP: Nausea Relief**

Acupressure points, liver 3, stomach 36, large intestine 4, and pericardium 6, may help alleviate nausea. The digestive tract reflexes, especially stomach and liver, also may be helpful. Many hospital massage therapists also report that the application of general relaxation strokes decrease nausea. Refer back to the nausea research in Chapter 2 for additional information.

A THERAPIST'S JOURNAL

I Don't Think I Could Have a Stranger Massage Me

For weeks, I had offered massage to one of the bone marrow transplant patients. He always politely refused. "My wife massages me," he would say. "I don't think I could have a stranger massage me." Eventually, I no longer stopped by to offer him my services.

One night, the man's wife approached me in the hall and asked if I would massage her husband's feet. He had been nauseated for days on end and was desperate for relief. He hadn't eaten for more than a week and was only getting nutrition from total parenteral nutrition (TPN).

I did nothing fancy to the patient's feet, just long, fluid strokes. His wife watched, surprised at how gentle my contact was. She complained that her hands and wrists hurt when she massaged him. I showed her what I was doing and how to position her hand so that the wrist was in alignment. Within a few minutes, her husband was asleep. I continued working for another 15 minutes. When he woke, the man said his stomach felt empty and he wanted to eat. His was another example of the power of simple touch.

Gayle MacDonald, MS, LMT

■ CLINICAL CONSIDERATIONS

Pressure considerations:
- Pressure or force that creates movement should be avoided.

Positioning adjustments:
- Self-limiting. Patients may prefer not to reposition.

PAIN

Pain is one of the most feared parts of illness. Anxiety, beliefs, and prior experience influence the way a person experiences it. At best, the management of pain is a complex and inexact science that cannot always be accomplished with pharmaceuticals. To add further complication, some physicians are still afraid of prescribing too much pain medication for fear of drug addiction or respiratory depression. Patients are frequently resistant to taking analgesics because they feel less alert.

Just as medications cannot control all pain, nondrug methods of pain management, such as hypnotherapy or massage, are not the complete answer either. Because pain is the result of a multitude of forces, the ideal pain-management regimen combines pharmaceutical and nonpharmaceutical interventions and is individually tailored to the patient. Despite the evidence that nondrug strategies are useful in the treatment of pain, healthcare providers seldom initiate these techniques. One study reported that audits of hospital charts show that as few as 2% of patients in pain received any type of nondrug intervention.[7]

Massage can be one part of a comprehensive pain-management program, but it is not a replacement for analgesics. In fact, massage tends to be more effective when patients have received an adequate amount of pain medication; they are then more fully able to relax. Paradoxically, as patients release the muscular tension used to guard a painful area, discomfort may increase if insufficiently medicated. Some patients understand that this is a temporary phenomenon and that the pain will subside as they fully relax. Others perceive the massage to be the source of pain and choose to stop or shorten the session.

People won't always admit to pain. Physical clues can be found in moans, sighs, breath holding, grimacing, rigid posture, restlessness, and insomnia. Withdrawing; acting out; exhibiting depression, anxiety, irritability, or confusion; or talking about death may be other indications of severe discomfort. If patients share feelings or report information during a massage session regarding pain, the nurse should be informed.

Pain is not always related to an incision, procedure, or trauma. A significant amount of discomfort has myofascial origins. This can be from lying in bed for an extended period, from the muscular holding that accompanies fear, or from being positioned in awkward ways during scans, procedures, or surgery (Fig. 7-4). Addressing myofascial pain will improve the discomfort caused by medical treatment or injury. These muscle-related pains do not require deep trigger-point techniques or heavy pressure. Gentle, noninvasive modalities can efficiently solve the myofascial problems of most patients.

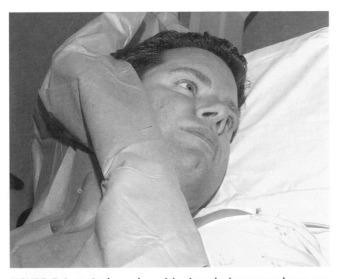

FIGURE 7-4. ■ Awkward positioning during procedures can cause myofascial pain. The patient in this photo is being prepared for a heart biopsy, a position he must hold for nearly 30 minutes. Massage is helpful in relieving the discomfort caused to the neck by the procedure. (Photo by Richard York, Oregon Health and Science University.)

■ CLINICAL CONSIDERATIONS

Pressure considerations:
- Pain medication.
- Take a gentle approach with guarded areas. They are best coaxed open.

Site restrictions:
- Painful areas often cannot be massaged directly but may be improved through attention to reflexology or acupressure points.

Positioning adjustments:
- Self-limiting. Patients in pain can surprise a bodyworker with their willingness to reposition, especially to receive a back massage.

Other:
- Remain focused on imparting comfort and nurturance. This will decrease anxiety. A reduction of muscular tension and pain will follow.

☞ TIP: Opening to Pain

Being in the presence of someone who is suffering, particularly from pain, is difficult. We want to either take away the pain or separate from the patient to avoid our own suffering. However, when we take either of these two approaches, we say to the patient, "I can't cope with you the way you are. I need you to be different than you are right now." Being ill, therefore, is a lonely experience because those around the ill therefore, person disconnect in the presence of suffering.

The pain of others forces us to explore our own pain. If we can stay open in the face of our own anguish instead of closing down, stay soft rather than hardening, trust instead of controlling, we will be more able to accompany the ill person on her journey, opening to her just as she is.

A Therapist's Journal
Asleep for Hours

Following a massage presentation at a day-long nurses' retreat, one of the CNAs put the new information to good use the next week. She was working with a patient who was very agitated and in chronic pain. He was somewhat confused and kept trying to get out of bed, saying that he had to move because he was so uncomfortable. The CNA asked him if he would like his feet rubbed. The man thought it was a bit strange but said "OK." Several minutes into the foot massage, he fell asleep and stayed that way for hours. Both the CNA and his family were astounded.

Gayle MacDonald, MS, LMT

PERIPHERAL NEUROPATHY

Peripheral neuropathy can accompany a number of conditions, most notably diabetes as a result of decreased circulation; chemotherapy treatment for cancer, which damages nerves; or spinal stenosis compressing nerves in the narrowed area. The common sensations are numbness, tingling, pins and needles, and stabbing in the hands and feet.

Some people with diabetic neuropathy find that massage improves the conditions to a certain degree. Chemo-induced neuropathy tends to diminish the most over time and benefits the most from touch therapies. Numbness due to spinal stenosis may partially improve.

■ CLINICAL CONSIDERATIONS

Pressure considerations:
- Massage is well tolerated by many neuropathy sufferers, but they are unable to give accurate feedback. The therapist must know when to adjust pressure.
- If the sensations are extremely painful, the pressure should be no more than the amount needed to apply lotion.
- Those affected by diabetic neuropathy also may have fragile tissue in the extremities.

Site restrictions:
- Some patients will prefer to not have neuropathic areas touched.

To have a successful oncology office, we need to provide services that enhance patient quality of life. Our goal in this office has always been to spoil our patients with information, expertise, attention, love, and kindness. Massage has added significantly to patient satisfaction. So much healing happens through simple touch. For patients living alone, massage provides healing touch in their lives. It also decreases the stress of patients and staff members. We also have been very impressed that massage helps with chemotherapy-induced neuropathies. Once or twice a week, I receive massage in my office. Massage therapy needs to become a technique that everyone does at least weekly for both relaxation and healing.

Judy L. Schmidt, MD, FACP
Hematology, Oncology, and Internal Medicine
Missoula, Montana

SKIN CONDITIONS

Private massage practitioners focus predominately on a client's musculature, observing its tone, flexibility, and tissue quality. Massage therapists who work with the medically frail must learn to move their primary attention to the skin. Not only will focusing on the skin help them to provide a comfort-oriented session, but will give bodyworkers hints about the person's health status.

The skin of a hospital patient is breached continuously and affected by medications and a lack of oxygenation and hydration. Touch therapists need to read the skin, noticing areas that are not intact or that are inflamed, swollen, bruised, thinned, discolored, scarred, pale, or dehydrated. Vast quantities of information are available by assessing this organ. The skin will give bodyworkers hints about how the massage session needs to be adjusted or will point them toward questions that should be asked of the nurse.

Rather than listing and providing photographs of specific skin conditions, which are difficult to recognize from black-and-white photos, qualities of unhealthy skin and their relationship to massage are described below.

■ CLINICAL CONSIDERATIONS

Pressure considerations:
- Dehydrated or parchment-like condition
- Evidence of bruising
- Evidence of swelling

Site restrictions:
- Skin that is not intact should not be touched, either with or without gloves.
- Areas with vesicles should not be touched. Herpes is an example.
- Because of the highly contagious nature of herpes, which also includes shingles, practitioners should glove. Even if practitioners are massaging well away from the affected area, gloves should be worn because exudate from the vesicles can spread virus into the bedding.
- Glove to massage an area affected by a fungal infection or other communicable condition.
- Glove when massaging over an area that is scabbed.
- Glove if blood or other body fluids are present on the skin.
- Avoid contact with inflamed areas that have been caused by infection, such as cellulitis or an abscess.
- Swollen areas require the practitioner to ask the nurse about the cause of swelling.
- Inquire about areas with raised, but intact, bumps on the skin.
- Inquire about rashes in which the skin remains intact. Some such conditions can be gently massaged. Petechiae, which are tiny hemorrhagic spots under the skin, are an example.

Other:
- A patient with shingles can cause chicken pox in others who have not previously been infected. Therefore, bodyworkers who have not had chicken

pox or been immunized for it should not administer touch to infected patients to reduce the possibility of contracting the virus and spreading it to other patients.

THROMBOPHLEBITIS AND DEEP VEIN THROMBOSIS

Thrombus comes from the Greek word for "clot," and **thrombosis** denotes the formation or presence of a thrombus. **Thrombophlebitis** and **deep vein thrombosis** (DVT) are the two common thrombosis-related conditions. Thrombophlebitis is the occurrence of a blood clot in conjunction with an inflamed vein. Sometimes, for the sake of convenience, the condition is referred to only as phlebitis. Thrombophlebitis is usually a superficial condition, generally formed in the saphenous veins of the legs. It can be recognized by localized heat, redness, swelling, pain, or tenderness. The affected vein may be rope-like and hard to the touch.

Superficial thrombophlebitis rarely leads to serious complications. However, if the same condition occurs in the deeper veins, it is known as DVT, and the potential side effect is very dangerous. A blood clot could break free and lodge in a smaller vessel, blocking the flow of blood and oxygen to the tissue fed by that vessel. If one of these **emboli**, blood clots that have broken free, gets stuck in the lungs, the consequence can be fatal.

DVT is sometimes asymptomatic and other times presents with edema distal to the site, often a dusky discoloration, and pain that is exacerbated by activity or standing still for too long. For the most part, thrombophlebitis can be diagnosed visually and through palpation. Diagnosing DVT requires an ultrasound or **venogram.**

Three factors are thought to lead up to thrombosis. The first is venous stasis, which can happen following surgery, childbirth, or extended bedrest. Injury to the vessel wall, particularly to the pelvis or lower extremities, is another influence. Injuries can occur as a result of a hip fracture, trauma to the body, insertion of IV catheters, infusion of medications, or infection in the tissues surrounding the vessel. Abnormal coagulation can also lead to clot formation. Obesity, varicose veins, previous heart disease such as a myocardial infarction (MI) or CHF, previous lung disease, a tumor, pregnancy, advanced age, or estrogen replacement therapy or other medications are also risk factors.[2,3,8]

There is no standard of practice within the nursing profession or among hospital massage therapists regarding this subject. Each institution must create protocols in conjunction with nursing and medical administrators and the massage therapy team. Many factors, such as the age of the patient, ambulatory status, type of surgery, and previous history of blood clots, go into the decision. Many hospitals will choose to avoid massaging the lower limbs

of someone at risk of developing a thrombus. Other hospitals may elect just to massage hands and feet as a precautionary measure, or to administer those modalities, such as Jin Shin Jyutsu®, that involve no pressure or stroking.

■ CLINICAL CONSIDERATIONS

Pressure considerations:
- When massaging patients at risk for but with no known DVT, the pressure should be very light to avoid dislodging a possible clot.
- The patient may be taking anticoagulant or thrombolytic medications, which cause easy bruising and/or bleeding.

Site restrictions:
- When massaging patients being treated for DVT, the affected limb should not receive any touch therapy that includes stroking or pressure. Resting the hands on the limb is permissible.
- Central IV catheters and femoral catheters increase the risk of clot formation. Apply very gentle pressure to an arm with a PICC or to a chest with a central line. If the catheter is in the inguinal space, stroking can be administered to the foot and the hands can rest on the leg, but no stroking movements should be performed on the leg.
- Those who are in danger of developing a thrombus usually have either an elastic or pneumatic compression device on the extremity (see Figure 8-7). Do not remove these unless the nurse approves.

Positioning adjustments:
- Elevation of the limb may be required to enhance venous return and decrease swelling.

VARICOSE VEINS

Varicose veins occur when the one-way valves inside blood vessels weaken, causing blood to pool. The veins become distended and elevated, appearing ropey and knotted. A slightly bluish color will be obvious. Practitioners should be especially watchful for varicosities in obstetrical patients and among the elderly, women, and the obese.

The same guidelines that are used in private massage practice apply in the hospital. Care needs to be taken when massaging extremities with varices because the tissue is sometimes more fragile as a result of impaired circulation. There is also an increased risk of clot formation because platelets aggregate in the pooled blood. However, clots that form in varicose veins are superficial and tend to resolve more easily than those that develop in the deep veins of the leg. Despite this, caution should still be employed.[3,9,10]

Ms. T

Ms. T is 48 years old with end-stage liver disease related to alcohol abuse and hepatitis C. She was admitted to the hospital with shortness of breath (SOB) and a 15-lb weight gain during the 2 weeks before entering the hospital. The patient also has a history of diabetes, renal disease, cardiomyopathy, and hypertension. Her presenting problem of fluid overload is multifactorial due to the liver, renal, and heart disease. Ms. T is thrombocytopenic with a platelet level of 50,000. Hematocrit is 35 (normal range is 40–53) and red blood count is 3.5 (normal is 4.5–6.2). The patient is on multiple medications: Lasix, a diuretic to rid the body of excess fluid; Epogen to support hematocrit levels; Digoxin for the heart; Nifedipine, an antihypertensive; Zofran for chronic gastrointestinal problems; insulin; vitamin K to assist coagulation; and a multivitamin (Nephro-Vite).

The nurse states that the patient is prone to bleeding due to coagulopathies related to the liver disease. She has been in the hospital for 5 days, mostly on bedrest. Edema in the limbs, SOB, and discomfort associated with ascites have made ambulation difficult. According to the patient herself and the unit staff, who spend a great deal of time responding to her needs, the patient has a high level of discomfort.

Ms. T is feeling depressed and the nurse thinks that skilled touch might bring her some comfort. However, the nurse is against the patient receiving vigorous massage due to low platelet levels, extended bedrest, and the edema in her limbs. The massage therapist explains to the nurse that rather than administering any bodywork that involves stroking or pressure, she could perform a modality that only uses static holding. After the touch practitioner demonstrates what she means, the nurse whole-heartedly approves, adding that gentle stroking to the face, head, and upper shoulders would also be OK. The nurse instructs the therapist to wear gloves because of the patient's history of hepatitis.

A 40-minute session in semireclining position was given. Because of the ascites, positioning even on the side was uncomfortable. The therapist started with holding the feet and then progressed up the leg with holds at each joint—ankle and knee, knee and hip, hip and shoulder, shoulder and wrist. The same progression was repeated on the other side. The patient slept off and on. With the patient's approval, her face and head were massaged with gentle circular strokes and light acupressure. Light lotioning was given to the neck and upper shoulders. To finish, the practitioner returned to the starting place—the feet—and held them once again.

The patient reported less anxiety, increased physical comfort, and slept much better that night. When this was relayed to the doctor, she ordered massage therapy three times a week for Ms. T.

■ CLINICAL CONSIDERATIONS

Pressure considerations:
- Use gentle pressure on the entire extremity containing varicose veins that are visibly distended and bluish. This includes the area distal to the varices. Even if the vein is only mildly discolored and not raised or painful, control the amount of pressure.
- When massaging directly over a visible varicosity, use only the amount of pressure necessary to apply lotion.
- Use a lubricant with good glide to limit friction over the affected area.
- Do not perform cross-fiber friction over the varice or wringing to the affected limb.
- Spider veins are slightly dilated venules that require minimal pressure restriction.
- Edema may be present in a limb with varices.

Site restrictions:
- Chronically impaired circulation may result in varicose ulcers or phlebitis. These would be reasons to avoid massaging the affected area.

Positioning adjustments:
- Elevate the legs to aid venous return.

Other:
- All strokes on the affected limb should be made toward the heart.

SUMMARY

Each new chapter presents more factors that must be taken into account when planning a massage session. To the new practitioner, it might seem as if all of the necessary calculations would feel confining and unnatural, thereby overriding the pleasure of giving and receiving simple touch. While the major emphasis in this chapter, as well as in the book, is on "Doing No Harm," there should be no doubt that despite all of the precautions that must be observed when working with people who are seriously ill, massage is a joyful event to both therapist and patient.

TEST YOURSELF

1. Which of the following conditions require close attention to the amount of pressure?
   A. Edema
   B. Fever
   C. Thrombocytopenia
   D. Herpes

2. Which of the following platelet counts demand ultralight pressure?
   A. 112
   B. 78
   C. 19
   D. 6

3. Which of the following conditions require the practitioner to perform strokes only toward the heart?
   A. Constipation
   B. Edema
   C. Varicose veins
   D. Lymphedema

4. Immunosuppression is an indication for:
   A. Pressure restriction
   B. Site restriction
   C. Positioning restriction
   D. Attention to Standard Precautions

5. Which of the following patients are most at risk for developing lymphedema?
   A. Those with chronic bowel obstruction
   B. Those who had lymph node removal from the axilla
   C. Those who are neutropenic
   D. Those who had radiation therapy to the major clusters of lymph nodes

6. Which is the single most important massage adjustment for the patient with lymphedema or at risk for it?
   A. Elevating the affected limb
   B. Decreasing the pressure
   C. Avoiding the shoulders
   D. No prone positioning

7. Which of the following situations is often accompanied by peripheral neuropathy?
   A. Varicose veins
   B. Nausea
   C. Diabetes
   D. Certain cancer drugs

8. Which of the following conditions require gloving?
   A. DVT
   B. Herpes
   C. Constipation
   D. Phlebitis

9. Which of the following sites should never receive direct touch?
   A. Skin that is not intact
   B. Edema due to a blood clot
   C. Peripheral neuropathy
   D. Varicose veins

10. Which of the following puts a patient at risk for DVT?
    A. Extended bedrest
    B. Insertion of an inguinal catheter
    C. Easy bruising
    D. Pregnancy

REFERENCES

1. Otto S. Oncology Nursing. 4th Ed. St. Louis, MO: Mosby, 2001.
2. Nettina S. The Lippincott Manual of Nursing Practice. Philadelphia, PA: Lippincott Williams & Wilkins, 2001.
3. Werner R. A Massage Therapist's Guide to Pathology. Philadelphia, PA: Lippincott Williams & Wilkins, 2002.
4. Zuther J. Traditional Massage Therapy in the Treatment and Management of Lymphedema. Massage Today June 2002:1.
5. Burt J, White G. Lymphedema: A Breast Cancer Patient's Guide to Prevention and Healing. Alameda, CA: Hunter House Publishers, 1999.
6. Swirsky J, Diane Sackett Nannery. Coping With Lymphedema. Garden City Park, NY: Avery Publishing, 1998.
7. Rhiner M, Ferrell BR, Ferrell BA, et al. A Structured Nondrug Intervention Program for Cancer Patients. Cancer Practice 1993;1(2):137–143.
8. Mayo Clinic Family Healthbook. New York, NY: William Morrow and Company, 1990.
9. Jordan K. What About Varicose Veins? Massage Today May 2001:1.
10. Osborne-Sheets C. Pre- and Perinatal Massage Therapy. San Diego, CA: Body Therapy Associates, 1998.

ADDITIONAL RESOURCES

Academy of Lymphatic Studies, www.acols.com or (800) 863-5935.

Dr. Vodder School—North America, (800) 522-9862 or www.vodderschool.com.

Lymph Drainage Therapy. Upledger Institute, www.upledger.com or (800) 233-5880.

MacDonald G. Cancer, Radiation, and Massage. Massage and Bodywork. August–September 2001:16–32.

Rattray F, Ludwig L. Clinical Massage Therapy: Understanding, Assessing and Treating Over 70 Conditions. Toronto, Canada: Talas Inc., 2000.

Turchaninov R, Cox C. Medical Massage. Phoenix, AZ: Aesculapius Books, 1998.

COMMON MEDICAL DEVICES AND PROCEDURES

8

Hospitals are mystifying to the uninitiated. Unknown procedures and foreign-looking machinery can contribute to bodyworkers feeling hesitant or even fearful when approaching a patient. Familiarity with medical apparatus allows therapists to relax and be more present to the person beneath their hands. Knowledge of these devices and procedures is also necessary for safety, and by being able to speak the same language and exhibit familiarity with common reference points, the bodyworker is more likely to be treated as a credible member of the healthcare team.

The purpose of this chapter is to acquaint touch therapists with common medical devices and procedures and their relationship to massage. Common sense will tell a therapist that medical devices and procedures are site restrictions and also may require positioning adjustments. However, pressure also may need to be reduced around certain devices and after specific procedures. In addition, alterations will be necessary based on the person's diagnosis, severity of illness, or age, to name just some of the possible influences. That information is presented in other parts of the book.

MEDICAL DEVICES

The massage adjustments required by medical devices are mostly common sense. Without much instruction, therapists will figure out that positioning adjustments are often necessary. Also, they will instinctively know that the immediate area around many devices should be avoided both as an infection control practice and to ensure that the piece of apparatus is not dislodged. However, other devices necessitate specific guidelines to protect against harming the patient. For instance, some intravenous (IV) catheters and the accompanying procedures call for gentle touch because of the possibility of bleeding or blood clots.

The importance of this section is not only in the safety guidelines given, but also in learning the names and functions of commonly encountered devices. Familiarity with these pieces of apparatus contributes to the ability to speak the same language as other care providers.

BEDPAN, URINAL, AND EMESIS BASIN

These items are the most basic hospital equipment. The bedpan and **urinal** are used for patients who are unable to get out of bed to use the toilet or **commode**—a portable toilet placed near the bed. An emesis basin is an open, plastic container that patients use when they need to vomit or expel oral secretions.

■ CLINICAL CONSIDERATIONS

These pieces of equipment do not impact the massage per se, but the touch therapist may need to move them. If the piece of equipment has been used, the practitioner must glove the hand that will be in contact with the receptacle (see Figure 4-5). Be sure to wash the hands after removing the glove.

Bedpans and urinals should be set on the back of the toilet. As was mentioned in Chapter 4, nothing should be set on the floor. Do not empty these collection containers into the toilet in case the nursing staff are monitoring the contents of the bedpan or emesis basin or the output of urine.

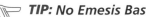

TIP: No Emesis Basin

If a patient is suddenly on the verge of vomiting and there is no emesis basin in the room, grab the garbage can for him to use.

CATHETERS

A **catheter** is a hollow, flexible tube that can be inserted into the body for a variety of purposes. The process of inserting a catheter is referred to as **catheterization.** The most common uses are administrating medications and fluids, collecting body fluids, monitoring physiological functions, and performing medical procedures.

Catheters have a variety of designs depending on their purpose. Some, such as the Foley and the Swan-Ganz, are referred to as balloon-tipped catheters because they have an inflatable sac at the end that holds the device in place. Catheters used during a procedure to remove plaque from coronary vessels have a blade tip that cuts and shaves. IV catheters have openings to the exterior that allow blood to be drawn or medications to be given without the skin being punctured each time. Other catheters come equipped with an electrical cautery wire, which can be used for such procedures as opening the bile duct to allow extraction of kidney stones.[1]

Foley Catheter

The Foley catheter is a balloon-tipped catheter. It is inserted into the patient's bladder to allow the drainage and collection of urine into a bag that hangs off the side of the bed, usually near the floor. The balloon, which is filled with sterile water, holds the tube in place. Most commonly, a Foley is used to drain urine before and after surgery.

■ CLINICAL CONSIDERATIONS

Site restrictions:
- Mindfulness is needed around the drainage bag that is connected to the Foley catheter. This bag will hang off the side of the bed below the level of the bladder.
- To be certain that the catheter does not accidentally dislodge from the bladder, only ultra gentle touch should be applied to the abdomen.

Positioning adjustments:
- Self-limiting

IV Catheters

IV equipment allows the administration of fluid directly into a patient's veins. This fluid might contain medications, nutrients, water, electrolytes, or blood products. IVs are also used to withdraw blood.

There are a variety of IV catheters depending on the type of use that is needed. A **peripheral line** is inserted by needle into a vein on an extremity. The most common insertion sites are the lower arm, hand, or antecubital space. Peripheral lines are used in situations in which a temporary IV catheter is needed, such as postoperatively. Practitioners may hear the term **"hep lock"** in relation to peripheral lines. They are sometimes referred to in this way because a heparin solution is placed in the catheter to prevent it from closing up when the catheter is not in use.

The **central IV catheter,** also known as a **central line** or a **central venous access device,** is another type of IV catheter. It is inserted into a central vein, such as the subclavian or superior vena cava and is usually left in place for an extended period of time. Oncology, organ transplant, and intensive care unit (ICU) patients often have central lines.

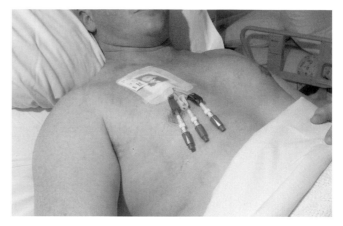

FIGURE 8-1 ■ Central IV catheter. (Photo by Richard York, Oregon Health and Science University.)

There are several types of central lines. Tunneled devices, such as a Hickman, Broviac, and Groshong, are inserted into a central vein, usually the subclavian, by tunneling under the skin. The insertion site may be in the chest, usually on the right side (Fig. 8-1), in the upper arm, or the antecubital space. Central IV catheters inserted into the arm are referred to as peripherally inserted central catheters (PICCs). PICCs are placed into one of the central veins in the upper arm (basilic, brachial, or cephalic) that flows into the subclavian vein (Fig. 8-2).

Implanted IV devices, such as a **Port-A-Cath** (also known as a **port**), are reservoirs that are placed under the skin and hooked to a catheter that travels **subcutaneously** to the vein. They aren't visible from the outside, although the therapist will see a bulge at the placement site. The nurse accesses these devices with a special needle that has a 90° angle.

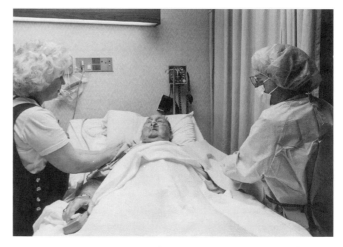

FIGURE 8-2 ■ Massage contributes to a patient's comfort during a PICC placement. The massage therapist (left side of photo) applies gentle touch to the patient's right arm and shoulder while the nurse is inserting a PICC line in the left arm. (Photo by Jacque Corey, MacKenzie-Willamette Medical Center.)

A THERAPIST'S JOURNAL
A Dying Man's Tears

I was rushing. It's like that a lot in the hospital . . . urgency . . . move quickly. We were conducting an ongoing study of patients' perceptions of their pain and anxiety levels during PICC placement. Two massage students had asked to observe today's procedure. The nurse placing the line, the two students, and I quickly located the patient.

I stepped behind the curtain to ask the patient's permission for the students' observation. I approached a painfully thin man with long dark hair, sunken eyes, and lots of visible tattoos. He was in the last stages of cancer. I couldn't determine his age . . . 40 . . . 60? This PICC line was to provide him nourishment. He was having difficulty taking in solids. I asked if he would mind two students observing the procedure, and to my surprise, he simply shook his head and said, "No, I don't want anyone watching." I excused myself, notified the students, then stepped back in and began to engage with the patient. At first, he was hesitant about massage, but he agreed to allow his hands, arms, and shoulders to be touched. The nurse began to set up for the procedure, and with his permission, I sat in a chair next to the bed and began to massage his hand.

Time seemed to stop when I saw the tears fill his eyes. I gently held his gaze and told him that his tears were welcome here. I continued to hold his hand. He cried quietly and told me he had originally decided to refuse food, but changed his mind and was willing to have the PICC line placed so that he could travel to the Midwest to say goodbye to his children. He proceeded to talk about his life, his tattoos, his dying. His tears came and went. I simply held his hand and listened. I spoke occasionally, but mostly I listened, and for a little while we were the only two people in the world.

Moments later, the nurse announced that the line had been successfully placed. Although it could have been a difficult placement, it had gone smoothly and quickly. I squeezed his hand gently, and we said our good-byes. I no longer felt rushed. The urgency of the day had dissolved in a dying man's tears.

Later, his sister came to me in the hallway and gave me a big hug. She said that it was the first time that he had cried throughout his entire ordeal with cancer. She felt that it was the "tender touch," the compassionate connection, that helped him access his emotional pain and begin his emotional healing. I was left with a deep sense of humility and gratitude . . . gratitude for the gift of each moment with each patient.

—Jan Locke, LMT,

McKenzie-Willamette Hospital, Springfield, Oregon

IV fluids can be infused into the patient through external or internal means. The traditional external method is to hang the bags of solution on an **IV pole,** allowing them to be fed by gravity. Computerized pumps attached to the IV pole (see Figure 11-3, upper right-hand corner, for an example) are another method of delivery. These pumps allow fluids to be infused at a certain volume per hour. Pumps also can be implanted under the skin, usually in the lower left quadrant of the abdomen, to continuously deliver pain medications or chemotherapy.[1]

■ CLINICAL CONSIDERATIONS

Pressure considerations:
- Only use gentle pressure on the extremity containing an IV due to the increased risk of clot formation. This is true more often of central lines, including ports, where the development of a blood clot in the arm is not an unusual occurrence. Swelling and warmth are common signs.
- Bodyworkers must make it part of their intake routine to ask the nurse if patients have an IV, what type, and whether they are exhibiting any signs of a thrombus.

Site restrictions:
- Do not touch IVs or the area several inches around them. This will help to prevent the introduction of bacteria into the area and to avoid accidentally dislodging the catheter or causing discomfort to the patient.
- Massage distal to central lines or ports.
- Limbs containing peripheral lines can be massaged lightly over the entire extremity, but avoid the area around the insertion point.
- Phlebitis, which presents as a red streak on the skin, can develop in the limb containing an IV. Not only can the catheter itself be irritating to the vein but so too can the medications. The hands can rest on a phlebitic limb, but modalities that require stroking movements, such as effleurage, should not be performed in the affected area.

Positioning adjustments:
- Usually, patient comfort will be the guiding influence on positioning. Some people are comfortable lying on their IV catheters; others are not.
- A small towel or washcloth placed just above the proximal border of a port can allow the patient to comfortably lie prone. Do not place the padding directly under the Port-A-Cath, as this compresses the catheter into the chest wall.
- For catheters such as Groshongs and Hickmans that have tubing external to the body (see Figure 8-1), a small towel positioned between the catheter and the body may create enough comfort to allow the patient to lie prone.

■ Care must be taken of IV tubing, which often is quite long. When moving bedrails or repositioning the patient, be certain the lines don't become wedged in the bedrails, occluded, or create a tugging sensation to the patient at the insertion site.

Cardiac Catheters and Devices

The heart may be catheterized for a number of reasons. One is to perform diagnostic procedures that measure its functioning. Information such as cardiac output and pulmonary blood flow, pressures in the heart chambers, oxygen saturation, and health of the heart's valves is gathered. Catheterization also may be employed as part of a treatment intervention, such as an **angioplasty** or **atherectomy,** to improve blood flow in the coronary vessels.

The heart catheter is introduced either into a vein in the groin, the antecubital space, the radial side of the wrist, or the neck. Before inserting the catheter, a short tube called a sheath is sometimes placed in the blood vessel at the insertion site. The catheter is then threaded into the sheath and gently guided to the heart.

An **angiogram** is usually performed in conjunction with heart catheterization. During this part of the process, an x-ray contrast fluid is injected into the coronary blood vessels, which allows the cardiologist to view the heart's anatomy on a fluoroscopic screen. If narrowing, also known as **stenosis,** has occurred, the doctor may perform a balloon angioplasty to compress the plaque against the vessel wall or an atherectomy to grind the plaque into small bits. Laser angioplasty is also an option. During this procedure, amplified light waves are transmitted via a fiberoptic catheter. The laser beam heats the catheter tip and vaporizes the plaque.

A small metal coil or mesh tube called a **stent** may then be placed in the affected area to prevent the artery from narrowing again. The stent is mounted on a balloon-tipped catheter. When it has been placed in the area that was treated with angioplasty or atherectomy, the balloon is inflated to open the stent.[1,2] The use of stents is not limited to cardiology. They also are used in other areas that have a tendency to constrict, such as the bile duct or the femoral artery.

■ CLINICAL CONSIDERATIONS

Pressure considerations:
■ Patients are at risk of bleeding, especially if a femoral catheter was used and because of anticoagulant or thrombolytic medications. Therefore, no deep pressure should be applied anywhere on the body.
■ If a femoral catheter was used, do not administer massage to the leg that may cause a circulatory effect. Apply only noncirculatory techniques to the

legs, lower back, and gluteals. Catheters inserted at the groin can potentially cause bleeding into the back, known as retroperitoneal bleeding. The patient affected by a retroperitoneal bleed may complain of back, thigh, or groin pain. However, it is a problem that cannot be addressed by massage.
■ Several areas usually can be massaged safely—the feet, neck, shoulders, arms (except in the case of a radial catheter), and hands. (Personal interviews with Barbara Estes, LPN, LMT, on June 25, 2002, and April 12, 2003.)

Site restrictions:
■ Patients lie on an examining table for a prolonged period during this procedure, which takes a toll on the back. Special attention to this area is often appreciated.

Positioning adjustments:
■ To prevent bleeding or dislodgment of the catheter, the affected extremity is immobilized for up to 24 hours following the procedure. If the arm was involved, it will be placed in a sling. Side-lying on the opposite arm will be possible in some instances.
■ Catheterization into the groin requires immobilization in a supine position for at least 4 to 6 hours.[1] After that time has ended, side-lying may be possible. However, the puncture site will be tender for days, possibly eliminating the use of prone position.

Swan-Ganz Catheter

A Swan-Ganz catheter, commonly referred to as a "swan," is a balloon-tipped catheter that monitors heart function. Most commonly, it is used in patients with congestive heart failure or those who have had a severe myocardial infarction (MI) or heart surgery. The device is threaded into the heart and ultimately wedged into a pulmonary artery where it can measure heart rate, pressures in the heart chambers, cardiac output, and blood volume. The entrance site most often is at the side of the neck (Fig. 8-3) but can also be at the antecubital space. These devices are left in for about a week or less. The risk of infection is higher with catheters, such as the Swan-Ganz or a central line, that have an external opening. In this situation, an infection would be serious because the catheter leads directly into the heart.[1]

■ CLINICAL CONSIDERATIONS

Pressure considerations:
■ Massage the neck gently to avoid dislodging the IV.

Site restrictions:
■ Massage to the unaffected parts of the neck may be very welcome since the patient must lie for an ex-

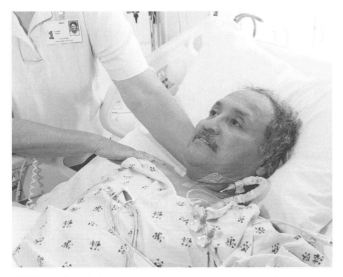

FIGURE 8-3 ■ Patient with a Swan-Ganz catheter receives shoulder massage. (Photo by Don Hamilton.)

A Patient's Story
The Hands of an Angel

The previous day, a "swan" catheter was placed in my neck. For 30 minutes, I had to keep my head and neck turned to the side while the doctor threaded the catheter in. This irritated an old disk problem in my neck. The pain is so bad today that my nurse gave me a shot of morphine and a hot pack, neither of which worked. When the nurse asked if I would like to be seen by the massage therapist, I was willing to try anything. What a difference the massage made! I told the therapist she had the hands of an angel.

—Peter S, hospitalized for congestive heart failure

---

tended period with the head turned to the side in a static posture while the catheter is placed.

■ The site of the catheter should be avoided. If it is placed in the neck, the back of the neck on the side containing the catheter, as well as the entire opposite side of the neck, can be gently massaged. The remainder of the body also can be massaged with relevant adjustments for other conditions.

Positioning adjustments:

■ Positioning will be restricted to supine and side-lying on the side opposite the catheter.

Pacemakers and Implanted Defibrillators

Two common medical devices that are used to maintain heart function are **pacemakers** and **implanted defibrillators.** A pacemaker is implanted if the patient's own heart is unable to beat at a steady rate. Pacemakers, which may be temporary or permanent, are placed in a surgically created pouch just under the skin, preferably on the left side of the chest because of the shorter distance to the heart. However, under certain circumstances, they may be positioned in the abdomen or on the right side of the chest. Temporary devices most often have an external pulse generator that attaches to a belt around the waist. Internal pacemakers tend to be permanent and are surgically placed into the chest or the abdomen. In either case, an electrode is inserted into the heart and attached to the pulse generator, which sends an electrical signal to stimulate the heart.

An automatic implantable defibrillator is used to stop the heart when it goes into ventricular **fibrillation** or **tachycardia.** Like a pacemaker, it can be placed under the skin on either side of the chest or abdomen, although the left side of the chest is preferable. It too has a pulse generator and system of electrodes. One set of electrodes is used to sense an **arrhythmia** in the heart. The other set is used to transmit an electric shock, which acts to stop the heart briefly, allowing its rhythm to be "reset."[1] (Personal interview with Karen Griffith, RN, on April 9, 2003.)

■ CLINICAL CONSIDERATIONS

Pressure considerations:

■ Gentle massage is generally permissible to the unaffected area of the upper body. For instance, if the device is placed in the left side of the chest, gentle massage to the right side is permissible. Moderate or deep force is not advisable to ensure that the leads will not be dislodged. Two months are needed for them to become embedded in the body.

■ Within reason, the patient can have self-limiting pressure from below the rib cage to the lower extremities.

■ Pain medication will affect the ability of the patient to give accurate feedback.

Site restrictions:

■ The entire affected area (shoulder, upper back, and arm) should be avoided for the first day or two.

■ If the device is placed on the right side, do not massage either side of the upper body. When devices are implanted in the right side of the body, the lead wires are still brought across to the left side, so the entire upper body needs to remain stable.

Positioning adjustments:

■ Following the placement of these pieces of apparatus, patients are on bedrest for 24 to 48 hours, and the extremity nearest to the device must be immobilized. This allows the leads in the heart to stabilize, thereby preventing dislodgment.

- Even after the initial 24 hours, movement of the affected extremity is limited, especially over-the-head motions, which are not allowed for the first week.[1]
- No prone positioning will be possible. The care team may allow side-lying on the unaffected side.

COLOSTOMY BAG AND OTHER COLLECTION DEVICES

Following colon surgery, perhaps to remove a tumor or because of an **ischemic** or inflamed bowel, the two ends of the colon may be brought up to the abdominal surface and **sutured** into place. The opening formed by these two ends is called a **stoma**. Fecal matter then eliminates through this opening into a colostomy bag.

A similar surgical process can be performed to other areas of the bowel and urinary tract. If the affected area is the **ileum**, an **ileostomy** bag collects waste from that part of the bowel; a **J-pouch** is used to collect the contents of the **jejunum**. When surgery is performed to divert the flow of urine from the bladder to a path outside the body, a **urostomy** bag is placed over the stoma to collect urine. Often, these procedures are temporary and serve to allow the affected area to heal. When this has been accomplished, the two ends of the stoma are "taken down" and reunited inside the body.[1]

■ CLINICAL CONSIDERATIONS

Pressure considerations:
- Generally self-limiting unless there are other health conditions

Site restrictions:
- If the patient is comfortable with it, there is no medical reason not to give gentle touch in the area containing the collection bag.
- Leakage may occur around the stoma, causing irritation and possibly breakdown to the surrounding skin. Colostomies on the far right side of the colon and ileostomies tend to have more leakage because the fecal matter is looser and more watery in these areas. If leakage has occurred, practitioners should glove when massaging the site.

Positioning adjustments:
- Patients differ in their comfort level with regard to lying on or near their collection bag. Many people who have had a colostomy for a number of years are at ease lying in all positions. Others will want to minimize repositioning. The neck, feet, and hands are good starting places because no repositioning is required.
- Patients with a collection bag on the far side of the abdomen may need to confine their positioning to the opposite side and supine.

- As patients become more trusting of the bag and familiar with the accompanying sensations, they will be more apt to try a variety of positions.

Other:
- Invariably, people with a collection bag suffer initially from body-image issues. The acceptance of touch therapy may be difficult but can go a long way toward healing the emotional impact of their medical condition.

COMPRESSION DEVICES

Compression devices are used to prevent edema or to promote circulation in the extremities. Sometimes they are simple, elastic garments that fit tightly on the arms or legs; in other cases, an air-filled tube is used to create the compression. The latter are generically referred to as pneumatic compression devices (Fig. 8-4). The air can be maintained at either a constant low pressure or be rhythmically inflated and deflated. Rhythmic inflation/deflation promotes circulation and prevents deep vein thrombi from forming in the legs.[1]

■ CLINICAL CONSIDERATIONS

Pressure considerations:
- Compression devices can be taken off in order to massage the legs if the nurse is in agreement. As was stated in the previous chapter in the section on deep vein thrombosis, there is no standard of practice within the massage or nursing professions with regard to rubbing the legs of patients at risk for developing a blood clot. The decision to massage patients with compression devices must be made on a case-by-case basis. If approval is given, the pressure should be light.

Site restrictions:
- While it is possible to remove elasticized compression hose, a great deal of effort is required, which is fatiguing to the patient. Although skin-to-skin contact is beneficial, it is often better to leave the stockings on and stroke over them without lotion, assuming, of course, that the nurse has given approval.
- Pneumatic devices, on the other hand, are removed easily. However, since these devices must be replaced in a certain way, have the nurse put them back onto the patient's leg or foot.
- If the nurse does not want the pneumatic compression device removed from the legs, it is sometimes all right to massage the feet, which extend beyond the apparatus as in Figure 8-4.

Positioning adjustments:
- Generally self-limiting

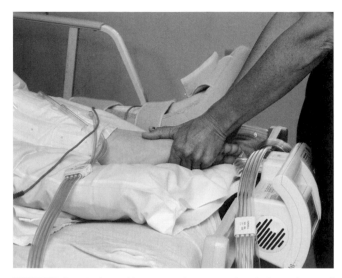

FIGURE 8-4 ■ Patient with pneumatic compression device on legs and feet receives foot massage. (Photo by Don Hamilton.)

DRAINS, TUBES, AND SHUNTS

Besides being used as catheters, tubes are also used as drains, feeding tubes, and shunts. A drain is used to remove fluid that collects in a cavity or wound. It can be as simple as a wick of gauze, or it can be made of tubing attached to a suctioning machine. The drained fluids are then collected in a bag or other container. The Jackson-Pratt (or J-P tube) and Pleur-evac are commonly encountered drainage systems. (Figure 11-3, on p. 151, lower right-hand corner at the base of the IV pole, illustrates a Pleur-evac drainage system.)

Drains may be used following surgery to allow drainage from an internal organ to the outside. The **T-tube**, which drains bile, is an example, along with the **gastrostomy, jejunostomy,** and **nephrostomy** tubes. These last three drain the stomach, middle portion of the small intestine, and kidneys, respectively.

Some tubes are employed as both a drain and a feeding tube. The nasogastric (NG) tube is an example of this. (Notice the patient in Figure 8-2; he has an NG tube. The NG tube is the single tube in his nose secured by adhesive tape. He also has a nasal cannula, the double-pronged tube, from which he receives oxygen.) The patient who is unable to eat may have an NG tube, which is inserted into the nose, guided down the esophagus, and into the stomach. Food and medications can then be delivered through this passageway. The NG tube also can be used to suction out irritating stomach secretions that cause nausea or ulcers. An **orogastric** tube is similar, but the tubing is inserted into the mouth instead of the nose. Several drains mentioned earlier, such as the gastrostomy and jejunostomy tubes, are also used to administer nutrition. They often are referred to simply as "feeding tubes."

Other tubes assist the breathing process. An endotracheal tube creates a passage from the mouth or nose into the trachea and is used to provide an open airway, to prevent aspiration of intestinal contents, and to suction out secretions. A **tracheotomy** tube is surgically inserted directly into the trachea from the outside and is used when there is an obstruction in or damage to the airway (Fig. 8-5).

A **shunt** is a tube that diverts fluid from one compartment of the body to another. It, therefore, is unseen. For example, an arteriovenous shunt is placed in the arm of a person needing hemodialysis. The device connects an artery to a vein, usually in the forearm. In patients with **hydrocephalus,** a shunt is used to divert cerebrospinal fluid away from a blocked area in the brain. Extracranial shunts divert cerebrospinal fluid to another part of the body, such as the **peritoneum** or the right ventricle of the heart.[1]

■ CLINICAL CONSIDERATIONS

Pressure considerations:
■ Force or movement that places pressure on the tube should be avoided.

Site restrictions:
■ The site of the tube and surrounding area should be avoided. One reason is that tubes opening to the outside are susceptible to bacterial infections. Avoiding contact with the site will decrease the chance of introducing further bacteria into the area.
■ When working around drains, bodyworkers must be mindful of the possibility of leakage onto the bedding or gown and apply the appropriate Standard Precautions.
■ Patients often complain about significant throat irritation from NG or tracheal tubes. Of course the throat cannot be directly touched when these devices are in, but holding the hands several inches above the throat, as is done with Therapeutic Touch

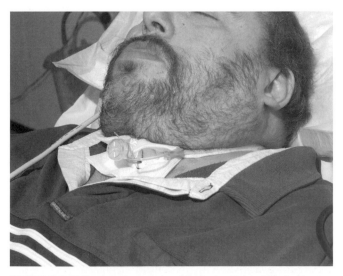

FIGURE 8-5 ■ Tracheostomy tube. (Photo by Richard York, Oregon Health and Sciences University.)

or Reiki, often reduces the discomfort. This in turn increases the patient's overall comfort level.

Positioning adjustments:

- Most drains and tubes preclude using the prone position.
- Side-lying may be acceptable if there are no other influencing factors with regard to the patient's general health.

MONITORS

When continuous measurement of some aspect of a patient's health is necessary, an electronic monitor might be used. Some monitors use telemetry, which transmits information by wire or radio signals to another location, such as the nurses' station. An example of this is cardiac telemetry, in which data from the heart's pressures and electrical activity is sent to a monitor somewhere distant from the patient (see Figure 6-2). The information about pressures is gathered by a Swan-Ganz catheter, which was mentioned earlier in the chapter. An **electrocardiograph** (ECG) monitors the electrical activity of the heart via electrodes attached to the patient's chest.

The amount of oxygen in the blood is monitored by a **pulse oximeter,** known as a "pulse ox." A pulse oximeter works by passing a specific wavelength of light through a vascular bed, usually a finger, and measuring the absorption of light by oxygenated (red) and deoxygenated (blue) blood. (Notice the device on the middle fingertip of the patient's left hand in Figure 6-2. That is a pulse ox.) The relationship between these two can be used to determine if the blood is carrying enough oxygen. Practitioners can see the digital readout of the monitor, which is near the patient's bed. Oxygen saturation above 90% is the desired level.

In childbirth, a fetal monitor is used to measure the child's heartbeat and the mother's abdominal tension during uterine contractions. Fetal monitors can be external (Fig. 8-6) or internal. Internal types, which are inserted into the uterus, are more accurate than external ones, which are placed on the outside around the woman's abdomen.

Massage practitioners may encounter many other types of monitors. The **electroencephalograph,** or EEG, measures the electrical activity in the brain. Respiratory monitors are frequently used for children, especially those at risk for sleep apnea. A variety of cranial monitors are used to measure pressure inside the skull if the person has suffered head trauma.[1]

■ CLINICAL CONSIDERATIONS

Pressure considerations:

- Force or movement that could displace the monitor should be avoided.

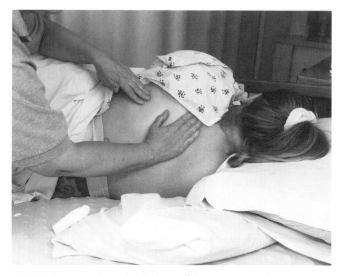

FIGURE 8-6 ■ Patient attached to a fetal monitor receives massage. The monitor belt is visible on the lower back. (Photo by Don Hamilton.)

Site restrictions:

- Monitors require the touch therapist to be mindful when massaging around the sites containing a measurement device, such as the belly of a woman connected to a fetal monitor, the neck of someone with a Swan-Ganz catheter, the chest of a person with ECG electrodes, or the finger containing a pulse ox monitor.

Positioning adjustments:

- Positioning will be affected by most of these medical apparatus. However, repositioning is nearly always possible. The necessary adjustments are usually apparent by using common sense.

TIP: Stay Focused on the Patient

When working with patients attached to medical machinery, stay focused on the patient instead of the monitors.

ORTHOPEDIC DEVICES AND EQUIPMENT

When a patient has disease or trauma to the musculoskeletal system, it may be necessary to immobilize the affected body part(s) to allow bones and other connective tissue to heal. This is accomplished through the use of splints, braces, casts, slings, fixators, and traction devices.

There are a variety of relatively simple devices that stabilize an area. **Splints** act to immobilize a joint or joints through the use of a rigid framework bound to the body. A **brace** is similar to a splint, but it usually allows some movement of the joint, often with the use of hinges. A **cast** can be made of plaster, plastic, or fiberglass and is molded to fit the body part that needs to be immobilized. A **sling** is a supporting bandage used to immobilize a limb, most commonly a loop suspended from the neck to support the forearm.

Another group of apparatus is more complex and often involves surgery. A **fixator** uses a combination of pins, nails, screws, and plates to hold bones together and can be either internal or external. An example of an external fixator can be found in Figure 8-7. **Traction** devices, which are a system of ropes, pulleys, and weights, bring injured body parts into alignment by pulling on them and holding them in place. A **continuous passive motion device** is sometimes used to passively move a joint after surgery, to maintain its range of motion.[1]

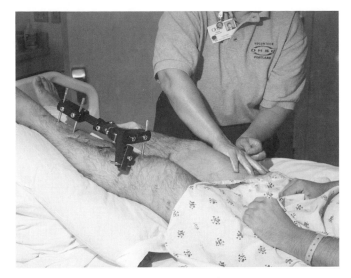

FIGURE 8-7 ■ Patient with an external fixator receives massage. (Photo by Don Hamilton.)

■ CLINICAL CONSIDERATIONS

Pressure considerations:
- Force or movement that could displace the body's alignment must be avoided.

Site restrictions:
- Casts must be protected from becoming soiled or wet. Moisture causes plaster to soften, which can then cause skin breakdown.
- The skin at the edge of a cast or other orthopedic devices can become irritated.

Positioning adjustments:
- Orthopedic apparatus severely limits the positioning possibilities for a massage session.
- Maintaining proper alignment of the affected areas is vital. Practitioners should work closely with the nursing staff to ensure that this happens. Any touch technique that affects alignment must be avoided.

Other:
- Study the "Orthopedic" section in Chapter 6 for further massage adjustments related to the patient's general condition.

OXYGEN-DELIVERY DEVICES

If the patient's blood oxygen level is low, oxygen will be given from an external source. This can be through a simple face mask that fits over the nose and mouth or through a pronged tube in the nose known as a **nasal cannula.** (Notice the patient in Figure 8-2; he has a nasal cannula as well as an NG tube.) The latter device delivers a low oxygen flow. If this amount of extra oxygen does not keep the saturation levels high enough, masks that deliver a higher concentration of oxygen are used.

When patients don't have the energy to breathe, but the doctor does not want them on a mechanical ventilator, they may be put on a **continuous positive airway pres-**sure (CPAP) mask. This provides positive airway pressure during both inhalation and exhalation. With a CPAP mask, the patient often has an NG tube that can be used to suction out excess air that might enter the digestive system. The CPAP mask is not well tolerated by some patients because it must be sealed tightly against the face.

Oxygen is sometimes administered directly to the trachea through an endotracheal tube, a **tracheotomy tube,** or a catheter that is placed directly into the trachea. The placement of an endotracheal tube is referred to as **intubation.** Removal of the tube is **extubation.** If a patient is unable to breathe on his or her own, a **mechanical ventilator,** or **vent,** is attached to the endotracheal tubing. Patients on ventilators are nearly always placed in the ICU due to the high amount of expertise required to monitor these devices.[1] (Personal interview with Janey Slunaker, RN, on April 8, 2003.)

■ CLINICAL CONSIDERATIONS

Positioning considerations:
- Positioning will be the main adjustment needed. However, this is not caused so much by the oxygen-delivery devices in and of themselves. It is the general condition of the patient that will dictate positioning restrictions.
- Those with a nasal canula, face mask, or tracheal device may be able to lie on their side for a back massage.
- The mechanical ventilator does not prevent the patient from side-lying, but the overall condition of this group of patients usually is very acute. Often, they are in a comatose or semicomatose state.
- Repositioning, whenever possible, will help maintain skin integrity.

Other:

- Massage is beneficial, for both the health of the skin and breathing difficulties. Relaxation can create greater openness in the chest and, therefore, increase the delivery of oxygen.
- Patients with tracheal devices or on a ventilator will be unable to speak. Several of the communication suggestions in Chapter 6 will help touch therapists in their interactions with this group.

PAIN-MANAGEMENT DEVICES

Pain is most often managed pharmacologically and is delivered via IV and epidural devices. Some systems allow the patient to control the amount of pain medication given, a method called patient-controlled analgesia (PCA). The person with a PCA pump can press a button when pain relief is needed. The PCA system is computerized, which controls the maximum amount of medication that the patient can receive in a given time period. Pain medication can also be injected into the epidural space in the lumbar spine for pain in the lower extremities and abdomen. Epidural anesthesia is frequently used during childbirth and spinal surgery.

Electrical stimulation is sometimes used to relieve pain. **Transcutaneous electrical nerve stimulation (TENS)** is a system that delivers electric currents to the surface of the skin, relieving pain in underlying areas. A TENS unit can be worn continuously to relieve chronic pain. For deeper stimulation, a **percutaneous** electrical nerve stimulator can be surgically placed around a nerve. An internal receiver is implanted under the skin, and the patient activates an external transmitter when pain relief is needed. In similar systems, electrodes can also be placed in the spinal cord or brain.[1]

A PATIENT'S STORY

Someone to Pay Attention to Me

My husband and daughters had left for home after being at the hospital all day. Our home was 160 miles away, and I was a bit lonely. When I was offered a massage, anxiety turned to relief. Here was someone to pay attention just to ME, not my disease, not my treatment, not the machines I was attached to, just to ME.

Toni B, admitted for cancer treatment

■ CLINICAL CONSIDERATIONS

Pressure considerations:

- Massage strokes administered to people receiving systemic pain relief should not be forceful because the medication will affect the ability of the patient to give accurate feedback about the pressure.

- When the pain-control system treats only a localized area, gentle pressure should be applied to that area.

Site restrictions:

- IV and epidural catheter sites and the area surrounding them should be avoided. This is especially true of an epidural catheter, which is placed near spinal nerves and the spinal canal.
- Any stroke that creates excessive movement also should be avoided to prevent any displacement of the epidural. This is also true for electrical stimulation devices.

Positioning adjustments:

- Generally self-limiting

A THERAPIST'S JOURNAL

Calling on My Massage Skills

An oncology patient presented to our PICC room one afternoon to have a central line placed. A PICC line is just a fancy IV line that allows medications such as chemotherapy, which can be caustic to the smaller peripheral veins, to be administered. PICCs are the least invasive central lines that a patient can receive. Other lines require a surgical procedure, which is much more intrusive and costly.

The patient was being prepared for a bone marrow transplantation and was very agitated. She had been through many medical procedures and at times was overwhelmed with pain. She stated emphatically that she suffered from needle phobia.

Fortunately, there were two nurses in the room that day, which allowed us to give her extra emotional support. My colleague and I worked for nearly an hour trying to place the PICC. We wanted to be successful so that the patient would not have to have the line placed surgically. However, our attempts were not meeting with success. Finally, I decided to call upon my massage therapy skills. I put on some soothing music, dimmed the lights, and sat at her feet giving light massage. I continued to reinforce the patient with soft words of encouragement. This allowed her to relax, and my colleague was able to place the device. Perhaps best of all was the outcome of the patient's mental status. She amazed herself by being able to become so calm and relaxed during the placement. I felt that we helped empower the patient to believe that she could handle other medical procedures with less fear. The result was rewarding for all of us.

Lana Adair, RN, LMT,
Oregon Health and Science University, Portland, Oregon

PROCEDURES

This section will familiarize the touch therapist with common medical procedures and the equipment used during them. Some procedures are part of the treatment process; others are diagnostic in nature. Massage therapy can be helpful as the patient undergoes certain procedures, such as hemodialysis or a PICC placement, or following other procedures, such as a heart biopsy (see Figure 7-4), positron emission tomography (PET) scan, or endoscopic procedure. It is also useful for practitioners to understand the basics of procedures to better know what the patient has experienced.

BIOPSY

A biopsy is most commonly used as a diagnostic assessment. Tissue from the area in question is removed and then sent for analysis by a pathologist. The pathologist treats the sample chemically, slices it in thin sections, and then examines it under a microscope.

Most often, the procedure is performed with a needle that aspirates a small portion of the desired tissue. Needle biopsies are frequently employed for assessing lumps in the breast and lesions in the thyroid, liver, kidney, and lungs. Tissue also can be excised surgically, but this is not preferred unless necessary due to the greater invasiveness of surgical procedures.

The needle often can be inserted directly into the questionable area. In other instances, such as a tumor deep in the body, an x-ray is used to locate the lesion and then guide placement of the needle into the biopsy area. Fiberoptic instruments, such as bronchoscopes or colonoscopes, also can be used to collect tissue samples.

Bone marrow is also biopsied in the diagnosis of blood disorders, such as leukemia or **aplastic anemia,** or to monitor the course of an illness, such as **multiple myeloma,** and its response to treatment. Usually, bone marrow is aspirated with a needle from the iliac crest or sternum. This particular biopsy is painful because the doctor must pass a somewhat large outer metal sleeve through bone before entering the cavity that produces the marrow. The needle that removes the bone marrow sample is inserted into the outer sleeve.[1,3]

■ CLINICAL CONSIDERATIONS

Pressure considerations:
■ Risk of clot formation due to insertion of needles, especially the large bore type.

Site restrictions:
■ Biopsy site due to tenderness or bruising.
■ Be mindful of bleeding at the biopsy site, and observe appropriate Standard Precautions.

Positioning adjustments:
■ Most often, they will be self-limiting.
■ Biopsies of certain organs, such as the kidney and liver, may require positioning adjustments away from the biopsied area.

LUMBAR PUNCTURE

A lumbar puncture, also known as a spinal tap, is performed between two lumbar vertebrae, usually the third and fourth, with a thin, hollow needle that is inserted into the spinal canal. It usually takes about 30 minutes. Two common purposes for a spinal tap are to measure pressure in the cerebrospinal fluid (CSF) or to take a sample of spinal fluid for analysis. A number of diseases or conditions may be diagnosed from the sample: **multiple sclerosis, Guillain-Barré syndrome,** meningitis, encephalitis, a brain abscess, **Reye's syndrome,** and AIDS-related conditions. The presence of blood in the spinal fluid also can be determined through a sample of spinal fluid.

A lumbar puncture may also be performed to inject a contrasting dye or radioactive substance as part of creating a diagnostic image of the CSF. Antibiotics and anti-cancer drugs, as well as spinal anesthesia, may be placed in the spine by this process. A new use of the procedure is to determine levels of the "tau" protein and beta-amyloid, two substances associated with Alzheimer's disease.[1]

■ CLINICAL CONSIDERATIONS

Pressure considerations:
■ Patients usually feel unwell afterward and have increased muscular tension. Headaches are not uncommon. Therefore, soothing pressure is called for.
■ Pain medication will interfere with the ability to give accurate feedback.

Site restrictions:
■ The puncture site will be very tender.
■ Bleeding or CSF leakage may occur at the puncture site following the procedure.
■ The patient may have sore muscles as a result of the position that must be maintained to open the lumbar vertebrae—side-lying, curled into a tight ball with the knees pulled to the chest.

Positioning adjustments:
■ The patient must lie flat for 2 hours following the procedure.

ENDOSCOPY

Endoscopy is a method of examining internal organs that are hollow or have a cavity, such as the lungs or stomach. The instruments, generically referred to as **endoscopes,** are made of a hollow tube that may be flexible or rigid. A lighted optical system allows the tissues to be seen through a video screen or telescopic eyepiece.

Each scope is unique and geared toward the part of the body to be viewed. Pulmonary specialists employ a bronchoscope to examine the trachea and bronchial tree for such conditions as tumors, constrictions, bleeding, or pulmonary diseases such as tuberculosis. A **gastroenterologist** uses a gastroscope to view into the stomach, intestines, and other digestive organs. A **sigmoidoscope** allows the sigmoid portion of the colon to be inspected, while a colonoscope allows visual examination of the entire colon. The doctor can inspect for such conditions as tumors, polyps, ulcerative colitis, or bleeding.

These scopes also have the capacity to provide treatment. For example, a laser beam can be directed through a channel of the scope to stop bleeding from a lesion. Another channel in the scope allows the passage of instruments that can take a biopsy, remove a foreign object, or excise polyps. Narrowed areas, such as in the esophagus, can be stretched to ease swallowing.

A number of other endoscopes are available for use in other areas of the body. A **cystoscope** is used to inspect the bladder and prostate gland, an **arthroscope** allows a view into joints, a **laparoscope** provides a way to inspect the abdomen, and the **colposcope** examines the vagina and cervix.[1]

As we take massage therapy into the welcoming and heady atmosphere of "integrative medicine," let's not be hesitant to promote the most important aspect of our work: touch for the sake of touching. Touch comforts patients and caregivers. Touch makes invasive procedures more tolerable for patients who may be afraid, restless, out-of-control, in pain, and/or doubting their very touchableness. The undivided attention and compassionate human touch we bring to them is the most important "stroke" in the massage therapist's repertoire.[4]

Tedi Dunn, *Massage Therapy Guidelines for Hospital and Home Care,* 4th ed.

■ CLINICAL CONSIDERATIONS

Pressure considerations:
- Pain medication or sedatives will interfere with the ability to give accurate feedback.

Site restrictions:
- Usually, the scope is inserted through an orifice, so there are no site restrictions. One exception is a laparoscopic procedure in which a small incision is made near the umbilicus.
- Depending on the type of procedure, the positioning may have created discomfort, especially in the neck or back.

Positioning adjustments:
- Generally self-limiting
- As part of some scoping procedures, such as a laparoscopy and esophagogastroduodenoscopy, air is inserted to permit better visualization or to separate the intestines from the pelvic organs. This manipulation of the intestines can cause bloating, abdominal discomfort, and difficulty passing gas or having a bowel movement.

SCANS

Body scans allow the examination of internal organs and structures. The x-ray has been used for nearly a century, while computed tomography (CT) scans, magnetic resonance imaging (MRI) scans, and ultrasound are more recent methods of assessment. Even newer still are nuclear scans.

X-rays

X-rays are high-energy electromagnetic waves that have the ability to penetrate most solid matter and to act on photographic film. These rays often are used to assess the health of the skeletal structure but can be used for certain soft-tissue areas. A mammogram is an example.

Special procedures combine the use of a contrasting dye and x-rays to obtain a clearer picture of the affected area. For instance, to better see the functioning of a joint, dye that is opaque to x-rays is placed in the joint and then x-rayed, a process called **arthrography.** This same process can be used to examine arteries in the brain, which is known as a cerebral **arteriograph** or **angiography.** Kidneys, bile and pancreatic ducts, and the space around the spinal cord also can be assessed using this procedure.[1]

■ CLINICAL CONSIDERATIONS

Pressure considerations:
- Adjustments to pressure will not be necessary because of a simple x-ray but may be required when dye is injected into the body.
- Some patients have a reaction to the dye, such as nausea, headache, dyspnea, hives, increased heart rate, and numbness in the extremities.
- Sedatives will interfere with the ability to give accurate feedback.

- The process of threading a catheter through the veins can dislodge a clot or plaque deposit. In light of that risk, only superficial massage should be administered.

Site restrictions:
- Bleeding at the catheter site
- Certain parts of the body may feel strained from lying in awkward positions. Massage to them might be helpful.

- Certain procedures require the use of a catheter in the inguinal area. Massage should be avoided to that extremity due to the increased risk for a thrombus. The patient may have groin pain from the use of this type of catheter.
- IV catheter sites
- Pain at the site where dye was injected

Positioning adjustments:
- Generally self-limiting

CT and MRI Scans

Many of the x-ray techniques have become supplemental with the advent of less invasive CT and MRI scans. CT scans employ ultrathin x-rays to analyze soft-tissue structures. The x-rays are beamed through segments of the body and picked up by the CT equipment to create a three-dimensional composite representation of the body. The information is fed into a computer that converts the data into a video or photographs. Contrasting dyes are sometimes used to enhance the contrast of the image. CT scans are particularly useful for imaging brain disorders such as strokes, hemorrhages, injuries, tumors, swelling, and fluid accumulation.

An MRI is also a computerized scanning technique. Unlike a CT scan, which uses x-rays, the MRI machine employs a strong magnetic field that measures the response of the body's hydrogen atoms, which are abundantly present in water. MRIs, because of their ability to give high-resolution pictures, are useful for assessing the spinal cord and nerve fiber disorders such as multiple sclerosis.[1,4]

A touch practitioner cannot be in the room during a CT scan because of the use of x-rays. However, it is possible during an MRI. An MRI tube is extremely confining and, despite the use of sedatives, very anxiety producing. For some patients, the presence of a family member or massage therapist who is holding their feet can be reassuring as they lay for lengthy periods of time inside this machine (Fig. 8-8).

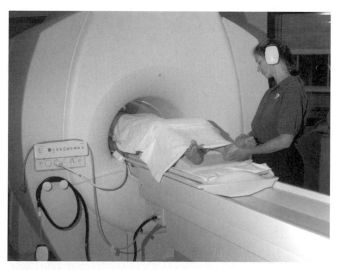

FIGURE 8-8 ■ Foot massage provides comfort during an MRI scan. (Photo by Don Hamilton.)

■ CLINICAL CONSIDERATIONS

Pressure considerations:
■ Pain medication or sedatives will interfere with the ability to give accurate feedback.

Site restrictions:
■ If contrasting dye was administered, there will be an IV site.
■ Patients are required to lie flat on their back during the scan, sometimes for hours. Attention to the back will soothe tensed musculature.

Positioning adjustments:
■ Self-limiting

Other:
The contrasting dyes are absorbed into the bloodstream and eliminated through urine. They pose no risk to practitioners. Patients must, however, be well hydrated before and after procedures using contrasting agents to protect the kidneys. Therefore, they may need to make frequent trips to the bathroom. (Personal interview with Miles Hassell, MD, on April 14, 2003.)

Ultrasound

This technology uses sound waves to create an image of the body. A wand-like device sends high-frequency sound waves into the tissue, which reflect back and form an image that can be displayed on a screen. Most people are familiar with the use of **ultrasound** to monitor the progress of a fetus in utero (see Figure 6-3). It also can be used to detect tumors, examine abdominal organs, the thyroid, and prostate gland. IV nurses who specialize in the placement of PICC lines use ultrasound to locate a vein suitable for inserting the catheter. Additionally, it can measure the flow of blood in veins and arteries.[1]

■ CLINICAL CONSIDERATIONS

Usually, there are no adjustments necessary as a result of an ultrasound.

Nuclear Scans

Nuclear imaging employs small amounts of **radioactive isotopes** that are attached to a drug or chemical. The two together are referred to as **radiopharmaceuticals.** These substances, which can be swallowed, inhaled, or injected into the body, are designed to concentrate in a certain organ. The radioisotope gives off radioactive energy that in turn produces an image of the organ showing its size, shape, and functioning. Some damaged tissue will have an increased uptake of the radioactive material, suggesting an abnormality, while other tissue will show an irregular distribution. Bones, lungs, liver, brain, thyroid, heart, and blood can be scanned in this way.

PET scans are one particular type of a nuclear scan. They are still a fairly new and expensive technology and therefore only available at a limited number of hospitals. A PET scan, or **positron emission tomography,** combines the use of radioisotopes, called **positrons,** with computer imaging techniques. A glucose-like solution is mixed with mildly radioactive tracers, which are injected or inhaled into the body. The PET scanner measures how quickly tissues absorb the radioactive isotopes, an indication of cellular metabolism based on patterns of glucose utilization. In the brain, areas of decreased metabolism indicate dysfunction. However, when testing for a cancer, just the opposite is true. Quick absorption of the solution indicates an area containing cancer because tumors need increased nutrition to remain viable, greedily absorbing the sugary solution.[1,4]

The multiple gated acquisition (MUGA) scan is another diagnostic procedure that employs nuclear technology. It assesses the function of the heart by withdrawing a small amount of blood from the patient, inserting a radioactive substance into the sample that attaches to the red blood cells, and then reinjecting the cells back into the bloodstream. A gamma camera placed above the patient detects the low-level radiation being given off by the radiolabeled cells and is able to produce an outline of the heart's chambers and accurately measure the output of the left ventricle.[6]

■ CLINICAL CONSIDERATIONS

Pressure considerations:
■ Generally self-limiting
■ Some people have a sense of malaise or slight fatigue afterward.
■ Some scans, such as a PET, require the patient to lie very still for more than an hour while the nuclear material circulates through the body. Generalized muscular tension will be evident. Gently coaxing the muscles into relaxation is the best approach.

Site restrictions:
■ Usually, when the nuclear material is injected, it is done through a peripheral IV catheter. Tenderness will be present at the site.
■ Depending on the part of the body that requires scanning, the patient may have to lie in an awkward position, such as with the arms over the head, for a prolonged period. Attention to the affected areas will be welcomed.

Positioning adjustments:
■ Generally self-limiting

HEMODIALYSIS

Hemodialysis, a process that artificially cleanses the blood of accumulated waste products, is used for people with chronic, end-stage renal failure or temporarily for patients whose acute illness has shut down the kidneys. If the patient's general health is good enough, the procedure can take place in the hemodialysis unit (Fig. 8-9). Other patients, often those in the ICU, are dialyzed with a portable machine at the bedside. Those with stable kidney problems will receive dialysis in an outpatient center.

Blood is accessed in several different ways. An oversized central line called a Perma-cath may be placed in either the subclavian, internal jugular, or femoral vein. Another method of creating an access point is via an arteriovenous **fistula** (Fig. 8-10). A fistula is created by suturing an artery and a vein, usually the radial artery and cephalic vein in the nondominant arm. Another term for this connection is an **anastomosis.** Two large-bore needles are then inserted into the vessel, one to obtain blood, the other to reinfuse it. A synthetic tube can also be grafted between an artery and vein to serve as an access point.

Blood is pulled from one of these access points and directed through a semipermeable dialyzer, which performs the filtering function of the kidneys. When the process is finished, usually in about 4 hours, the blood is returned to the body through the patient's access.

The hemodialysis patient requires close monitoring. Any time a large quantity of blood is removed from the body, homeostasis is put at risk. The patient can easily "crash" due to a drop in blood pressure, electrolyte imbalance, or a change in the pH.

Potential complications from this process are severe. Infection can occur at the vascular access point, or the catheter can clot off. Also possible are stroke, cardiovascular conditions, anemia, fatigue, psychological problems, and bone problems as a result of improper calcium metabolism.[1,3] (Personal interview with Linda Hughes, RN, LMT, on March 23, 2003.)

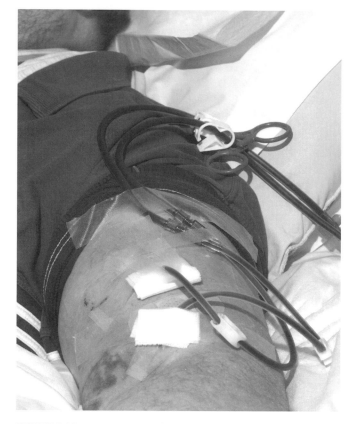

FIGURE 8-10 ■ Arteriovenous fistula. (Photo by Richard York, Oregon Health and Science University.)

It must be remembered that the person undergoing hemodialysis usually has a complex medical history. Many of these patients are diabetic or have heart conditions. Touch therapists should also study the sections in the book related to those subjects.

■ CLINICAL CONSIDERATIONS

Pressure considerations:

- Potential for homeostatic disequilibrium. Massage should not be demanding to the body.
- Fatigue
- Easing bruising
- Fragile skin
- Heparin
- Hypertension
- Neuropathy
- Central line catheters, such as a Perma-cath, or shunts increase the risk of clot formation. Massage the extremity nearest to the central line or shunt very gently. For instance, if the Perma-cath is in the subclavian, massage the arm on the side very lightly.

Site restrictions:

- Do not perform circulatory touch techniques to the arm containing a shunt because of the possibility of clot formation. Also, it is important not to risk dis-

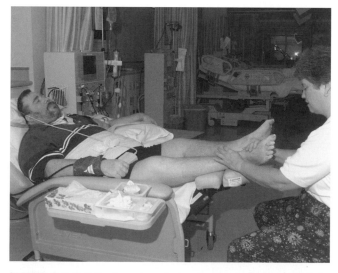

FIGURE 8-9 ■ Patient receives foot massage during hemodialysis. (Photo by Richard York, Oregon Health and Science University.)

lodging or damaging the shunt. Lotioning the hand is usually permissible.

- Avoid Perma-cath site.
- Blood pressure cuff on opposite arm.

Positioning adjustments:

- Because of the potential for hemodialysis patients to crash, do not have them sit at the side of the bed.
- No prone positioning.
- Side-lying only on the opposite side from the access device.

A THERAPIST'S JOURNAL
Failed Kidneys

The patient is a 41-year-old man whose body is rejecting his own—and anyone else's—kidneys. Nothing has worked. Even a kidney from a living donor and a deceased accident victim have been rejected. His system is slowly and irrevocably shutting down. He is admitted to the hospital every few weeks for a several day regimen of kidney dialysis. I always see him with the same complaint—extraordinarily tight shoulders and an aching back. Putting my hands on him, I am always amazed at the railroad tracks on his back, sides and chest. The capsule around his heart has been infected more than once; physicians have gone into his back and chest several times for his many systemic failures.

He is becoming shrunken, leathery, an odd color. His hands are becoming proportionately larger and harder than the rest of his body. The doctors can't tell him why.

He was handsome a few years ago. He's dark, Italian, with big dark eyes that are half closed. His face is swollen from his own toxic backup. When he comes into the hospital to begin the round of dialysis, he is always just a bit jaunty; he wears a baseball cap, lots of gold chains, flirts with the nurses. He has a lot of money, he says; he drives a fast car, he says. And when he sleeps, he looks like a child.

Today, during the massage, he falls asleep half a dozen times in a period of 30 minutes. The sleep is fitful. He jerks, twitches, shivers, grabs at an imaginary bug, scratches. His long eyelashes flutter. His hands open and close quickly. At one point his entire body jerks so violently that it leaves the bed completely and plunks back down, and yet this does not wake him.

The massage he receives each day is per his request. One day, it's his hands; the next, he says his shoulders are killing him. Once, the focus was his forehead alone. The massage is careful, slow, as deep as he can tolerate with a lot of lubrication. Working on his skin is a lot like applying lotion to an old leather purse—you can't be sure it's doing

any good but it seems to soften a little in the process. The toxicity of his body has turned normal tissue to almost-intolerable stiffness, so the massage must be thoughtful, almost tentative, gentle yet probing. His face must be watched constantly for any wincing, since to create any more pain in this man would be unforgivable. There is no hacking, no tapotement, no jostling. The touch, the act of touch with loving intent at this point, matters as much as any physiological outcome.

The failure in his blood circulation is affecting his brain function. He repeats himself, forgets easily. Yet, his speech is always positive. When he wakes he tells me the massage is the best one he has ever had, how it's the best thing about the hospital stay. I hear him tell the nurses they are the best he has ever seen, how this stay is the best he has ever had.

One nurse enters and places five pills in a little paper cup onto the bedside table. He is to take them with dinner. He knows what they are, what they do, and he smiles and nods at her.

I ask when he's due to go home. "Well, I was supposed to go home yesterday, but here I am. If I don't go home tomorrow, why don't you come back and give me one of those great massages?"

And as the last word is out of his mouth, he is asleep again. Twitching, grabbing at himself in the fitful sleep of a body that is slowly poisoning itself.

The next day when I visit him, he has just endured several hours of dialysis. He says it doesn't hurt; it just feels funny and takes a long time. I remark at the number of railroad track scars over his body. He points to each one in turn, his forearm, his groin, his upper arm and says, "These are all the ports they used to use, where they put the tubes and wires to do the dialysis. But I keep clotting them off." He's on blood thinners now in an effort to stop his blood from creating deadly clots. One could be "thrown" and go to his heart, brain, or lungs and kill him.

"This is my last chance," he says, pointing to the one in his upper arm. This is the last place they can get in. "If this one clots off," he shakes his head and looks down, "it doesn't look very good for me."

The next day I visit, and he says there are no more places for them to start the dialysis. All of his veins have shut down or thrown clots, and he's got to go to the Mayo Clinic to find a specialist.

"It doesn't look good," he says, rubbing his forehead.

Today, he gets a massage focused on his very hard and stiff hands. He can barely make a fist. As his hands are massaged slowly and deeply, he begins to moan like a man who is experiencing great pleasure. He wants to stay sitting up because he wants to stay awake for this massage. He knows if he lies down he will fall asleep, and he doesn't want to miss this sensation. He hunches over, holding his head up with his elbow on his knee as his hands are worked on. Every muscle in his hand, every joint is massaged slowly and carefully, and he continues to moan. He rocks a little and moans more.

Suddenly he says, "If Hitler would have had this done to his hands, he could have never held a gun." He chuckles at his own comment, closes his eyes, and continues to rock.

—*Charlotte Versagi, LMT, NCTMB, Royal Oak, Michigan, excerpted from a book in progress, Men Who Carry Purses: Portraits of Patients and Those Who Love Them*

(Copyright © 2004 Charlotte Versagi)

Mrs. B

CASE HISTORY

Mrs. B was a 67-year-old woman who had been flown into a large urban hospital from an outlying rural care center. She had experienced a dissecting aortic aneurysm and an MI. Immediately upon arrival, she was taken to surgery, where vascular surgeons attempted to repair the aneurysm. Essentially, it was deteriorating before their eyes, and they were only able to clamp the aneurysm at both ends and send Mrs. B to the ICU, where she was expected to die.

The patient awoke from the surgery intubated but alert. To everyone's astonishment, she started to get better. However, the vascularization to everything below her waist was compromised, if not devastated, by the aneurysm and surgery. This was evidenced by the need for a colostomy as well as dialysis three times a week. The dialysis was needed due to decreased blood flow to the renal arteries.

The most acute and brutal consequence of her compromised vascularization was an enormous sacral wound that began as a result of limited blood flow to that area. The wound took up an area that covered her entire sacrum, not just superficially, but deep, revealing the bone itself. This was documented in photos at the front of the progress notes. Mrs. B also had decubitus ulcers forming on both legs and feet resulting from decreased blood flow. An abdominal wound from both surgeries required a VAC (vacuum-assisted closure) dressing, a device that pulls out fluid, pus, and cellular debris from the wound in hopes of improving healing to the area.

When I saw her for the first time, the patient was off the mechanical ventilator and was on a T-piece with oxygen. She had many medical devices, such as a colostomy, a trach, an arteriovenous fistula for dialysis, the VAC dressing to the abdominal wound, and piles and piles of dressing over the sacral wound. She was on a nursing unit that accepted only intubated patients with pathogens that required isolation. In Mrs. B's case, the pathogen was an antibiotic-resistant bacteria, which required that I glove, gown, mask, and wear shoe covers to enter the room.

The patient had many position, site, and pressure restrictions. Repositioning was a major occurrence due to pain. She could lie only on her back, tilted slightly to one side. There was minimal surface area available on the body to work with, so there were few options available to massage. Since she had been through so much for such a long time, the patient was compromised on many levels, including nutritionally, which caused her skin to be fragile, so the pressure had to be adjusted.

Mrs. B enthusiastically agreed to a touch-therapy treatment. Before beginning the session, we talked about her desires and goals for the time together. She was excited about massage to her back and shoulders, which were very tense and sore. I explained the therapies that I could provide to her, which included Swedish massage, Reiki, Healing Touch, and guided imagery.

Her nurse helped me to turn Mrs. B onto her right side so that I could massage the back and shoulders. This position was tolerable for only a few minutes, so I rolled her onto her back and stood behind her. From there, I massaged her head and neck and performed Reiki to the head, neck, and shoulders. My intention was centered on comfort and relaxation. After I started the Reiki, Mrs. B entered a deep sleep and was still sleeping when I left.

Later that week, the nurse reported Mrs. B had enjoyed the treatment; the feeling of relaxation lasted all day. It was the first time since entering the hospital that she had felt deeply relaxed. She spoke frequently about the treatment and wanted a repeat visit.

The next visit was cut short, however. The patient was experiencing too much pain to tolerate any form of therapy, no matter how light. She asked me to leave with tears streaming down her face. As I left, I spoke to the nurse regarding Mrs. B's pain control.

(continued)

CASE HISTORY

The following visit was very difficult for me as the sacral wound had spread farther over the back side and now had a terrible odor. I tried to do some massage and Reiki but was quite nauseated and overwhelmed by the smell of rotting flesh. Fifteen minutes was all I could tolerate. By this time, she was off dialysis and off the T-piece and, therefore, able to talk. Mrs. B was still in significant pain from the nonhealing wound and spoke of dying. Her husband wanted all effort made to save her. Consults were made with the ethics team and palliative care unit, to no avail. Eventually, an axillary-femoral artery bypass was offered to encourage vascularization to the lower half of the body.

Following the surgery, she was brought back to the ICU, where she was again on the vent for several days. Eventually, medication was required to maintain blood pressure. At that time, it was decided to take her off the vent and transfer her to the palliative care unit, where she would be supported with comfort measures only. Several hours after being extubated, Mrs. B died.

Being part of Mrs. B's struggle and pain was a profound experience. I was conflicted about issues and judgments of what is right for another. Questions arose, such as, "What does life, or more importantly, living, really mean?" I struggled with the deterioration of her body and the all-too-real sensory experiences that accompany the dying process. I felt sorrow for her journey as well as disgrace at my inability to be present to her during the various stages of death and disintegration. I was humbled by the experience.

Tina Ferner, St. Vincent Mercy Hospital, Toledo, Ohio

SUMMARY

Medical devices and procedures add yet another dimension when planning a massage session with a person who is hospitalized. The main medical devices have been presented in this chapter, along with a cross section of procedures. Space limitations do not allow for coverage of every piece of apparatus or procedure. However, by extrapolating from this sampling, touch therapists will be able to calculate the necessary massage adjustments.

TEST YOURSELF

Circle the correct answer. There may be more than one.

1. Which of the following can cause clot formation?
    A. Use of a nasal cannula
    B. A central IV catheter
    C. Insertion of a Foley catheter
    D. An inguinal catheter

2. The purpose of a shunt is to:
    A. Collect urine
    B. Allow nurses to give medications
    C. Divert fluid from one compartment of the body to another
    D. To drain fluid that collects in a cavity or wound out of the body

3. Pressure should be very gentle when massaging:
    A. The upper body of a person who has just had a pacemaker implanted

B. An extremity that contains or is near a central IV catheter
    C. A patient who is connected to a pulse oximeter
    D. A patient who has just had an MRI

4. Which of the following reasons are an indication for gentle pressure when massaging a person undergoing hemodialysis?
    A. The potential for a complex medical history that often includes heart disease or diabetes
    B. The potential for clot formation around the access device
    C. The potential for homeostatic disequilibrium
    D. The possibility of disturbing the Swan-Ganz catheter inserted into the neck

5. Which of the following devices or procedures are used in the diagnosing process?
    A. Endotracheal tube
    B. CT scan
    C. Nuclear imaging
    D. J-P tube

6. Which of the following devices require that the patient remain supine?
    A. PCA pump
    B. Nasal cannula
    C. Traction device
    D. Fetal monitor

7. Which of the following pieces of medical equipment might also require the use of Standard Precautions?
    A. Moving a urinal
    B. Massaging in the vicinity of a drain

C. Massaging near a fetal monitor

D. Massaging near a nasal cannula

8. A massage therapist could safely be in attendance during which of the following procedures?
   A. Biopsy
   B. CT scan
   C. MRI
   D. Placement of a peripheral IV catheter

Matching

____ **1.** Angiogram

____ **2.** Telemetry

____ **3.** Swan-Ganz catheter

____ **4.** Implantable defibrillator

____ **5.** PET scan

____ **6.** Port-A-Cath

____ **7.** Stenosis

A. A procedure that examines blood vessels

B. A device that a patient may have following open-heart surgery

C. Combines the use of radioisotopes with computer imaging

D. A device that transmits information by wire or radio signals

E. Used by nurses to draw blood or give medication

F. A narrowing

G. A device that stops the heart

REFERENCES

1. Nettina S. The Lippincott Manual of Nursing Practice. Philadelphia, PA: Lippincott Williams & Wilkins, 2001.
2. Understanding Coronary Artery Procedures. Krames Health and Safety Education, The Stay Well Company, 2000.
3. Mayo Clinic Family Healthbook. New York, NY: William Morrow and Company, 1990.
4. Dunn T, Williams M. Massage Therapy Guidelines for Hospital and Home Care. 4th ed. Olympia, WA: Information for People, 2000.
5. Chabner DE. The Language of Medicine. Philadelphia, PA: W.B. Saunders, 1996.
6. The MUGA Scan. Available at: http://heartdisease.about.com/cs/cardiactests/a/muga.htm. Accessed November 27, 2003.

ADDITIONAL RESOURCES

Hospitals have nursing education centers that usually have samples of some medical devices.

Various labs within the hospital, such as the heart catheterization lab, may have out-of-date catheters that are going to be thrown away. These make excellent teaching aids.

Check with the various nursing units to see if they have posterboard displays of medical devices relevant to their patient population. For instance, the oncology unit may have a display of central IV catheters.

Contact some of the procedural labs or treatment clinics, such as nuclear imaging, heart catheterization, or radiation oncology, and ask to observe.

MEDICATIONS

9

Massage therapists are trained to ask clients what medications they are taking. Many dutifully do this but don't then know what to do with the information because of a lack of pharmacology training. However, because touch therapies given to acutely ill people are inherently gentle, the need for massage therapists to master the knowledge about medications before embarking on a hospital massage training or career is not crucial.

Touch therapists not yet familiar with drug-related massage precautions can still practice safely in the acute care setting or with the medically frail by building the massage precautions into the intake process. Most of the massage adjustments required by pharmaceuticals are in the Massage Patient Data form being used in this book. These include such side effects as easy bruising, which can be caused by prednisone, heparin, or anticancer therapies; rashes, which happen because of many, many medications; or "fall precautions," the possible result of narcotics or sedatives.

Perhaps more important than in the acute care setting, where therapists can turn to nurses for advice, outpatient or private practice settings require the massage therapist to have a rudimentary knowledge of medications. It is these patients who more often push therapists for vigorous bodywork, not realizing that their health condition places a demand on the body that precludes forceful massage. Many of the drugs taken by outpatients, such as analgesics, corticosteroids, and heart medications, are examples of pharmaceuticals that require the implementation of massage precautions.

As they spend more time in healthcare settings, bodyworkers will slowly accumulate knowledge about frequently encountered drugs, such as Lasix, Ativan, or heparin. The purpose of this chapter is to present frequently prescribed categories of drugs, their common uses, and their side effects. The side effects are then categorized into the clinical framework that revolves around pressure considerations, site restrictions, and positioning adjustments.

BOX 9–1	*Of Special Interest*

TOP 25 MOST OFTEN PRESCRIBED DRUGS

1. hydrocodone	14. Paxil
2. Lipitor	15. Zocor
3. atenolol	16. Prevacid
4. Synthroid	17. ibuprofen
5. Premarin	18. triamterene
6. Zithromax	19. Toprol
7. furosemide	20. cephalexin
8. amoxicillin	21. Celebrex
9. Norvasc	22. Zyrtec
10. hydrochlorothiazide	23. Levoxyl
11. alprazolam	24. Allegra
12. albuterol	25. Ortho Tri-Cyclen
13. Zoloft	

From The Top 200 Prescriptions for 2002 by Number of U.S. Prescriptions Dispensed. Available at: www.rxlist.com/top200.htm. Accessed July 17, 2003.

Information on drugs could fill volumes. This chapter only aspires to present a broad overview rather than a lengthy listing of minute details. Pharmacology is a complex field requiring years of study on the part of pharmacists. The average hospital massage therapist can only be expected to know a finite amount of drug information. A drug reference manual can supply the remaining information.

Each hospital or healthcare organization has a **formulary** from which physicians must prescribe drugs. Differences will exist from institution to institution. Presented in the "Selected Drug Names" sections are the more frequently used medications.

Most often, brand names are used because they are easier to pronounce and remember than the generic names. For instance, docusate is a generic stool softener, but doctors and nurses most often use Colace, the brand drug. Another example is nabumetone, a therapy prescribed for rheumatoid arthritis. However, the drug a therapist might hear more often is Relafen. When the name of a drug is capitalized, it reflects a brand-name medication. Those beginning with a lowercase letter are generic names. Coumadin, for instance, is a brand-name anticoagulant; warfarin, on the other hand, is the generic medication. In this text, the generic drug is listed first with the brand name in parentheses; for example, docusate (Colace) and warfarin (Coumadin).

People are often on medications from more than one category. For instance, someone who has cardiac problems may not only be on medications to support the heart, but also on medications to control blood pressure and cholesterol, anticoagulants, and anxiety. To help illustrate the number of drugs a patient may be on at one time, several examples are given in "Of Special Interest" boxes throughout the chapter.

The massage precautions presented in this chapter relate only to drugs. The patient's health condition, medical devices, age, and other variables will also impact the touch-therapy session. Additionally, the focus is on massage adjustments that may occur with some regularity rather than on an infrequent basis. The study of drug reactions in a pharmacological handbook might lead a touch practitioner to believe that the person on medications is so complex and fragile that massage would always be contraindicated. However, the majority of drug side effects listed in reference manuals occur on a limited basis. Dizziness is a good example. It is commonly listed as a drug reaction to scores of medications. In reality, dizziness is not a widespread phenomenon, which is also true of many other symptoms. The Tip Box titled "The Main Side Effects" outlines the most common side effects of medications in general.

One final note—many touch practitioners gravitate toward natural healing concepts, and a few may have a bias against drugs. However, it is imperative to honor a patient's treatment choices. It is the massage therapist's job to provide only massage. Advising the patient to alter the dosage or stop a medication is outside the bodyworker's scope of practice, as is making suggestions about herbs, vitamins, or other supplements.

ANALGESICS

Analgesics are prescribed for pain reduction. The type of pain reliever administered is dependent mostly on the severity of pain. **Narcotics,** which are derived from opium or opiate-like substances, provide the strongest pain relief, but are also addictive. The other two categories, nonnarcotic analgesics and nonsteroidal anti-inflammatory drugs, control pain by decreasing inflammation.

NARCOTICS

PURPOSE: Relief of severe pain and anesthesia

USES: Induces sleep and tranquilizes the central nervous system (CNS) before invasive procedures such as surgery, provision of local anesthesia, relief of severe or chronic pain, cough suppression, narcotic withdrawal (methadone), and labor pain

BASIC MECHANISM: Binds with opiate receptors in the CNS, altering perception and emotional response to pain. Local anesthesia is caused by the inhibition of nerve impulses from sensory nerves. The cough reflex is suppressed by action on the cough center in the brain.

SELECTED DRUG NAMES: morphine, codeine, hydromorphone (Dilaudid), methadone, oxycodone (OxyContin), fentanyl (anesthesia); combination products—Darvon, Demerol, Darvocet

COMMON SIDE EFFECTS: Sedation, dizziness, light-headedness, gastrointestinal (GI) reactions, respiratory depression, constipation, euphoria, hallucinations, anxiety, decreased mental alertness, confusion, weakness, hypotonic muscles, and depressed neural responses. Anesthesia can also cause tremors, restlessness, hypotension, and flatulence.

A PATIENT'S STORY
Willing to Try Anything

It was a brand new year, 1999, when I found out I had cancer of the colon. Surgery was recommended, which I did not hesitate to say yes to. When I awoke after the surgery, I was in a lot of pain. The good news was they got all the cancer, but in order to do that, I was sliced open with a 12-inch-long incision over my belly. I was on a morphine pump, which was supposed to help with the pain but seemed only to make me terribly nauseous and left me with the dry heaves. I was anxious and in too much pain to relax, so I couldn't sleep.

Mary, my partner, came to visit that evening and asked if I would like her to do some Therapeutic Touch (TT). My experience with TT was brief prior to that day, but I knew about it and wanted to try anything that might help. I lay on my back with my eyes closed while Mary moved her hands just above my incision area. She said it felt hot. As she continued to stroke her open palms over my body, I began to feel very relaxed, and a calmness set in, which relieved the anxiety. I don't know if I said anything to her, but I very quickly went into a deep state of peaceful relaxation, the pain receded, and I went to sleep. I think this took maybe 10 or 15 minutes. When I awoke, I was amazed. I had believed before that TT worked, but this was so powerfully effective that all I could say was "wow!" Through the weeks of recovery, I received many more TT sessions and every time received that wonderful peaceful state of deep relaxation.

—John Welander

■ CLINICAL CONSIDERATIONS

Pressure considerations:
- Analgesic effect makes feedback about pressure inaccurate.
- Apply stretching techniques carefully due to hypotonic muscles and decreased neural responses. It is easy to overstretch joints and muscles during this time.

Site restrictions:
- GI reactions are common from narcotics and may require avoiding the abdomen.
- If tolerated, attention to abdominal reflexes may help diminish nausea and constipation.
- Narcotics are sometimes delivered via a **transdermal patch.** Avoid massaging the area containing a patch. Also, heat caused by fever or environmental influences, such as heating pads or hot tubs, can increase the delivery of the analgesic in a transdermal patch and cause toxicity.

Positioning adjustments:
- Narcotics cause a number of side effects that make the patient a fall precaution risk. Information concerning fall precautions is presented in Chapter 10.
- Weakness, confusion, or constipation may make repositioning difficult.

Other:
- Encourage deep breathing following surgery. It promotes the elimination of anesthesia.
- Drugs that cause CNS suppression can make a patient "less communicative and seemingly indifferent to supplying"[6] complete information during intake or during the massage session. The bodyworker must be more assertive to get the necessary information.[1-6]

NONNARCOTIC ANALGESICS AND ANTIPYRETICS

PURPOSE: These drugs have mild pain-relieving, anti-inflammatory, and fever-reducing effects. **Antipyretic** is the medical term for the ability to reduce a fever.

USES: Mild to moderate pain from arthritis, prevention of thrombosis, reduction of myocardial infarction (MI) risk in patients with previous MI or angina, inflammatory conditions, fever

A PATIENT'S STORY
Better Than Morphine
I've been given a variety of pain medications, including morphine, to help with the discomfort from liver disease. But the thing that's been most effective in alleviating the pain is massage, both the physical pain and the emotional discomfort.

BASIC MECHANISM: These drugs are thought to block pain impulses by inhibiting **prostaglandin** synthesis in the CNS. Prostaglandins contribute to the inflammatory response by causing vasodilation and by intensifying the effect of histamines and kinins, other chemicals that are part of the inflammatory response. By inhibiting prostaglandins, inflammation is decreased. Fevers are believed to be reduced by acting on the heat-regulating center of the **hypothalamus** to produce **vasodilation,** which allows heat to dissipate.

SELECTED DRUG NAMES: aspirin, acetaminophen (Tylenol)

COMMON SIDE EFFECTS: Easy bruising, mild GI reactions, rash[1,2,3,7]

■ CLINICAL CONSIDERATIONS

Pressure considerations:
- Patient will not give accurate feedback due to analgesic effect.
- Easy bruising

NONSTEROIDAL ANTI-INFLAMMATORY DRUGS (NSAIDS)

PURPOSE: Reduction of inflammation, pain, and fever

USES: Mild to moderate relief from osteoarthritis, rheumatoid arthritis, pain, ankylosing spondylitis, gout, bursitis, tendonitis, **dysmenorrhea**

BASIC MECHANISM: NSAIDs inhibit an enzyme that decreases prostaglandin synthesis.

SELECTED DRUG NAMES: celecoxib (Celebrex), ibuprofen (Advil), naproxen (Aleve), nabumetone (Relafen), rofecoxib (Vioxx)

COMMON SIDE EFFECTS: GI reactions, including bleeding and ulcers[1,2,3,6,7]

■ CLINICAL CONSIDERATIONS

Pressure considerations:
- Patient will not give accurate feedback due to analgesic effect.
- If the patient is under treatment for GI side effects, she will most likely prefer gentler pressure.

Site restriction:
- If the patient is under treatment for GI side effects, refrain from abdominal massage.

ANTIANXIETY DRUGS

PURPOSE: To control anxiety

USES: Anxiety, panic disorders, acute alcohol withdrawal, preoperative apprehension, conscious sedation before short diagnostic or endoscopic procedures, sedation of in-tubated patients in critical care settings

BASIC MECHANISM: They are thought to most likely poten-tiate the effects of **gamma-aminobutyric acid (GABA),** an inhibitory transmitter that depresses the CNS.

SELECTED DRUG NAMES: Long-lasting—diazepam (Valium), lorazepam (Ativan), midazolam (Versed), clonazepam (Klonopin); short-lasting—chlordiazepoxide (Librium), alprazolam (Xanax). Antianxiety medications are also re-ferred to as **anxiolytics** or **benzodiazepines.**

COMMON SIDE EFFECTS: Sedation, lethargy, dizziness, GI re-actions, ataxia, confusion, memory impairment[1,2,3] (Per-sonal interview with Doug Beal, adult nurse practitioner, on July 21, 2003.)

■ **CLINICAL CONSIDERATIONS**

Pressure consideration:
■ Patient may not give accurate feedback if drowsy or lethargic.

Positioning adjustment:
■ If the patient is dizzy, take care during reposition-ing or when the patient is rising from the table or bed.

ANTIBIOTICS

PURPOSE: To prevent and treat bacterial infections

USES: Sinus infections, pneumonia, **otitis media,** urinary tract infections (UTIs), respiratory infections, acne, bac-terial infections such as meningococcus, staphylococcus, *Escherichia coli*, gonorrhea, and syphilis

BASIC MECHANISMS: Each group of antibiotics acts differ-ently to inhibit the growth of bacteria. They can act to disrupt bacterial cell walls or cell membranes, inhibit bac-terial protein synthesis, or block specific steps in bacterial metabolism.

SELECTED DRUG NAMES: There are several groups of antibiotics, including (1) penicillins—penicillin, amoxi-cillin, ampicillin, cloxacillin, nafcillin, oxacillin; (2) amino-glycosides—streptomycin, gentamicin, neomycin; (3) cephalosporins—cefaclor (Ceclor), cefotaxime (Claforan), cefotetan (Cefotan), cefoxitin (Mefoxin), ceftazidime (Fortaz), ceftriaxone (Rocephin); (4) the sulfonamides—co-trimoxazole (Bactrim, Septra); (5) the tetracyclines; and (6) the fluoroquinolones—ciprofloxacin (Cipro), lev-ofloxacin (Levaquin). Other miscellaneous antibiotics are erythromycin, vancomycin, and bacitracin. Most antibi-otics are derived from a living organism (e.g., penicillin is derived from mold). Others, such as the sulfonamides, are derived from organic chemicals.

COMMON SIDE EFFECTS: GI reactions[1,2]

■ **CLINICAL CONSIDERATIONS**
■ The side effects of antibiotics are seldom severe enough on their own to force any adjustments in a touch-therapy session.

ANTICOAGULANTS

PURPOSE: To prevent the formation of blood clots

USES: Deep-vein thrombosis (DVT), pulmonary em-bolism, various cardiac conditions, surgery, dialysis, **apheresis,** prevention of clot formation related to central IV catheters

BASIC MECHANISM: Inhibits conversion of **prothrombin** to **thrombin** or lowers levels of prothrombin. This ulti-mately interferes with the production of fibrin, which forms a delicate net that entangles red blood cells, white blood cells, and platelets. These trapped cells can then be-come a clot. Anticoagulants are often referred to as "blood thinners," which is a misnomer. More accurately, they de-fend against platelet aggregation or dissolve thrombus.

SELECTED DRUG NAMES: heparin, warfarin (Coumadin), aspirin

COMMON SIDE EFFECTS: Bruising, GI reactions, [headache and dizziness (Plavix)][1,2,3,7] (Personal interview with Janey Slunaker, RN, on July 22, 2003, and Joe Bubalo, oncology pharmacist, on June 25 and July 21, 2003.)

■ **CLINICAL CONSIDERATIONS**

Pressure consideration:
■ People on a therapeutic dose of anticoagulants are at increased risk for bruising. Those on a **prophylactic** dose are at no more risk of bruising than people not on the drugs. The elderly are an exception to this. They are at risk even on a preventive dose.

☞ **TIP: Bring a List of Your Medications**

When working with patients in private practice, ask them when they call to set up their first ap-pointment to bring a list of their medications. Many people can recall them without effort when doing intake; others cannot.

ANTICONVULSANTS

PURPOSE: Inhibiting or decreasing the amplitude, fre-quency, and duration of seizures

USES: Epileptic and nonepileptic seizures, **Bell's palsy,** migraines, diabetic neuropathy, **trigeminal** neuralgia, ventricular dysrhythmias

BASIC MECHANISM: Inhibits nerve impulses by limiting the transport of sodium ions across the cell membrane in the motor cortex. Sodium is necessary for the transmission of nerve impulses.

SELECTED DRUG NAMES: phenytoin (Dilantin), fosphenytoin (Cerebyx), carbamazepine, gabapentin (Neurontin). Barbiturates and benzodiazepines are also used as anticonvulsants. Information about barbiturates is given in the "Sedatives and Hypnotics" section. Benzodiazepines are listed under the "Antianxiety Drugs" heading.

COMMON SIDE EFFECTS: GI symptoms, rashes, CNS effects such as **nystagmus, ataxia,** slurred speech, mental confusion, and drowsiness[1,2,3,7]

■ CLINICAL CONSIDERATIONS

Pressure consideration:
■ Patient may be unable to give reliable feedback.

Positioning adjustment:
■ Patient may need extra assistance with positioning or ambulation.

ANTIDEPRESSANTS

PURPOSE: Generally used to treat depression and anxiety

USES: Obsessive-compulsive disorder, panic disorders, posttraumatic stress disorder, migraines, chronic headaches, chronic pain, peripheral neuropathy, attention deficit disorder, bedwetting in children, narcolepsy, insomnia, bulimia, cocaine withdrawal

BASIC MECHANISM: Affects the level of serotonin and other neurotransmitters

SELECTED DRUG NAMES: The commonly prescribed antidepressants are divided into tricyclics—amitriptyline (Elavil), imipramine (Tofranil), nortriptyline (Pamelor), and doxepin (Sinequan)—and selective serotonin reuptake inhibitors (SSRIs)—fluoxetine (Prozac), paroxetine (Paxil), sertraline (Zoloft), citalopram (Celexa), venlafaxine (Effexor), and fluvoxamine (Luvox). Two miscellaneous antidepressants are trazodone and bupropion (Wellbutrin).

COMMON SIDE EFFECTS: Tricyclics—sedation, dry mouth, orthostatic hypotension; SSRIs—sexual dysfunction, GI reactions, mild sedation, overstimulation of CNS[1,2,3] (Personal interview with Doug Beal, adult nurse practitioner, on July 21, 2003.)

■ CLINICAL CONSIDERATIONS:

Pressure consideration:
■ Patient may not be able to give reliable feedback.

Positioning adjustments:
■ Patient may need extra assistance with positioning and ambulation.
■ Be aware of the patient's need to rise slowly out of bed.

ANTIDIABETICS

PURPOSE: Stabilization of blood glucose level

USES: Diabetes

BASIC MECHANISM: Insulins decrease blood sugar by accelerating the transport of glucose into cells. Usually, the oral hypoglycemics also contribute to lowering blood sugar levels, but in a variety of ways. Sulfonylureas stimulate the **beta-cells** in the pancreas to release insulin; biguanides act on the liver to decrease glucose production and on the intestinal absorption of glucose; TZDs promote the increase of glucose uptake in the muscles and in the liver; and starch blockers inhibit the enzyme alpha-glucosidase, which delays the digestion and absorption of complex carbohydrates, resulting in a smaller rise in blood glucose.

SELECTED DRUG NAMES: There are two groups of antidiabetic drugs, insulins and oral hypoglycemic drugs. The latter group is composed of four groups of drugs—sulfonylureas, biguanides, alpha-glucosidase inhibitors, and thiazolidinediones (TZDs). Sulfonylureas include chlorpropamide (Diabinese) and glipizide (Glucotrol). Metformin (Glucophage) is a common biguanides drug. Acarbose (Precose) is a frequently prescribed alpha-glucosidase drug, also known as a starch blocker. The class of TZDs commonly includes rosiglitazone (Avandia) and pioglitazone (Actos).

COMMON SIDE EFFECTS: Hypoglycemia is the most common side effect in both groups of drugs. Other possible side effects from various drugs are fatigue, edema, headaches, thrombocytopenia, skin conditions and sensitivities, and paresthesia.[1,2,3,7] (Personal interview with Janey Slunaker, RN, on July 22, 2003.)

BOX 9-2	*Of Special Interest*
DIABETES DRUG COMBINATIONS (FOR SEVERE CASES)	
antianxiety or antidepressant	diuretic
	digoxin
anticoagulants	insulin or oral
antihypertensives	sedative hypoglycemics

■ CLINICAL CONSIDERATIONS

Pressure considerations:
- Easy bruising
- Edema
- General fatigue and weakness
- Muscle cramps, weakness, numbness, and tingling

Site restrictions:
- Rashes and other skin sensitivities (sulfonylureas)
- Be mindful of injection or testing sites that may be sensitive or painful.

Other:
- Be aware of the possibility of metabolic instability due to hypoglycemia. Commons signs are headache, tingling in the fingers, blurred vision, and increased perspiration. Discuss with the patient ahead of time the action that should be taken if hypoglycemia occurs.

ANTIEMETICS

PURPOSE: To control nausea and vomiting

USES: Nausea and vomiting associated with cancer treatment or surgery, motion sickness, vestibular disorders, GI disorders, Parkinson symptoms, reduction of secretions before surgery

BASIC MECHANISMS: Most antiemetics act by blocking neurotransmitter receptors for serotonin or dopamine in regions of the brain or the periphery, such as the small intestine, that are involved in the control of vomiting. For instance, serotonin, which is released from certain cells in the GI mucosa, causes **afferent** transmission to the CNS via the vagal and spinal sympathetic nerves. Blockage of these receptor sites inhibits the stimulation of these peripheral nerves.

SELECTED DRUG NAMES: Two main groups: (1) Drugs that block dopamine receptors (dopaminergic antagonists)—prochlorperazine (Compazine), chlorpromazine, droperidol, haloperidol, metoclopramide (Reglan), promethazine (Phenergan); (2) drugs that block serotonin receptors (5-HT3 antagonists)—ondansetron (Zofran), granisetron (Kytril), dolasetron (Anzemet). Drugs from other categories are also used to control nausea or are used in conjunction with other antiemetics: cannabinoids (marijuana, Dronabinol, Marinol); Decadron, a glucosteroid, benzodiazepines such as Ativan, antihistamines such as Dramamine, and scopolamine, an anticholinergic, are examples. Anticholinergics reduce the effect of acetylcholine, a neurotransmitter that stimulates skeletal muscle contraction.

COMMON SIDE EFFECTS: Sedation is the most common, followed by restlessness, headache, constipation, and **dysphoria.** Prolonged use of corticosteroids can cause many adverse side effects (see "Corticosteroids"). Cannabinoids can cause distorted perceptions, such as **euphoria** and dysphoria.[1,2,3,7,8] (Personal interview with Joe Bubalo, oncology pharmacist, on July 21, 2003.)

■ CLINICAL CONSIDERATIONS

Pressure considerations:
- Distorted perceptions (cannabinoids)
- Sedation

ANTIFUNGALS (SYSTEMIC)

PURPOSE: To destroy fungal infections

USES: Histoplasmosis, cryptococcal meningitis, blastomycosis, phycomycosis, aspergillosis, candida, skin infections

BASIC MECHANISM: Antifungals perform their job by binding to **sterol** in the fungal cell membrane. This alters cell permeability, which allows potassium, sodium, and cell nutrients to leak out, causing fungal cell death. Sterols, such as cholesterol, are in the lipid family.

SELECTED DRUG NAMES: nystatin, fluconazole (Diflucan), itraconazole (Sporanox), amphotericin, ketoconazole

COMMON SIDE EFFECTS: Fatigue, GI reactions (can be moderate to severe), itching, rash, headache, dizziness, edema[1,2,4]

■ CLINICAL CONSIDERATIONS

Pressure considerations:
- During fungal cell die-off, clients do not feel well.
- Edema
- GI reactions

Site restriction:
- Rashes

ANTISPASMODICS (SKELETAL MUSCLE RELAXANTS)

PURPOSE: Reduction of muscle tone in skeletal muscles

USES: Muscle hypertonicity and pain in musculoskeletal conditions (injury, inflammation, fibromyalgia); spasticity in multiple sclerosis, stroke, spinal cord injury, and cerebral palsy; during surgery to prevent muscle spasms; facilitation of endotracheal intubation and orthopedic manipulations

BASIC MECHANISM: Centrally acting muscle relaxants work on the brain and/or spinal cord to suppress nerve impulses on motor pathways. Peripherally acting muscle relaxants act either on the muscle cell itself by blocking calcium channels or on the neuromuscular junction by blocking the effects of acetylcholine, a neurotransmitter that stimulates skeletal muscle contraction.

SELECTED DRUG NAMES: dantrolene (Dantrium), cyclobenzaprine (Flexeril), succinylcholine, diazepam (Valium)

COMMON SIDE EFFECTS: Sedation, dizziness, weakness, fatigue, hypotonicity of muscles, GI reactions, respiratory depression[1,2,6,7] (Personal interview with Joe Bubalo, oncology pharmacist, on July 21, 2003.)

■ CLINICAL CONSIDERATIONS

Pressure considerations:
- Drowsiness
- Weakness and fatigue
- Hypotonic muscles can be easily overstretched. Range-of-motion techniques should be performed with slow tenderness, taking care not to overstretch joints and muscles.

Positioning adjustment:
- Fall precaution if dizzy

ANTITUMOR (ANTINEOPLASTIC) DRUGS

PURPOSE: To destroy cancer cells and/or prevent tumor growth

USES: Tumors, leukemias, lymphomas

BASIC MECHANISM: There are several different mechanisms of action: (1) **alkylating** drugs, **antimetabolites,** and antitumor antibiotics disrupt the synthesis and function of DNA and RNA; (2) mitotic spindle drugs impair cell division by preventing formation of the mitotic spindle; (3) hormonal agents affect tumor growth in cancers dependent on hormones; (4) interferons help activate the body's immune system against cancer cells.

SELECTED DRUG NAMES: Antineoplastics are grouped by: (1) alkylating agents—busulfan, carmustine, cisplatin, cyclophosphamide (Cytoxan); (2) antimetabolites—doxorubicin, etoposide, fluorouracil (5FU); (3) antibiotic agents—bleomycin, dactinomycin, methotrexate; (4) mitotic impairment agents—vinblastine, vincristine; (5) hormonal agents—breast cancer: tamoxifen, letrozole, anastrazole; prostate cancer: Lupron, goserelin; (6) miscellaneous agents—rituximab (Rituxan), thalidomide, arsenic trioxide, gemcitabine.

COMMON SIDE EFFECTS: Most cancer drugs cause thrombocytopenia, leukopenia or neutropenia, anemia, and fatigue. Other common side effects are nausea, vomiting, diarrhea, hair loss, peripheral neuropathy, rashes, skin sensitivity, skin fragility, edema, anorexia, seizures, cardiotoxicity, kidney toxicity, liver toxicity, osteoporosis, fever, and chills.[1,2]

A THERAPIST'S JOURNAL
Getting Things Moving

Annie was in the hospital because the various medications she was taking weren't interacting well. In addition, the chemo prescribed for her throat cancer left Annie severely constipated. On a scale of 0 to 10, with 10 being severe, Annie rated her pain at a 9. When she was offered a massage, the patient didn't think she could. Her abdomen was painful from gas and blocked bowels, and a central IV catheter prevented her from lying facedown. The massage student explained that there was no need for moving or turning, that she could massage whatever was accessible without repositioning. Annie agreed to this.

Kendra, the massage student, applied Polarity Therapy techniques to the painful areas of Annie's abdomen. The Polarity quickly started movement in the bowel. Peristaltic activity increased, gurgling sounds started, and Annie burped several times. Her husband, Bill, questioned Kendra about what he could do to help his wife relax. Kendra talked to him about breathing techniques and the effectiveness of simple touch. Together they each held one of Annie's feet for several minutes. Kendra then showed him ways to position his hands on his wife's head.

Following the session, Annie's pain dropped to a 3. But, best of all, she had a bowel movement 10 minutes after the session ended.

—Gayle MacDonald, MS, LMT

■ CLINICAL CONSIDERATIONS

Pressure considerations:
- Edema
- Fatigue
- Fever
- GI symptoms
- Leukopenia/neutropenia
- Organ damage and toxicity
- Osteoporosis

BOX 9-3 *Of Special Interest*

CANCER DRUG COMBINATIONS

analgesics	antitumor drugs
antianxiety or	(usually several)
antidepressant	diuretic
antibiotic	hematopoietic drugs
antifungal	laxative
	prednisone

- Peripheral neuropathy
- Skin problems (sensitivity and fragility)
- Thrombocytopenia

Site restrictions:
- Areas affected by osteoporosis
- Peripheral neuropathy
- Rashes and other skin disorders

Positioning adjustment:
- Nausea

Other:
- Be sensitive to the patient's feelings regarding hair loss.
- The antitumor drugs Cytoxan and thiotepa are excreted through the skin. Therapists should glove within 24 hours of treatment.
- Sessions may need to be shortened if fatigue is severe.

ANTIVIRAL DRUGS

PURPOSE: To prevent replication of viruses

USES: HIV/AIDS, herpes, encephalomyelitis, influenza, shingles, cytomegalovirus, chronic hepatitis B

BASIC MECHANISM: Antivirals disrupt the enzymes that cause the DNA synthesis necessary for viral replication. Antiretrovirals, a specific type of antivirals, are used primarily in the treatment of HIV. Two of the main groups of antiretrovirals interfere with an enzyme known as reverse transcriptase. This enzyme is needed by HIV to infect healthy cells and reproduce itself in a person's body.

A THERAPIST'S JOURNAL

Making Patients Feel Beautiful

I started something new in the chemo room this week: painting toe nails before a foot massage and finishing off with a toe ring. Dr. Schmidt thinks it is great. It all started 2 weeks ago with one of my favorite patients who just turned 70 and is getting a divorce. She has neuropathy in both feet and her toenails are turning black, both as a result of chemo. She felt so upset and ugly. I figured "out of sight, out of mind," so I painted her toenails bright red. She was so happy and felt very sexy. She came back this week with a box of toe rings from Wal-Mart and wanted me to put one on her. She felt so spunky—it was great. Then another patient commented that she had never had a toe ring, so I bought a supply of toe rings. Now I not only massage their feet, but I paint their toenails and give them a ring. It has been a blast!

—Sue Lenander, Massage Therapist, Missoula, Montana

| BOX 9-4 | *Of Special Interest* |

HIV/AIDS DRUG COMBINATIONS

antianxiety	antifungal	antiretrovirals
antibiotic	antiparasitic	sedative

Protease inhibitors, another type of antiretroviral medication, block protease, an enzyme that breaks down protein. Protease also is one of the enzymes HIV uses to reproduce itself.

SELECTED DRUG NAMES: Antivirals (used for influenza, herpes, cytomegalovirus retinitis)—ganciclovir, foscarnet, famciclovir (Famvir), acyclovir (Zovirax), valacyclovir (Valtrex), cidofovir (Vistide), oseltamivir (Tamiflu), zanamivir (Relenza); antiretrovirals—(1) reverse transcriptase inhibitors: didanosine (Videx), zidovudine (Retrovir), AZT, nevirapine (Viramune), atevirdine [ATV], delavirdine (Rescriptor), lamivudine (Epivir), stavudine (Zerit), efavirenz (Sustiva), delavirdine (Rescriptor), (2) protease inhibitors: amprenavir (Agenerase), saquinavir (Invirase), indinavir (Crixivan), nelfinavir (Viracept), lopinavir/ritonavir (Kaletra)

COMMON SIDE EFFECTS: GI reactions, fatigue, headache, rash, yeast infections[1,2,3,9,10]

■ CLINICAL CONSIDERATIONS

Pressure consideration:
- General fatigue and weakness

Site restrictions:
- Rashes
- If treatment is for herpes, be aware of the possibility of herpes lesions as well as drug reactions.

CARDIAC GLYCOSIDES

PURPOSE: To reduce the workload of the heart by slowing the heart rate and increasing the efficiency of the cardiac cycle

USES: Congestive heart failure (CHF), atrial dysrhythmias

BASIC MECHANISM: Alters the sodium/potassium pump, resulting in influx of calcium into cardiac muscle cells, which causes more forceful contractions. Also reduces the conduction rate of electrical impulses at the AV node and increases vagus stimulation to slow the heart rate.

SELECTED DRUG NAMES: digitalis, digoxin (Lanoxin)

COMMON SIDE EFFECTS: Fatigue, general muscle weakness, GI reactions (usually mild), headache, hypotension[1,2,3]

Pressure consideration:
■ Fatigue and weakness

Positioning adjustment:
■ Hypotension is an indication for care when repositioning and rising from the table or bed.

ANTILIPEMICS

PURPOSE: To lower lipid levels

USES: Reduce the risk of coronary artery disease; reduce the risk of MI, cardiovascular accident (CVA), or transient ischemic attack (TIA) following MI or with familial hypercholesteremia

BASIC MECHANISM: Inhibition of an enzyme needed for cholesterol synthesis

SELECTED DRUG NAMES: atorvastatin (Lipitor), lovastatin (Mevacor), simvastatin (Zocor), pravastatin (Pravachol)

COMMON SIDE EFFECTS: Headache[1,2,3] (Personal interview with Barbara Estes, LPN, LMT, on July 6, 2003.)

■ **CLINICAL CONSIDERATIONS**

The side effects from anticholesterol medications are generally so benign that massage adjustments are not required due to the drugs themselves.

ANTIPLATELET MEDICATIONS

PURPOSE: Prevention of platelet aggregation

USES: Prevention of recurrent cardiovascular events such as an MI or stroke, unstable angina, angioplasty (Pletal)

BASIC MECHANISM: Platelet inhibition is sometimes described as a mild form of "blood thinning." The mechanism is slightly different for each drug. In general, the chemicals prevent adenosine diphosphate (ADP) from binding to its platelet receptor, inhibit the enzyme phosphodiesterase III, or bind to certain glycoprotein receptors, each of which inhibits platelet aggregation.

SELECTED DRUG NAMES: clopidogrel bisulfate (Plavix), aspirin, ticlopidine (Ticlid), cilostazol (Pletal), eptifibatide (Integrilin), tirofiban (Aggrastat)

COMMON SIDE EFFECTS: GI reactions, headache, dizziness, bleeding[1,2,11]

■ **CLINICAL CONSIDERATIONS**

Pressure consideration:
■ Bleeding

Positioning adjustment:
■ If the patient is dizzy, be prepared to assist with positioning or rising from the table.

VASODILATORS

PURPOSE: To decrease blood pressure by increasing vessel diameter of peripheral blood vessels, which decreases peripheral resistance

USES: Angina pectoris, hypertension, tachycardia, CHF, dysrhythmia

BASIC MECHANISM: (1) Nitroglycerin causes smooth muscle relaxation by forming nitrous oxide; (2) calcium channel blockers block the influx of calcium into smooth muscle cells, which then causes the muscle tone in the vessel walls to relax; (3) angiotensin-converting enzyme (ACE) inhibitors prevent the formation of angiotensin II, a substance that causes vasoconstriction; (4) alpha-receptor drugs act on alpha-sympathetic receptors to reduce the vasoconstrictive effects of sympathetic stimulation.

SELECTED DRUG NAMES: These drugs can be grouped into four categories: (1) vasodilators—nitroglycerin; (2) calcium channel blockers—nifedipine (Procardia, Nitro-Dur), verapamil (Isoptin), diltiazem (Cardizem); (3) ACE inhibitors—captopril (Capoten), enalapril (Vasotec), lisinopril (Zestril); and (4) alpha-receptor drugs—prazosin (Minipress), doxazosin (Cardura), clonidine (Catapres), methyldopa (Aldomet).

COMMON SIDE EFFECTS: Hypotension, dysrhythmia, headache, flushing, edema, mild GI reactions, drowsiness[1,2,3]

■ **CLINICAL CONSIDERATIONS**

Pressure considerations:
■ Drowsiness
■ Edema

Site restriction:
■ Nitroglycerin is sometimes administered via a transdermal patch. Therapists should avoid getting the ointment on their fingers, as it will cause vasodilation.

Positioning adjustment:
■ Hypotension (The patient should take care when repositioning or rising from the table.)

Other:
■ Interventions that cause vasodilation, such as heated stones, hydrocollators, or body wraps, should be greatly moderated or avoided with these patients.

CARDIOVASCULAR DRUGS

Several groups of medications support heart and vascular function. Some, such as the beta-blockers and cardiac glycosides, work directly on the heart. Others cause changes in the blood vessels either by relaxing them or by interrupting substances that contribute to constriction of the vessels. Increasing vessel diameter reduces peripheral resistance, thereby easing the heart's burden. Vasodilators and ACE inhibitors are examples of these. Anticholesterol medications are also prescribed for heart patients to reduce the risk of an MI or stroke. In addition, patients will take drugs from groups mentioned in other sections of the chapter, such as anticoagulants or diuretics.

BETA-BLOCKERS

PURPOSE: To relieve cardiac stress by slowing cardiac contractions, improving rhythm, and reducing blood vessel constriction

USES: Hypertension, angina pectoris, dysrhythmias, MI, migraines, anxiety and tremors

BASIC MECHANISM: Prevents sympathetic stimulation by competing with sympathetic neurotransmitters for beta-receptor sites

SELECTED DRUG NAMES: propranolol (Inderal), metoprolol (Lopressor), atenolol, labetalol

COMMON SIDE EFFECTS: Orthostatic hypotension, brachycardia, mild GI reactions. Individual drugs may cause cough, insomnia, dizziness, and dry mouth.[1,2,3,6]

■ CLINICAL CONSIDERATIONS

Positioning adjustment:
- Dizziness and orthostatic hypotension may require the patient to take care when repositioning and/or require the therapist to assist the patient in rising from the table. Encourage the person to move more slowly to allow the blood pressure to reestablish itself. When rising from the bed or table, the patient should stay sitting for a minute or so before standing.

Other:
- Interventions that cause vasodilation, such as hot stones, hydrocollators, or body wraps, should be greatly moderated or avoided with these patients.

BOX 9-5	*Of Special Interest*

CARDIAC DRUG COMBINATIONS

analgesic	antihypertensives
antianxiety or antidepressant	cardiac glycosides
anticholesterol	diuretic
anticoagulant	

CORTICOSTEROIDS

PURPOSE: Glucocorticoids reduce inflammation and suppress the immune response; mineralocorticoids affect fluid and electrolyte balance.

USES: Glucocorticoids are used to decrease inflammation and to suppress the immune system. The following are examples of this: Autoimmune disorders (rheumatoid arthritis, lupus), inflammatory disorders (arthritis, tendonitis, bursitis), allergic disorders and hypersensitivity reactions, GI disorders (ulcerative colitis, hepatitis, inflammatory bowel disease,) respiratory disorders (asthma, emphysema, tuberculosis), cancer, and tissue- and organ-transplant rejection. Mineralocorticoids are given for certain adrenal conditions.

BASIC MECHANISM: Corticosteroids act directly on the nucleus to stimulate the production of specific proteins. These proteins, primarily enzymes and messengers, cause a variety of effects, such as decreased production of prostaglandins, histamine, kinins, and other inflammatory substances. Capillary permeability is decreased, inhibiting the migration of white blood cells into injured areas and reducing the quantities of circulating white blood cells. This group of drugs causes increased breakdown of cell proteins and fat in order to increase blood glucose through gluconeogenesis in the liver. Fibroblast and osteoblast activity also are decreased, as is calcium absorption from the intestines.

SELECTED DRUG NAMES: glucocorticoids—cortisone, dexamethasone (Decadron), hydrocortisone (Solu-Cortef), prednisone, prednisolone, methylprednisone (Solu-Medrol), fludrocortisone

COMMON SIDE EFFECTS: GI irritation, changes in mood and behavior, euphoria, insomnia, poor wound healing, edema, flushing, sweating, easy bruising. Long-term use can cause osteoporosis, skin fragility, and weakened connective tissue.[1,2,3,6]

■ CLINICAL CONSIDERATIONS

Pressure considerations:
- Easy bruising
- Edema
- Osteoporosis
- Skin and connective tissue fragility
- Decreased inflammation can make an injury appear less acute. Patients can't give accurate feedback.

Site restrictions:
- Areas of fragile skin or poor wound healing
- Areas that have received cortisone injections over a period of time are susceptible to poor tissue integrity. Also, the area may be tender from receiving injections.

Other:

- Immune suppression makes the patient more susceptible to infection.
- These drugs cause mood swings, which the therapist needs to be sensitive to.
- Patients are often very talkative during massage sessions because of the drug.
- If the patient is being treated with topical corticosteroids, gloving is necessary when massaging a recently treated area because the medication can be absorbed through the therapist's skin.

DIURETICS

PURPOSE: To decrease fluid volume in the body by increasing the output of urine

USES: Hypertension, edema due to CHF, ascites, liver disease, pulmonary edema, diabetes insipidus, glaucoma

BASIC MECHANISM: Diuretics act in different places in the kidneys to increase urine output. Most act by increasing sodium and chloride excretion, which causes water to follow through osmosis.

SELECTED DRUG NAMES: chlorothiazide (Diuril), furosemide (Lasix), spironolactone, mannitol

COMMON SIDE EFFECTS: Urinary frequency, dehydration, electrolyte imbalance (particularly low potassium), dizziness, fatigue, rash, mild GI reactions, orthostatic hypotension[1,2,3]

■ CLINICAL CONSIDERATIONS

Pressure considerations:

- Dehydration
- Electrolyte imbalance
- Fatigue

Positioning adjustment:

- If affected by orthostatic hypotension or dizziness, the patient should take care when repositioning, especially when getting up and down from the table or bed. These side effects put the patient at risk for falling.

☞ TIP: Scheduling Around Diuretics

Patients who have just been given a diuretic, usually Lasix, will spend the next hour using the toilet every 10 to 15 minutes. Trying to give a massage during this time is really frustrating to the therapist and patient because it is impossible to develop continuity or rhythm. Either schedule the session before the administration of the diuretic or wait for at least an hour afterward.

BOX 9-6	*Of Special Interest*

CONGESTIVE HEART FAILURE DRUG COMBINATIONS

antianxiety or antidepressant	diuretic
antihypertensives	dobutamine
(sometimes several)	dopamine
digoxin	sedative

FLUID REPLACEMENT

PURPOSE: To balance the fluid levels in the body

USES: To maintain or replace stores of water, electrolytes, or blood components, or to restore acid–base balance

BASIC MECHANISM: These fluids work via osmotic pressure in which fluid or substances move from an area of stronger concentration to weaker concentration.

TYPES OF FLUIDS: saline, Ringer's (an electrolyte solution of calcium chloride, potassium chloride, sodium chloride, and sodium lactate in water), and blood components, most commonly whole blood, red blood cells, platelets, plasma, or plasma expanders (Albumin, Plasmanate). Individual electrolytes can also be given. (Personal interview with Julia Crooks, RN, LMT, on July 6, 2003.)

COMMON SIDE EFFECTS: Most often there are no side effects from receiving fluids. Infused blood products can cause reactions sometimes, often within 5 minutes of infusion. Itching is the most common symptom, but infused blood products can infrequently cause hives, a swollen throat, or fever.[1,5,12] (Personal interview with Shelda Holmes, RN, LMT, on July 7, 2003.)

■ CLINICAL CONSIDERATIONS

Generally, a massage session does not have to be adjusted due to fluid replacement. If a patient were having a severe reaction to blood products, she would not be allowed to have massage during that time.

HEMATOPOIETIC DRUGS

PURPOSE: Stimulation of blood cell growth

USES: Red blood cell stimulants are prescribed for anemia caused by antitumor, HIV-related, and immunosuppressive drug regimens, as well as end-stage renal disease and bone marrow disorders. Patients undergoing antitumor or other immunosuppressive therapies that decrease white blood cell levels, such as occurs with organ transplantation, may be given drugs to boost the white blood cell count to decrease the risk of infection. These same groups of patients may also need support to induce platelet production.

BASIC MECHANISM: Each of the different types of hematopoietic drugs stimulates tissue in the bone marrow to create the early precursors, or stem cells, of the various blood cells. For instance, Neupogen encourages proliferation of a certain type of white blood cell, the neutrophils. The drugs also act as a growth factor that enhances production of red blood cells, white blood cells, or platelets. Leukine, for instance, contains granulocyte-macrophage–colony-stimulating factor, a substance that supports white blood cell production.

SELECTED DRUG NAMES: red blood cell production—epoetin alfa (Procrit, Epogen); white blood cell production—filgrastim (Neupogen), sargramostim (Leukine); platelet production—oprelvekin (Neumega)

COMMON SIDE EFFECTS: The most common among all three types of hematopoietic drugs is bone pain. Others are fatigue, headaches, GI symptoms, rash, edema, and hypertension. Within 12 hours of the injection, chills and sweating can occur.[1,2]

■ CLINICAL CONSIDERATIONS

Pressure considerations:
- Bone pain
- Chills or sweating
- Fatigue

BOX 9-7 *Of Special Interest*

ORGAN-TRANSPLANTATION DRUG COMBINATIONS

BEFORE TRANSPLANTATION:

anticoagulant (heart)
antihypertensive
immunosuppressants
insulin (if diabetic)
lactulose (liver)
prednisone

AFTER TRANSPLANTATION:

analgesics
antibiotic
anticholesterol
anticoagulant
antifungal
antihypertensive
antiulcer
calcium supplements
diuretic
hematopoietic drugs
immunosuppressants (usually several)
laxative
magnesium supplements

IMMUNOSUPPRESSANTS

PURPOSE: To suppress the immune system

USES: To prevent rejection of organ transplants and bone marrow transplants, rheumatoid arthritis, and psoriasis

BASIC MECHANISM: These drugs inhibit proliferation and function of T lymphocytes and release of lymphokines.

SELECTED DRUG NAMES: cyclosporine (Gengraf), azathioprine (Imuran), tacrolimus (Prograf), muromonab-CD3, sirolimus, mycophenolate mofetil (Cell Cept). Prednisone, too, is often part of the immunosuppressive drug regimen.

COMMON SIDE EFFECTS: Common to many of the immunosuppressant drugs are candida, tremors, headache, **hirsutism,** risk of infection, leukopenia, thrombocytopenia, fever, GI reactions, increased blood pressure, and decrease in kidney and/or liver function. In addition to some of the above side effects, muromonab-CD3 commonly causes tachycardia and chest pain as well as vision problems and several ear disorders. Sirolimus can result in back and joint pain, myalgia, breathing and respiratory disorders, rash, and acne.[1,2]

■ CLINICAL CONSIDERATIONS

Pressure Considerations:
- Fever
- GI reactions
- Myalgia and joint pain
- Potential organ toxicity
- Tachycardia and chest pain
- Thrombocytopenia

Site restriction:
- Skin disorders

Positioning adjustments:
- Breathing difficulties
- Chest discomfort

Other:
- Perhaps most important is the need for strict observation of Standard Precautions due to the patient's immunosuppressed status.
- Patients may feel embarrassed if they have experienced increased hair growth generally throughout the body, known as hirsutism.
- Tremors are a universal byproduct of many immunosuppressants. Massage may slightly reduce them temporarily for an hour or two.

LAXATIVES

PURPOSE: To soften stools or increase peristaltic movement in the bowel

USES: Constipation, preparation for childbirth, surgery, colorectal exam, and stool softening

BASIC MECHANISM: Some laxatives increase water retention in the stool or draw water into the intestine, allowing for easier passage. Others promote peristalsis.

SELECTED DRUG NAMES: Castor oil, docusate (Colace), psyllium, methylcellulose, senna, cascara sagrada, glycerin, magnesium salts

COMMON SIDE EFFECTS: Nausea, abdominal cramping, and diarrhea[1,2]

■ CLINICAL CONSIDERATIONS

Pressure consideration:
■ Abdominal discomfort makes the entire body uncomfortable. Forceful pressure is not usually welcome.

Site restrictions:
■ Direct touch on the belly often will be refused.
■ Attention to the digestive reflex points may be helpful.

Positioning adjustment:
■ Abdominal discomfort

👉 **TIP: The Main Side Effects**

There are a number of drug side effects that occur with some frequency:
■ bruising
■ headache
■ fatigue
■ decreased pain sensations
■ skin disturbances
■ edema
■ GI problems, such as nausea, diarrhea, and vomiting.

While a number of others are listed in medication manuals, they occur rarely. Therapists should be aware of the above list and then use a reference manual to educate themselves about other medications on a case-by-case basis.

PREGNANCY-RELATED DRUGS

Drug reference books do not contain a category known as pregnancy-related drugs. This section presents information on a variety of drugs that are used during high-risk pregnancy or labor and delivery but that come from other drug categories.

Preterm labor: Preterm labor drugs act by interfering with smooth muscle contractions. During acute preterm labor, the patient is usually given terbutaline, a short, fast-acting drug. The side effects can be increased heart rate, shakiness, and hypersensitivity to the environment. Vistaril, an antianxiety medication, is given to counteract the side effects of terbutaline. Massage would probably not be approved during this acute event, which generally lasts a few hours.

Magnesium sulfate and nifedipine (Procardia), a calcium channel blocker, are used to quell less intense early labor. The side effects of magnesium sulfate can be muscle flaccidity, hypotension, depressed reflexes, difficulty moving, sedation, and GI symptoms. Potential massage adjustments would be a decrease in pressure due to sedation and muscle flaccidity and positioning adjustments due to hypotension and difficulty moving. Procardia has negligible side effects.

Bleeding: Methergine is administered to stop bleeding. It can trigger GI symptoms, headache, dizziness, and hypotension. These side effects call for the use of noninvasive pressure and care in repositioning.

Labor: Pitocin and Oxytocin are used to induce labor. Medically, there are no reasons to adjust the variables of a massage session. However, the drug triggers contractions that are harder and faster than normal, lessening the mother's ability to cope with the intensified situation.

Nausea: Nausea is often controlled with promethazine (Phenergan). It commonly has a sedating effect on people, which is an indication for gentle touch and care during repositioning.

Pain management: The narcotic fentanyl is used during labor, as is Nubain. Massage cautions for narcotics can be found in the "Analgesics" section earlier in the chapter. Patients with an epidural will have greatly diminished sensation distal to the epidural site, a pressure caution with regard to massage.[1,2,12] (Personal interview with Leslie Stager, RN, LMT, and Julia Vance, RN, certified nurse midwife, on July 7, 2003.)

SEDATIVES AND HYPNOTICS

These two drug categories have been grouped together because they function in a similar manner and are used for common reasons.

PURPOSE: To sedate, relieve anxiety or insomnia

USES: Insomnia, preoperative sedation, before endoscopic procedures or biopsies to calm the patient, muscle spasms, psychiatric disorders, seizures

BASIC MECHANISM: These medications work in a variety of ways. Some act on the limbic, thalamic, and hypothalamic regions to depress the CNS. Others, such as barbiturates, also depress brain cell activity in certain parts of the brain stem, thereby decreasing impulse transmission to the cerebral cortex.

SELECTED DRUG NAMES: triazolam (Halcion), lorazepam (Ativan), flurazepam (Dalmane), temazepam (Restoril), zolpidem (Ambien), zaleplon (Sonata); barbiturates—pentobarbital (Nembutal), secobarbital (Seconal), phenobarbital

COMMON SIDE EFFECTS: Sedation, CNS depression, ataxia, impaired coordination, decreased mental alertness, confusion, muscular weakness.[1,2] (Personal interview with Doug Beal, adult nurse practitioner, on July 21, 2003, and Janey Slunaker, RN, on July 22, 2003.)

Mr. L

Mr. L, 80 years old, was transferred from a nursing home to the hospital because of pneumonia. He is diabetic and takes insulin to control his blood sugar. The patient also has a medical history that includes chronic obstructive pulmonary disease (COPD), CHF, and a previous MI. His drug profile includes three antihypertensives, digoxin, and furosemide, a diuretic. He is on oxygen and must maintain a 45° upright position to ease his breathing.

Three different antibiotics are being administrated, two for the pneumonia and one for sepsis, which occurred when a Foley catheter was inserted. Mr. L's temperature is 101.9°F. The patient has no family and is extremely anxious, confused, and restless after being transferred from the nursing home. He is being restrained to prevent him from pulling out his IV. Ativan is being given to calm him, and Restoril is being given for sleep.

Despite the numerous conditions requiring care, gentle massage could be given to this gentleman. It might especially help calm him without the use of so much medication. In many ways, Mr. L's condition presents a straightforward case. The list of pressure cautions is long—diabetic side effects, COPD, CHF, sepsis, bacterial infection, fever, and drugs that impair his ability to give accurate feedback, for example. Positioning is affected by the need to remain in a 45° sitting position, and there will be a couple of obvious sites to be mindful of—the feet, because of possible diabetic neuropathy, and the IV site.

In this case, the massage therapist approached Mr. L slowly, sat by the bedside to begin with, spoke in a calm, unhurried voice, with the focus on the patient rather than on any agenda related to massage. Eventually, the bodyworker suggested to Mr. L that the nurse requested lotion be put on his feet or hands. She then waited for a response, which consisted only of a nod and eye contact.

The practitioner chose to start on the arm without the IV. She merely applied lotion to the man's hand and arm with languid strokes toward the heart. Mr. L closed his eyes, and his breathing slowed. The therapist quietly told the man that it might feel good to have lotion applied to the neck. She again waited for a response before continuing. He made eye contact again, which the practitioner took for positive feedback, and so she gently extended the strokes up the neck. They continued in this way over to the other side of the neck, the hand containing the IV, the feet, and the lower legs. When she finished, Mr. L was asleep. Even so, the therapist thanked the man quietly, told him the session was over, and that she was leaving.

■ CLINICAL CONSIDERATIONS

Pressure considerations:
■ CNS depression
■ Confusion or decreased mental alertness
■ Muscular weakness
■ Sedation

Positioning adjustment:
■ Take care when repositioning the sedated, confused, or person with the wobbles associated with ataxia.

TIP: A Starting Place

A place to start studying medications is with the following list of drugs, which are commonly prescribed to a variety of patient populations. Investigate their purpose, side effects, and necessary massage adjustments.

■ acetaminophen
■ Ativan
■ Benadryl
■ Coumadin and heparin
■ Colace
■ ibuprofen
■ Lasix
■ morphine and its derivatives
■ prednisone
■ Valium
■ Vicodin

THROMBOLYTICS

PURPOSE: To break down blood clots

USES: DVT, pulmonary embolism, arterial thrombus and embolism, break down coronary artery thrombi after MI, acute ischemic CVA, acute, evolving transmural MI. Thrombolytics are used infrequently due to cost and the need to administer them soon after the event.

BASIC MECHANISM: Thrombolytics convert plasminogen to plasmin, which then breaks down the clot.

SELECTED DRUG NAMES: streptokinase, urokinase, alteplase, anistreplase, reteplase, tenecteplase

COMMON SIDE EFFECTS: The most common side effects of these drugs are decreased hematocrit, **urticaria,** headache, and nausea. Several side effects therapists also need to be aware of are an increased risk of surface bleeding and GI, genitourinary, intracranial, and retroperitoneal bleeding. These effects are short-lived. Usually by the time the patient has been taken to his or her room, the serious risks have passed.

■ CLINICAL CONSIDERATIONS

Pressure consideration:
■ Risk of bleeding

Other:

- Most often, thrombolytics are administered in the emergency department during a highly acute event. If a massage therapist were to work during such a time, the touch would most likely be to hold a hand or stroke the head.

SUMMARY

The trend is toward an aging population that is on more and more medications. Medically frail people are not shut away but are out in the mainstream of society. Massage therapists in nearly every type of practice—sports massage, spa facilities, private practice in the home, or massage in a chiropractic setting—will cross paths with medically affected people. Not only do hospital massage therapists need to expand their background in the subjects of pharmacology, so, too, do all bodyworkers.

Possession of basic pharmaceutical knowledge deepens the touch practitioner's understanding of a patient's overall health. It especially brings greater awareness of the demands medications place on the body. There is no free lunch, as the saying goes. This includes the use of drugs, which commonly cause GI symptoms; skin problems; organ toxicity, in particular the liver and kidneys; sedation; and decreased mental acuity and alertness. When these new layers of information are factored into the massage plan, it gives an additional reason to take great care when working with people who are in poor health.

TABLE 9–1 DRUG GROUPS, COMMON SIDE EFFECTS, AND ASSOCIATED MASSAGE INDICATIONS

Drug Groups	Side Effects	Common Drug Names	Massage Indications
Antivirals	GI reactions, fatigue, headache, rash	acyclovir, Retrovir, AZT, foscarnet, ganciclovir	Pressure restriction
Beta-Blockers	Hypotension, brachycardia	propranolol (Inderal), metoprolol (Lopressor)	Positioning assistance Heat precautions
Cardiac Glycosides	Fatigue, weakness, hypotension	digitalis, digoxin (Lanoxin)	Pressure restriction Positioning assistance
Vasodilators	Hypotension, dysrhythmia, headache, drowsiness	Capoten, Vasotec, Zestril, Catapres, Cardura, Aldomet	Pressure restriction Positioning assistance Heat precautions
Antilipemics	Headache	Lipitor, Zocor, Pravachol, Mevacor	None
Antiplatelet Medications	GI reactions, headache, dizziness, bleeding	Plavix, Aggrastat, Integrilin, ReoPro, aspirin	Pressure restriction
Corticosteroids	Mood changes, euphoria, insomnia, skin problems, bruising, osteoporosis	prednisone, Decadron, Solu-Medrol	Pressure restrictions Site restrictions
Diuretics	Frequent urination, dehydration, electrolyte imbalance, dizziness, fatigue, hypotension	furosemide (Lasix), mannitol, Diuril	Pressure restriction Positioning assistance
Fluid Replacement	Itching, anaphylactic shock	saline, Ringer's, blood components	Normally, minimal restrictions
Hematopoietic Drugs	Bone pain, fatigue, headache, rash, edema	Procrit, Epogen, Neupogen, Leukine, Neumega	Self-limiting Pressure restrictions
Immunosuppressants	Tremor, risk of infection, fever, thrombocytopenia, neutropenia, increase in blood pressure, hirsutism	Prograf, Imuran, Gengraf, Cell Cept, prednisone, cyclosporine	Strict Standard Precautions Pressure restrictions Site restrictions Positioning restrictions
Laxatives	GI reactions	Colace, Fleet enema, Senokot, Metamucil	Self-limiting
Sedatives and Hypnotics	Sedation, weakness, confusion, CNS depression	Ativan, Dalmane, Restoril, Ambien, Sonata, barbiturates	Pressure restriction Positioning assistance
Narcotics	Sedation, hypotension, nausea, constipation	morphine, codeine, hydromorphone, oxycodone	Pressure restriction Fall precaution
Nonnarcotic Analgesics	GI reactions, easy bruising	aspirin, acetaminophen (Tylenol)	Pressure restriction
NSAIDS	GI reactions	Celebrex, ibuprofen (Advil), Aleve, Vioxx, Relafen	Pressure restriction

(continued)

TABLE 9–1 CONTINUED.

Drug Groups	Side Effects	Common Drug Names	Massage Indications
Antianxiety Drugs	Sedation, dizziness, GI reactions, confusion	Valium, Ativan, Xanax	Pressure restriction Positioning assistance
Antibiotics	GI reactions	amoxicillin, Bactrim, Cipro, Levaquin, erythromycin, Ceclor, vancomycin	Self-limiting
Anticoagulants	Bruising, GI reactions	heparin, warfarin (Coumadin), aspirin	Pressure restriction
Anticonvulsants	GI symptoms, drowsiness, CNS effects	carbamazepine, Neurontin, Dilantin	Pressure restriction Positioning assistance
Antidiabetics	Hypoglycemia	Glipizide, Glucotrol, Glucophage, Avandia, Actos, Diabinese	Pressure restriction
Antiemetics	Sedation, headache, constipation, depression	Compazine, Reglan, droperidol, Phenergan, haloperidol, Zofran	Pressure restriction Site restriction
Antifungals	GI reactions, fatigue, headache, dizziness, rash, itching	Diflucan, nystatin	Pressure restriction Positioning assistance
Antispasmodics	Sedation, dizziness, fatigue, hypotonicity, Gi reactions	Flexeril, Valium, Dantrium, succinylcholine	Pressure restriction Care when stretching Positioning assistance
Antitumor Drugs	Fatigue, thrombocytopenia, neutropenia, GI reactions, neuropathy, edema, organ toxicity, hair loss	Cytoxan, 5FU, cisplatin, carmustine, methotrexate, etoposide, vincristine, vinblastine	Pressure restriction Site restrictions Positioning considerations
Thrombolytics	Bleeding, urticaria, headache, GI reactions	streptokinase, urokinase, alteplase, anistreplase	Severe pressure restriction

CNS, central nervous system; GI, gastrointestinal.
The drug groups listed throughout the chapter are presented here in table format. However, a complete picture cannot be gleaned from the table. The reader is encouraged to study the material presented in the main body of the chapter in order to gain a deeper understanding of medications and their effect on the massage process.

TEST YOURSELF

Circle the correct answer. There may be more than one.

1. Which of the following group of drugs is prescribed for the purpose of decreasing the body's fluid volume?
   A. Immunosuppressants
   B. Corticosteroids
   C. Anticoagulants
   D. Diuretics

2. Which of the following group of drugs is prescribed for the purpose of inflammation?
   A. Narcotics
   B. Corticosteroids
   C. Beta-blockers
   D. Antibiotics

3. Which of the following group of drugs is prescribed for pain relief?
   A. Corticosteroids
   B. Narcotics
   C. NSAIDs
   D. Anticonvulsants

4. Patients taking which of the following group of drugs would be at risk for bleeding or bruising?
   A. High-dose chemotherapy
   B. Thrombolytics
   C. Immunosuppressants
   D. Antidepressants

5. Which of the following precautions would a body-worker take when working with people on immunosuppressants?
   A. No side-lying positioning
   B. Avoiding the abdomen
   C. Strict observance of Standard Precautions
   D. Gentle pressure to the extremities

6. Which of the following drugs or group of drugs is an indication for reduction in pressure?
   A. Barbiturates
   B. Morphine-related medications
   C. Amoxicillin
   D. Prednisone

7. Medications that cause a sedative effect, relieve pain, or alter a person's perceptions are an indication for:
   A. No supine positioning
   B. Avoiding the torso
   C. Special care around the neck and throat
   D. Reducing the amount of pressure

8. Which of the following symptoms are common to a significant number of drugs?
   A. Osteoporosis
   B. Tachycardia
   C. Skin problems
   D. Nausea

9. Which of the following group of drugs would indicate that a person has a cardiovascular disorder?
   A. Benzodiazepines
   B. Calcium channel blockers
   C. Sedatives
   D. Anticoagulants

10. Antiemetic drugs are prescribed for
    A. Nausca
    B. Anxiety
    C. Muscle fatigue
    D. Vomiting

REFERENCES

1. Nursing 2003 Drug Handbook. 23rd Ed. Philadelphia, PA: Springhouse Lippincott Williams & Wilkins, 2003.
2. Skidmore-Roth L. 2003 Mosby's Nursing Drug Reference. St. Louis, MO: Mosby, 2003.
3. Persad R. Massage Therapy and Medications. Toronto, ON: Curties-Overzet Publications, 2001.
4. Venes D, ed. Taber's Cyclopedic Medical Dictionary. 19th Ed. Philadelphia, PA: F. A. Davis, 2001.
5. Stedman's Medical Dictionary. 27th Ed. Philadelphia, PA: Lippincott Williams & Wilkins, 2000.
6. Persad R. Massage and Medications. Massage Bodywork April/May 2002:59–67.
7. Tortora G, Grabowski SR, Prezbindowski KS. Principles of Anatomy and Physiology. 10th Ed. John Wiley and Sons, 2002.
8. Nausea and Vomiting. Available at: www.cancer.gov/cancerinfo/pdq/supportivecare/nausea/healthprofessional. Accessed May 14, 2003.
9. Introduction to HIV & AIDS Treatment. Available at: www.avert.org/introtrt.htm. Accessed July 26, 2003.
10. Antiviral Medications. Available at: http://members.tripod.com/enotes/antiviral.htm. Accessed July 26, 2003.
11. Antiplatelet Agents. Available at: www.healthyhearts.com/antiplat.htm. Accessed July 27, 2003.
12. Nettina S. The Lippincott Manual of Nursing Practice. 7th Ed. Philadelphia, PA: Lippincott Williams & Wilkins, 2001.

ADDITIONAL RESOURCES

Deglin JH, Vallerand AH. Davis's Drug Guide for Nurses. 7th Ed. Philadelphia: F. A. Davis, 2001.
Griffith HW, Moore SW. Complete Guide to Prescription & Nonprescription Drugs: 2003. New York: Perigee Books, 2002.
Hodgson BB, Kizior RJ. Nursing Drug Handbook 2003. Philadelphia: W. B. Saunders, 2003.
The PDR Pocket Guide to Prescription Drugs. 5th Ed. Medical Economics Co. New York: Pocket Books.
Sifton D, ed. The PDR Family Guide to Prescription Drugs. 7th Ed. New York: Three Rivers Press, 1999.
Silverman H. The Pill Book. 10th Ed. New York: Bantam Books, 2002.

REFERRALS, ORDERS, AND INTAKE

10

The presentation of clinical material is complete, and the actual massage is nearly in sight. However, before being able to start the touch-therapy session, three more items must be addressed—referrals, doctor's orders, and collection of patient information. There is no right way to accomplish these tasks. Several methods are presented for each category.

REFERRALS

A massage might be requested by patients themselves, family, or staff members. When staff or family makes the request, the bodyworker must still obtain permission from the patient. Massage should not be forced or undue pressure exerted on anyone to try massage if he or she is obviously not interested. The only exception is the patient who is semiconscious or comatose. Consent should then be sought from the patient's legal representative. Interestingly, however, even people who are unable to communicate consciously will signal their acceptance or rejection of touch via nonverbal means. They may pull away when touched, become agitated, or their rate of breathing may speed up if they do not wish to be massaged.

☞ TIP: Someone to Practice On

Often after I introduce myself as a massage therapist, a patient or family member will laugh and say, "Let me know if you need someone to practice on." People like the idea of being helpful, despite being in the midst of great stress, such as hospitalization. Even though I've been licensed for years and have been giving massage in a hospital for nearly as long, when patients or family offer themselves as practice subjects, I say, "Thanks! I'd appreciate that." This approach of letting them help me is one way to get some people to try massage who might not ordinarily.

A variety of referral processes are used in the medical care setting. At one institution, patients most often self-refer. During the admission process, they are given an informational brochure about the massage program. Those patients desiring to book a session call a designated phone number within the hospital to place their massage order. Another hospital has a computerized system through which specified staff, such as doctors, nurses, rehabilitation therapists, and social workers, can place a referral. The requests are printed out in the staffing office and placed in the massage therapist's box. An alternative to computer-generated requests is the use of a fax machine in the touch therapist's office. And, not to be forgotten is referring via the telephone. (Personal interviews with Jan Locke on July 30, 2003, Toni Creazzo on August 3, 2003, and Patti Cadolino on August 6, 2003.)

Often, massage requests happen on the spur of the moment as the bodyworker passes by the nurses' station. "Do you have time to massage Mr. M's back?" a nurse will ask. When the hospital experience is part of an educational program rather than an ongoing service, the massage school supervisor will seek the referrals from the nursing staff just before the student's arrival. This method of gathering referrals also works well for facilities that have a limited, part-time massage program.

DOCTOR'S ORDERS

After the request for massage has been made, the touch practitioner must obtain permission to give it. This authorization, known as "orders," must come from a physician or nurse practitioner. It is these individuals who are responsible for the care of patients in a medical facility. This includes complex forms of care and treatment, such as medications and procedures, as well as simpler types, such as foot care or massage therapy.

☞ **TIP: Offer Massage to Everyone**

Nurses, when asked for massage referrals, often try to second guess which of their patients would want one. Many times I have been told that a certain patient wouldn't want a massage, only to ask them and receive an enthusiastic "Yes!" When gathering referrals from nurses, I now phrase the question in a couple of different ways:

■ Which of your patients can have massage if they want it?

■ Are there any of your patients that can't have massage due to medical reasons?

■ Can all of your patients have some sort of gentle touch?

Asking in this way shifts the nurse's focus to the medical condition of the patients rather than perceived subjective considerations, such as the patients' age, weight, gender, or personality characteristics. Therapists, too, must never form a judgment about which people might say "Yes" when offered a massage. Loss of hair, loss of a body part, odor, or prior experience cannot predict who will or won't want a massage. Offer touch to everyone!

OBTAINING ORDERS FROM WITHIN THE HOSPITAL

There are a variety of ways for those with hospital affiliation, such as a volunteer, employee, or official independent contractor, to procure the medical practitioner's approval. More important than the method used is the establishment of a system-wide protocol. Such a protocol will avoid confusion and speed up the process. The first two methods in the list below are the fastest and require the least amount of effort for the touch practitioner.

1. **Standing orders.** This system gives nurses the discretion to decide who is appropriate to receive massage.
2. **Admitting orders.** When a patient is admitted to a healthcare facility, the doctor places admitting orders in the chart. With some prompting from the nurse, orders for massage could be recorded at this time, saving the massage practitioner time and frustration.
3. **Faxing orders.** The signed order is faxed to the hospital massage office at the same time as the referral.
4. **Initiation by the nurse.** The nurse makes the request for massage orders when they see the doctor. This does not always produce quick results because the doctor is not on the unit every day or the nurse is busy during the doctor's visit.

5. **Leave a note in the medical chart.** The massage therapist can leave a note for the medical provider in the chart requesting orders for massage along with any pertinent instructions. The Physician's Orders section is a common place to attach the request. If possible, it is best to leave the note the day before the massage.
6. **Combination of methods.** At some hospitals, certain doctors allow standing orders while other doctors require their personal approval for each patient. This is a chaotic and frustrating system.
7. **Verbal orders.** When orders are needed on the spur of the moment, the nurse can phone the patient's personal physician to obtain verbal orders. However, some medical providers do not want to be bothered by phone calls for such requests, and so the massage must be postponed until the doctor is next at the hospital. Another way to obtain orders on the spur of the moment is to phone the hospital's attending physician for verbal orders.

There are different protocols for recording the order. Some institutions allow the nurse to take verbal orders over the phone and record them in the chart. Other hospitals require the medical practitioner to personally place the order in the record. Important to the touch practitioner is ascertaining that the orders are in place before setting out to see the patient. This will save valuable time and can be done by calling the nurses' station and speaking to either the unit secretary or the patient's nurse.

THE PRIVATE PRACTITIONER AND DOCTOR'S ORDERS

Patients or their families will sometimes make arrangements with a private massage therapist to come into a healthcare facility from outside the system or to go to the patient's home. Physician approval is required by many healthcare facilities before a private practitioner can provide complementary services to patients in their care. The private practitioner planning to work with a client who is on outpatient status should also get approval from the client's doctor before initiating bodywork. This accomplishes three things: First, the doctor and massage therapist have a chance to educate one another. Second, it documents the therapist's attempt to practice safely. Lastly, it empowers some clients to be in charge of their own healing process. (Personal interview with Tracy Walton on January 6, 2004.) Following are four methods of requesting physician approval:

1. **Initiation by the nurse.** The private practitioner should contact the nurse by phoning the nurses' station. Relay to him what the patient would like, and ask the nurse to obtain doctor's orders. Request that the order be noted in the chart. Before going to the hospital to give the massage, contact the nurse

again to be certain the task was fulfilled and the orders recorded.

2. **Initiation by the patient or family.** Ask the patient or a family member to initiate the process during doctor's rounds or a visit to the doctor. They should request that the doctor record the orders in the medical chart. Or, if the client is being seen in a private practice, the physician can write a script, which the patient or family member can present to the therapist at the first massage session.

3. **Faxed letter.** Another method of obtaining orders, especially for private practice clients, is a faxed letter to the physician explaining the tentative massage plan. Include a place in the letter for her written approval and any instructions. The letter can then be faxed back to the bodyworker, or the client can bring it with him to the massage appointment. This method requires that the massage therapist have the client sign a "Release of Information" form before the therapist contacts the physician for instructions.

4. **Verbal orders.** When working with private patients, the massage practitioner can seek verbal orders over the phone. Usually, the nurse will give the orders. The touch practitioner should record in the patient's massage chart which staff member she spoke to, the date, time, and instructions given. Clients will also need to sign a "Release of Information" form for this method of obtaining orders.

It is not unheard of for some private practice massage therapists, such as Reiki or Jin Shin Jyutsu® practitioners, to perform their modality in healthcare settings without receiving prior permission, especially when the patient is a friend, family member, or long-standing client. Granted, many modalities are inherently gentle, but the prudent action for all bodyworkers is to check with the patient's doctor or nurse before initiating any touch therapy. Obtaining permission from those responsible for the patient's overall safety and care shows respect for the job the bodyworker has been charged with. Everyone's best interests are taken into account through this action.

COLLECTING PATIENT DATA

When massaging healthy clients, bodyworkers gather the majority of health information from the clients themselves. With medically frail patients, especially those being cared for in medical facilities, this is not always possible or appropriate. Patients may be too sick to respond to intake questions; they often may not be knowledgeable about all aspects of their condition; and certain questions would be inappropriate to ask a patient. Information, therefore, is usually gleaned from one or more of the following sources: (1) the nurse (or sometimes the doctor), (2) the medical chart, (3) the patient, and occasionally (4) the family.

CONSULTING THE CHART VERSUS THE NURSE

One factor that influences how data is collected is whether massage therapists have access to the patient chart. Some hospitals do not allow their massage employees to consult this source, let alone hospital volunteers or massage students enrolled in a clinical training program. Private practitioners without hospital affiliation are never permitted to look in the patient chart and must find other means of gathering patient data.

Some therapists who have chart privileges rely on the chart as the main source for their information about a patient and use the nurse sparingly. The advantages to this method are that the nurse is seemingly inconvenienced to a lesser degree and the therapist has access to a greater amount of information. However, while some patient information, such as age, gender, reason for admission, and vital signs, can easily be found in the chart, reading a medical chart requires specialized training, and the average massage therapist is neither trained nor experienced enough to find everything needed from the written record. Therefore, consulting the chart takes a great deal of time and does not usually yield a complete picture of the patient's immediate health status.

Even those with years of experience in a medical setting often fail to unearth everything from the chart. For example, Jana, a nurse massage therapist with 25 years of hospital experience, was gathering the information she needed to massage a patient. She went to the patient's chart first to discover what she could from that source, but it was only by interviewing the nurse that Jana learned the patient had vesicles on her legs that were oozing fluid onto the bedding. Nowhere in the chart was this evident to the touch practitioner.

One of the reasons information may not be available from the chart is that nurses sometimes wait until the end of the shift to record their notes. Or, if charting is still done by hand rather than through a computerized system, poor handwriting hinders the touch therapist's understanding of the chart notes.

In light of the reasons presented above, a strong case can be made for relying on the nurse as the main source of information about a patient. Medical charts can be significant in size, requiring an immense amount of time to read. Obtaining patient data from the nurse is faster and therefore a better use of the massage therapist's time. Also, it is a more complete way to gather the necessary data. This will translate into a safer massage session for both the patient and the touch therapist.

Hospital-affiliated therapists can procure information from nurses in one of two common ways: a checklist that the nurse fills out ahead of time or a verbal interview. An example of a checklist is found in Appendix C.1B. This text will use the Massage Patient Data form as the basis for the verbal interview method. The system chosen will depend

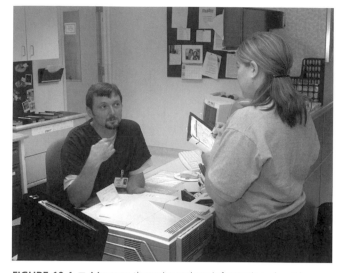

FIGURE 10-1 ■ Massage therapist gathers information about her patient from the nurse. (Photo by Don Hamilton.)

on staff or management preference. Both ways are useful; however, being able to directly gather information from the nurse through an interview will give the therapist a clearer image of the patient's present status (Fig. 10-1).

For those without prior healthcare experience, approaching the nursing staff directly can be the most daunting part of the massage process. Nurses are always busy, and novice practitioners are uncertain when to wait for them to finish a task or when to gently break into their current activity. Only experience will teach the novice when to hold back and when to politely interrupt. Sometimes the intake interview will need to be conducted as the nurse walks to or from a patient's room or while she is preparing to hang a bag of medications. If practitioners wait until the nurse "has a moment," they may be there all day.

Feeling like a burden to the nurses is one of the most common issues for touch practitioners learning to work in healthcare settings. However, for the sake of patients' well-being, the sense of being a bother must not stop a massage therapist from getting all of the information needed to give a safe bodywork session. Eventually, therapists will come to see the reality, which is that massage helps not only the patient, but nurses as well. By spending half an hour with one of their patients, the therapist frees up the nurse for that particular moment and usually, because the patient feels more relaxed, for a period of time afterward.

Each time a massage is given to a patient, it is important to obtain an update about the patient's status, even if the therapist has worked with him or her many times before. This is especially true in the acute care setting. Change occurs from hour to hour, let alone day to day or week to week. Libby, for example, was preparing to have a touch session with a patient she had massaged a number of weeks in succession. The patient's nurse, however, was hurried and unreceptive toward the therapist. Since she had massaged the woman a number of times over the past

month, Libby decided to sidestep the nurse and give the massage without updated information. However, the mental status of the patient had deteriorated since the last massage; the patient was confused, unsteady on her feet, and therefore had been rated as a fall precaution and was not allowed out of bed without staff assistance. To make matters worse, the patient had just been given Lasix, a diuretic, and needed to use the commode 15 minutes into the massage session. Libby had left the room to give the patient privacy during this time. The nurse just happened to enter the room and found the patient naked on the commode with the massage therapist out of the room. To say that the nurse was irate would be an understatement.

SKILLFUL INTERVIEWING

The importance of skillful interviewing cannot be overemphasized. Aside from the knowledge of massage precautions and infection control practices, precise questioning of the nurse or doctor is the next most important ability for the massage practitioner who works with seriously ill people. It is vital that bodyworkers perform not only a comprehensive interview, but also a quick one.

In the effort to be expeditious, it is tempting to ask the nurse open-ended questions such as, "Is there anything I

A THERAPIST'S JOURNAL

Learning to be Agreeable But Insistent

Therapists must learn to be agreeable but insistent about getting the necessary information from nurses rather than backing away because the nurses appear to be busy or in a brusque mood. Carl approached his nurse to do intake just as a shift change was occurring. The nurse's attention was on charting quickly so she could go home. The massage therapist was told only that the patient could have whatever she wanted. When he arrived in the room, Carl discovered that his patient had been on bedrest for a week and had pneumatic compression devices on her legs. Carl hadn't been in the room more than 2 minutes, with no time to assess the situation, when the patient's husband threw back the bedding and removed the compression devices so that his wife's legs could be massaged. Extended bedrest is a red flag for leg massage. When the touch therapist learned this piece of information, he should have gone immediately back to the nurse to get her input. Instead, not wanting to be a bother to the nurse who was trying to go home, he succumbed to the husband's request and massaged the patient's legs. The patient in this particular instance had no adverse outcome following the massage, but the potential was there.

—Gayle MacDonald, MS, LMT

need to know about the patient?" or "Tell me how the patient is doing." These inquiries are too vague and will not elicit the information the massage therapist needs to plan a safe massage session. One therapist who used this obscure line of questioning about a bone marrow transplant patient was cautioned only about the person's neutropenic status. However, when the therapist started conversing with the patient, she discovered that the woman was being treated for a blood clot in the arm, most likely due to a peripherally inserted central catheter (PICC) line. If the bodywork practitioner had been more specific with the nurse, the nurse would have remembered to mention the blood clot.

It cannot be said too often or too emphatically that the question, "Is there anything I need to know about the patient?" is grossly insufficient when gathering data from nurses. This is also true when the session is going to be a 5-minute neck and shoulder massage for a patient's family member or one of the hospital staff. An intake always needs to be performed using specific questions. Box 13-1, Chapter 13, lists questions to ask when preparing to give a seated massage to staff or family.

Nurses don't always know what information is important to massage therapists, or they may need the massage therapist's help in understanding the relevance of certain medications or conditions to the massage process. For instance, despite knowing that people on heparin bruise easily, a nurse told a massage therapist that the patient had no pressure restrictions. When the therapist specifically asked if the patient was on heparin, the nurse suddenly realized the significance of the questioning and then agreed that the pressure should be moderated. A handful of very specific questions will speed up the process and ensure that the bodyworker has the necessary information.

Throughout the book, three categories have been the anchor points in working with people who are hospitalized or otherwise medically fragile: pressure, site, and positioning adjustments. These classifications are also used in the collection of patient data. Figure 10-2 illustrates a sample intake form used for oncology patients in which the massage precautions are grouped by the three categories. This framework reminds bodyworkers of the questions they need to ask the nurse.

Private practitioners most likely will not be given detailed information about a patient if they enter a medical facility to perform a massage. In this day and age of HIPAA [Health Insurance Portability and Accountability Act] regulations, they will need to request that their clients sign a Release of Information form so they can make health status inquiries. However, in reality, most bodyworkers don't carry a Release of Information form in their back pocket A possible way of obtaining the data about the patient's medical status without official forms being signed is to ask the nurse to accompany the practitioner to the patient's room. There, the nurse, therapist, and patient can confer about

Oncology Massage Patient Data Form

PART A: (Nurse)

Patient Name Edward James   DOB 1/3/51 Sex M

Unit 5C   Room 17 Nurse John   Today's Date 7/10/03

Dx NHL   Chemo: Y N   Hx of Radiation: (Y) N

Surgery _____   Date of surgery _____

SENSORY IMPAIRMENT: ☐ Blind ☐ HOH ☐ speech   **FALL PRECAUTIONS:** Y (N)

PRESSURE RESTRICTIONS: (Y) N
☐ DVT   ☐ heparin   ☒ ↓ plt   ☒ ↓ WBC   ☒ fatigue   ☐ nodal dissection   ☒ central line

SITE RESTRICTIONS: (Y) N   **POSITION RESTRICTIONS:** (Y) N
_____ ostomy   _____ rash   ☐ no walking   ☐ lay flat   ☐ logroll
_____ incision   _____ tumor   _____ elevate extremity
_____ open wound   _____ infection   _____ posture limitations
(R) chest IV site   _____ drain   no prone – mucositis _____

GLOVING REQUIRED: (Y) N
☐ thiotepa or cytoxan (within 24 hours)   ☐ open wound (patient or LMT)   ☒ skin condition – back

CHECK IF THE PATIENT HAS ANY OF THE FOLLOWING CONDITIONS:
☐ hepatitis   ☐ herpes   ☐ other contagious disease   ☐ allergy to lotion
other: neutropenic fever – recent BMT _____

FIGURE 10-2 ■ Sample of Oncology Patient Data Form for Edward James.

necessary adjustments. Either way, the simplicity of the pressure, site, and position framework is particularly useful for those unaccustomed to gathering information from healthcare staff. Three simple questions can be used as the centerpiece for the interview:

Are there any

1. conditions that require light pressure?
2. sites to avoid?
3. position restrictions?

INTAKE DIALOGUE

Collecting patient data is seldom as linear and simplistic as the following two examples, especially once the therapist is more experienced. However, when learning to perform intake, the conversations with the nurse often sound formal and rigid. As bodyworkers gain more expertise, they are able to be succinct and fluid.

Be mindful of confidentiality when speaking to the nurse about a patient, and move to a private area whenever possible. If nurses are too busy to step into a private area, just show them the patient's name on the intake or referral form. In this way, if another patient or family overhears the nurse giving information to the touch practitioner, confidentiality about the patient's identity is not breached.

Example 1:

Imagine that before contacting the nurse, the touch therapist was only able to discover some of the patient's basic information from the bedside chart—room number (17), gender (M), age (62), diagnosis (NHL), and most recent vital signs. The practitioner will then need to begin the conversation by asking about the reason for admission. The dialogue might sound something like this:

MT: I'm here to massage Mr. James. Is this a good time to get some information about him?

RN: Sure. What do you need to know?

MT: Why has he been admitted to the hospital?

RN: He was discharged after a bone marrow transplant but brought back because of a neutropenic fever.

MT: Would it be OK to do some light massage strokes on him?

RN: Yes. I'm sure he'd love it.

MT: Has he had recent surgery or a procedure?

BOX 10–1 | *Of Special Interest*

SAMPLE "RELEASE OF INFORMATION" STATEMENT

I authorize the release of information between my physician (print physician's name) and massage therapist (print therapist's name) for the purpose of planning safe and effective massage therapy sessions. I understand that my medical records may be used in whole or part, but that only medical information relevant to massage therapy will be released.

> 👉 *TIP: Gauging the "Weather"*
>
> When first walking onto a hospital unit or into a medical facility, I teach my students to take a metaphorical "weather report," to put a finger into the air, so to speak, and gauge how hard the wind is blowing and from which direction. Stated another way, how busy does the floor feel? What is the level of stress? How fast are people walking? Are they smiling or making eye contact?
>
> These factors will influence how the massage therapist trying to collect referrals or patient information relates to the nurses. Massage therapists must adapt to their environment because it will rarely adapt to the therapist. If the "weather" is stormy and fast-moving, bodywork practitioners will need to be more assertive and obtain their information in a succinct, business-like manner. At other times, the atmosphere will be sedate, and therapists can move and speak with the staff in an unhurried manner.

RN: No.

MT: Are there any other reasons besides the neutropenic fever that I should be extremely cautious with my pressure, such as low platelets?

RN: His platelet count is a little low. I think it was 54 this morning. Light stroking is fine.

MT: Are there any sites you want me to avoid, such as a central line or skin problems?

RN: He has a Groshong on the right side of his chest. Check with him about the skin on his hands and feet. It peeled off after his transplant and may still be sensitive. He also has sores in his mouth that are a bit uncomfortable.

MT: Does he have any positioning restrictions?

RN: Whatever is comfortable for him is fine. The mouth sores might make it difficult to lie on his face, but it's up to him.

MT: Does he have any condition that I should glove for?

RN: He has a rash on his back that we just applied steroidal cream to. You should glove to massage in that area so that the cream isn't absorbed through the skin on your hands.

MT: One last thing, does Mr. James have any sensory impairments, or is he a fall precaution?

RN: No.

MT: Thanks for your time.

When seen in written form, the above conversation may appear to be lengthy and time consuming. However, it can be completed in just over a minute.

If the information regarding the above patient were recorded on the sample intake form, it would appear as in Figure 10-2.

Example 2:

Mrs. Kim requested a massage after delivering a baby girl by C-section. The nurse interview might sound something like this:

MT: Mrs. Kim has requested massage. Would that be OK with certain modifications?

RN: Massage to her back and neck would be OK, but stay away from the legs. She's just had a C-section. [This is because of increased risk of blood clots.]

MT: Should I reduce the pressure of my strokes for any reason?

RN: She can have whatever she wants on the back and neck.

MT: Is Mrs. Kim on pain medication?

RN: Yes. [This will then be a reason to reduce the pressure. It is an example of needing to ask specific questions to help the nurse help the massage therapist.]

MT: Are there any areas I should stay away from other than the legs?

RN: She has an epidural in the middle of her back. Stay away from that. And, of course, the abdominal incision.

MT: What about positioning? Is side-lying OK if she is comfortable with it?

RN: Whatever she is comfortable with. She may not want to move much.

MT: Is there any reason you know of that would require gloving?

RN: No.

MT: Does she have any sensory impairments or is she a fall precaution?

RN: No.

MT: Thanks for your time.

Figure 10-3 shows the completed Patient Data Form for Mrs. Kim.

Nurses will not be aware of some past health history, especially if the condition is unrelated to the patient's present diagnosis and treatment. If the patient is coherent enough, the touch therapist should also ask him or her about previous health history. For example, prior musculoskeletal ailments, such as back surgery or a serious injury, will be relevant to the massage plan.

Medical and nursing staff don't always have a grasp of how potent bodywork can be. They frequently tell bodyworkers during data collection that the patient can have whatever he wants. If this occurs, the therapist needs to clarify exactly what that means. Demonstrate on the nurse, with her permission, the amount of pressure that can be used, and ask about the length of the session. Massage therapists need to blend their own knowledge and experience with the nurse's instructions when planning the massage session.

To be sure, therapists should **NEVER** exceed the nurse's directions. They may, however, do far less if they feel, based on their education and experience, that the situation warrants it. For example, a nurse once told a bodyworker that she could give Swedish massage to the leg of a patient that contained a serious abscess. Based on her training, the therapist told the nurse she wasn't sure if that was a wise plan. Rather than performing Swedish massage, the practitioner chose to use static holds on the leg.

OB/GYN Massage Patient Data Form

PART A: (Nurse)

Patient Name _Anna Kim_ DOB _10/2/70_

Unit _MBU_ Room _42_ Nurse _Kathy_ Today's Date _7/8/03_

Dx _Postpartum_ Dx Procedure _____

Surgery _C-section_ Date of Surgery _7/8/03_

SENSORY IMPAIRMENT: ☐ blind ☐ HOH ☐ speech

PRESSURE RESTRICTIONS: (Y) N ☒ pain meds

☐ DVT ☐ phlebitis ☐ varicose veins ☐ long-term bedrest ☐ easy bruising ☒ recent surgery

SITE RESTRICTIONS: (Y) N   **POSITION RESTRICTIONS:** (Y) N

_____ skin condition   _X_ epidural   ☐ no walking   ☐ lay flat

Abd. incision   _____ diagnostic monitor   ☐ no prone   ☐ no side-lying

_____ infection   _____ labor stim points   _____ elevate extremity or head

(L) wrist IV site   _____ severe varicosity   _____

No massage to legs _____

GLOVING REQUIRED: Y (N)

☐ open wound (patient or LMT) ☐ skin condition ☐ presence of body fluids

CHECK IF THE PATIENT HAS ANY OF THE FOLLOWING CONDITIONS:

☐ hepatitis ☐ herpes ☐ other contagious disease ☐ allergy to lotion

other: _____

FIGURE 10-3 ■ Sample of OB/GYN Patient Data Form for Anna Kim.

SUMMARY

Sometimes the methods of procuring referrals and doctor's orders and gathering patient information are haphazardly organized. By creating institutional protocols for these parts of the process, patients will be served in a timely and safe manner. And touch therapists will have a system in place that utilizes their time wisely, integrates them into the healthcare team, and guarantees that legal protocols are observed.

TEST YOURSELF

1. Practicing With the Patient Data Form

Read the following case history. On a photocopy of Appendix C.1C, Patient Data Form, place the information from this patient's medical history. (See Appendix D to view a sample of how this patient's intake form would appear.)

The patient is on Unit 10A, Room 12, Nurse—Manny, Today's date—1/12/04:

Katherine Sonora, 56 (DOB 6/30/47), is recovering from a left knee replacement 2 days ago. The nurse reported the following information: The patient has been up sitting in a chair today but is not yet ambulatory. A passive motion device is being used on the treated knee to maintain mobility. The patient has being weaned off morphine and is now on hydromorphone. The doctor has approved massage to both feet, the back, neck, and arms, however, the legs should be avoided due to the risk of deep vein thrombosis. Positioning can be supine or on either side depending on the patient's comfort.

The therapist learned from Mrs. Sonora that she had a stroke 3 years ago that affected the right side of her body. She reported that the sensation in her right arm and shoulder is still diminished and the arm is significantly weaker than the other.

2. Intake Practice

Practice doing intake with a partner before doing it with a nurse. One person plays the role of the massage therapist; the other plays the nurse. The nurse will use the following patient profile to answer the massage therapist's intake questions. Touch practitioners should make a copy of Appendix C.1D, or use an intake form created by their instructor or the hospital, and practice recording the information given by the nurse.

Patient Profile (to be used by the person playing the nurse's role):

DOB 6/10/73, Unit 5A, Room 32, Nurse—John, Today's date—7/4/03:

Bill Nguyen is a 30-year-old man with testicular cancer. Three months ago, the right testicle was removed. The cancer has reoccurred in the other testicle. He is receiving chemo through a PICC in his left arm. He is experiencing fatigue. An outbreak of herpes has occurred in the pelvic area due to immunosuppression from chemo. His white blood cell count is 1.1 and platelets are 69. His skin is good except in the area of the herpes. He has no history of radiation therapy.

(See Appendix D for an example of how this patient's intake form would look.)

ADDITIONAL RESOURCES

Sohnen-Moe C. Business Mastery: A Guide for Creating a Fulfilling and Thriving Business and Keeping It Successful. 3rd Ed. Tucson, AZ: Sohnen-Moe Associates, Inc., 1997.

Thompson D. Hands Heal: Communication, Documentation, and Insurance Billing for Manual Therapists. 2nd Ed. Philadelphia, PA: Lippincott Williams & Wilkins, 2002.

Walton T. Communicating With the Client's Clinician. Massage Ther J 1999;38(3):40–48.

11

THE MASSAGE SESSION

Finally, all of the preliminaries are over. The doctor's orders have been given and verified, the nurse has been contacted, the patient data obtained, and materials gathered. The therapist can now get to the business at hand: being with the patient. This is the part that many novices think will be the most difficult, but it is by far the easiest and most rewarding part of the experience.

The focus of this chapter is on the components of the bodywork session and the steps leading up to and following it. The reader is reminded that it is not the purpose of this book or chapter to teach massage techniques. It is assumed that the practitioner already possesses basic massage skills.

BEFORE THE SESSION

The following tasks are usually performed in more or less the sequence listed:

1. On the way into the room, hang the "Massage in Session" sign on the door. This doesn't guarantee that there will be no interruptions, only that they might be made more gently.
2. The massage begins the moment the therapist enters the room. Irene Smith teaches touch therapists that "Every cell in the human body has consciousness, and therefore needs to be treated with the utmost respect and dignity. Everything about you is touching the person: Your eyes, voice, thought, feelings, breath, and hands."[1] Movements should be calm, slow, and gentle as the practitioner steps through the door, moves hospital furniture, or adjusts the bedding. Tedi Dunn advises therapists to "Match your movements to the patient's energy level, which is generally slower than the world outside the room."[2]

We have been told by many patients in hospitals that their fatigue and illness highly sensitized them to their environment—every sound, every smell, every word penetrated through the frail and sensitive outer layers. Illness had left them raw and alert. Many said that among those who visited during the day—hospice workers, doctors, nurses, relatives, and friendly droppers-by—it was noticeable after they left that some gave energy and some took energy. With some the patient felt more whole and confident and well-grounded after the visit. When others left, the patient's body felt jangled and tense and self-protective. . . . It may well be that the experience that these patients had was in part the difference between one's pain being touched with fear and one's pain being touched by love.

Stephen Levine, Healing Into Life and Death. Reprinted with permission from Random House.

3. Discuss with patients what they would like from the massage, taking into account any instructions given by the nurse. Also inquire about health conditions unrelated to their present treatment.
4. Identify all intravenous (IV) sites, dressings, open areas, lesions, and sore, painful areas.
5. Arrange the room so there is a path around the bed. The session will flow better if the therapist doesn't have to stop in midstream to move furniture, IV stands, or stacks of newspapers. Gently move the bedside table or chairs toward the wall, and push the IV stand slightly up toward the head of the bed.
6. Generally there will be sufficient pillows, linen, and bedding in the patient's room. If this is not the case, housekeepers or nursing assistants are helpful in finding additional items.
7. Practitioners new to hospital work must release their expectations of establishing the perfect environment. As Tedi Dunn points out in *Massage Therapy Guidelines for Hospital and Home Care*, "The physical and emotional environments in which hospital-based massage is practiced are often antithetical to the quiet sanctuary. . .usually associate[d] with massage."[2] Controlling all of the noise and chaos is impossible. However, it is

possible to help the patient create an atmosphere more conducive to relaxation. Suggest that the television be turned down or off and the phone be unplugged if no calls are expected. Dim the lights, but not so much that the person's condition cannot be easily assessed. If the light is too low, the therapist may miss areas of skin that are problematic, swelling or inflammation, or sites containing body fluids.

8. Close the privacy curtain if the patient is in a shared room. Before closing the curtain, acknowledge the roommates. Dunn points out that, "This supports privacy because when the roommates are acknowledged, included, and not ignored, they can more comfortably allow the patient and the massage therapist to be alone."[2]

9. Take time to help the patient position comfortably. Return to Chapter 5 for information on positioning. If patients need significant help with positioning, ask the nursing staff for assistance.

10. Lower the bedrails. IV tubing, surgical drains, or catheters are often in the vicinity of the bedrails. Be mindful when lowering or raising them so as not to catch the tubing, thereby occluding it or causing it to pull at the insertion site.

11. Raise the bed to a height comfortable to the therapist's back. Figures 5-1, 6-3, and 6-5 give excellent examples of this.

COMPONENTS OF THE MASSAGE SESSION

Providing comfort is the primary goal of most hospital massage programs. There is no one way to accomplish this. Comfort might come in the form of myofascial release to ease a sore back, acupressure points to relieve nausea, shiatsu to increase energy, or the repetitive rhythm of Swedish massage to induce relaxation. The important point is not the bodywork technique but the way in which the practitioner uses it. The focus is on being restful, simple, and nurturing rather than forceful, heroic, and ambitious. Mary Kathleen Rose, a hospice massage therapist, writes that, "In working with the elderly, the chronically ill and the terminally ill, do not underestimate the power of simplicity."[3]

The hands of those I meet are dumbly eloquent to me. The touch of some hands is an impertinence. I have met people so empty of joy, that when I clasped their frosty finger-tips, it seemed as if I were shaking hands with a northeast storm. Others there are whose hands have sunbeams in them, so that their grasp warms my heart.

Helen Keller

The hallmark of a massage session with an ill person is "less is better." The effort level is less, the length of the session is shorter, draping is simpler, and body mechanics are based on ease. The hands and very being of the hospital massage therapist are:

- Gentle
- Soothing
- Nurturing
- Comforting
- Undemanding
- Restful
- Calming
- Effortless
- Unambitious
- Simple
- Slow
- Nonjudgmental
- Spacious

Generally, the rhythm of the massage strokes is slower, more repetitive, and predictable. When using a stroking motion, direct the focus of the movement toward the center of the body. Being ill is a fragmenting experience; moving toward the torso of the body gives people a sense of being pieced back together.

☞ **TIP: A Taste of Your Own Medicine**

Many therapists have worked for years giving nurturing, compassionate touch to the ill. And yet, they themselves have never received such a session. If you are in that category, make an appointment with a practitioner who performs this type of bodywork. Go experience what it is you have been giving to patients and clients. It will reinforce and reaffirm the tremendous gift you are to others. Massage therapists who have never had a taste of their own medicine are stunned at how supportive and powerful gentle bodywork is.

The hands make full, broad contact rather than pointed, digging contact or light, feathery touch with just the fingers. Many patients find light and feathery to be ticklish and annoying. Often, when therapists first encounter ill people, they become fearful and pull away, causing part of the hand to raise off the body. Allow the entire hand—fingers, thumb, and palm—to settle onto the patient's body. People report that this type of touch feels the most nurturing and secure and gives a sense of more pressure than is actually being provided. Try the touch exercise in Box 11-1 to test the effect of various types of touch.

TOUCH EXERCISE

With a partner, perform effleurage strokes, experimenting with the following three ways of making contact: (1) full-finger contact with the palm slightly raised off the body; (2) full-finger and palm contact with the thumb raised, something that therapists often do unconsciously; and (3) full-hand contact, with fingers, palms, and thumbs completely relaxed into the partner's body.

Often I have settled the warm palm of my hand over a frightful looking scar and silently been with the person as they descended into the darkened tomb of that wound in search of its healing power. Repeatedly, I am amazed that the most wondrous of all the massage strokes is that of the "laying on of hands," of simply resting my hands, my intentions, my heart in the other as one would in contemplative prayer.

Mary Ann Finch, Care Through Touch:
Massage as the Art of Anointing

STARTING THE SESSION

Therapists commonly ask, "Which part of the body do I start with?" There is no right answer or recipe. One place to start is with the feet. The idea behind this is that massaging the feet first prepares the entire body to be massaged. However, some patients don't like their feet touched, so the therapist can't plan on this being a consistent starting place.

It also makes sense to start with the back, a place that commonly becomes painful when bed-bound. Also, the nightly back rub is familiar to patients who were hospitalized when it was part of standard evening care. Some patients, however, cannot position themselves for a back massage. Just as with healthy clients, there is no one way to start.

Perhaps more important than asking, "Where do I start?" A therapist could ask, "How does the patient want to end?" Touch therapy often puts people to sleep or makes them drowsy. If they want to continue to sleep, it makes sense to end in the position people prefer for sleeping. If they want to end on their side, then the session could start in supine position and end by massaging the back from the side-lying position. Patients who prefer to sleep on their back could be started side-lying or sometimes prone.

Another aspect of the massage session that is more important than the physical starting point is the way in which the session is started and ended. An opening and closing activity that involves the patient gives a sense of completeness, of beginning, middle, and end. For instance, the session could start with the therapist resting her hands on the patient and the two of them taking three breaths together. Other practitioners start by holding the feet and having the patient systematically relax each part of the body, beginning with the feet and working up to the head. There are any number of ways to start the session.

Ending with a similar exercise brings closure and completeness to the session and tells the patient that the massage is over. The bodyworker may end with the same activity she began with or something comparable. If the person has fallen asleep, therapists may incorrectly suppose that the patient is no longer able to hear them. However, since hearing is the last sense to go, practitioners should assume that patients can hear at some level and tell them the session is ending as the hands are slowly removed from the body.

LUBRICANTS

For several reasons, massage lotion is preferable to oil when working with people who are bed-bound. Petroleum-based products clog the pores of the skin, thereby inhibiting elimination through this route. Lotion absorbs more fully than oil, so that patients aren't left with the sense of needing to shower away the greasy residue. Additionally, oil causes both latex and vinyl gloves to stretch grossly out of proportion, which decreases their protective capacity and makes it difficult to perform a smooth massage. Lotion also has the advantage of being easier to control, resulting in fewer spills and greasy fingerprints in the patient's room and minimal staining to the bedding.

A few basic guidelines should be observed with all patients regarding the use of lotion:

■ Describe the lubricant so that patients can approve or decline if they have allergies or personal preferences.[2]

A THERAPIST'S JOURNAL
Bringing Wholeness

A patient once commented after her massage that it was a pleasure to have an interaction that had a beginning, middle, and end. Usually, she explained, her encounters felt more like punches or stabs. People lunged in and out to administer drugs, deliver food trays, or consult about discharge plans. The massage session smoothed over the frayed ends created by these inevitable, but necessary interactions. "I feel put back together again," she offered.

—Gayle MacDonald, MS, LMT

- If therapists are using their own personal container of lotion, the bottle and top must be washed with antiseptic soap for 30 seconds between each client. In the hospital setting, it is recommended that a new bottle of lotion be used for each patient.
- Use unscented products. Illness and its treatments can trigger a sensitivity to odors.

👉 TIP: Cup Holsters

The use of a holster for lotion bottles is especially helpful in the hospital setting. There are not usually convenient places to set the lotion bottle or, if there are, the surfaces are filled with patients' personal items. Lotion containers easily get lost among the debris of a hospital room. The holster allows the session to flow more smoothly because the therapist has immediate access to the lotion. Premade holsters are available for lotion bottles, but if therapists are transferring lubricant into a small cup, they will want a holder that is wider and shallower. (The therapist in Figure 3-2 is wearing such a holster on her right hip.) Refer to the Additional Resources in this chapter for ordering information on the latter type of holster.

Special Considerations Regarding Lubricants

Casts

When using lubricants near casts and other orthotic devices, be careful not to lotion under or near the devices. The skin in splinted areas should be kept dry. Also, some lubricants can soften plaster cast materials.

Chemotherapy

The skin of chemotherapy patients is often sensitive and dry; therefore, lotions containing alcohol or metals are poor choices. Alcohol further dries the skin, and metals, such as zinc oxide or aluminum stearate, can cause rashes to tender skin.

Radiation

Before using any type of lubricant on areas receiving radiation, check with the patient or staff to be certain it is allowed. Most are contraindicated during this time because they intensify the effects of the radiation to the skin. After a radiation session, pure aloe vera gel, which rehydrates the skin and decreases inflammation, is beneficial.

Immunosuppression

Use lotion supplied by the hospital during periods of immunosuppression. Lotion in bottles brought from outside the hospital have been carried in book bags, been used on other clients and patients, or been in the refrigerator and may contain potentially harmful germs. Unfortunately, some lotions supplied by hospitals lack "good glide" and are frustrating to use. When this is the case, the massage strokes can easily be performed without lubricant over the sheets so that the massage is smooth and flowing.

Thrombocytopenia

Lotion should have good glide to avoid creating friction, which might cause bruising.

DRAPING

By gently pulling the bedding out from the foot of the bed, draping can be performed in much the same way as when working with a client on a massage table. One of the differences is in how the sheet is secured. Rather than lifting limbs to tuck in the drape or firmly shoving the drape under the body, simply lay the bedding aside without tucking it in (Fig. 11-1). People who have just had surgery, are in pain, or are feeling fragile do not want to be handled in a rough manner.

Hospital patients invariably lose much of their modesty after the myriad procedures in which the body is exposed. This does not mean normal draping procedures should be abandoned. Just as in other massage settings, only expose the part of the body being massaged. An exception to this would be patients who are overly warm and have been lying on top of the bed in their gown. Proceed with the massage, moving the gown aside when necessary (Fig. 11-2). Some patients who have been in the hospital for weeks prefer to wear personal clothing, such as a sweat suit. Undressing for a massage can be difficult because of IV tubes threaded into the arm or neck of the garment. It is often easier in these situations to administer bodywork over the clothing.

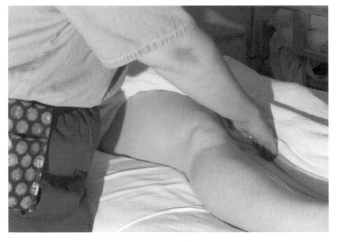

FIGURE 11-1 ■ When undraping, lay the bedding aside without tucking it in. (Photo by Richard York, Oregon Health and Science University.)

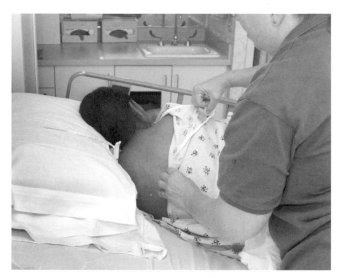

FIGURE 11-2 ■ The gown can be untied and moved aside to allow greater access to the back. (Photo by Don Hamilton.)

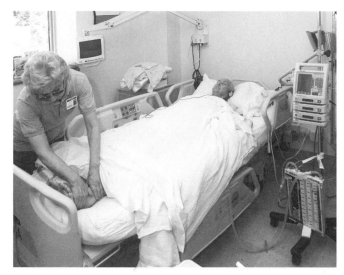

FIGURE 11-3 ■ The therapist demonstrates awkward body mechanics. The bed should be raised and the therapist positioned on the other side of the bed. (Photo by Don Hamilton.)

BODY MECHANICS

Although giving massage to the seriously ill is physically less strenuous than massaging a healthy client, working on people who are bed-bound forces the therapist to learn a whole new style of body mechanics. The following suggestions, combined with those generally taught to bodyworkers, such as do not bend and twist simultaneously, will help the therapist's physical comfort:

- When working with clients on a massage table or on patients in a hospital bed, raise the height so that the stance is almost completely erect. Many bodyworkers are accustomed to setting their tables lower to gain leverage. Leverage is not needed with medically fragile people, as the desired outcome is usually a comfort-oriented session. Raising the bed or table will not only ensure that the pressure is lighter, but it will also be comfortable to the practitioner's back, head, and shoulders. (Figures 5-1, 6-3, and 6-5 are excellent examples of this.) The therapist in Figure 11-3 demonstrates awkward body mechanics. For her own comfort, the bed needs to be raised, and she should move to the other side of the bed to massage the patient's left foot.
- Therapists should stop and readjust the bed if the height is incorrectly set rather than continuing on in discomfort. Patients will not mind, and they will be glad for the therapist to take care of her back.
- Lower the bedrails on the side being massaged to avoid lifting the shoulders to reach over.
- The footboards on many beds can be removed (Fig. 11-4), which will decrease shoulder strain caused by reaching over the board. Massage the feet from the side if the footboard cannot be removed.

- Headboards, too, often can be removed, which allows the practitioner a comfortable position from which to massage the face and head. If the headboard is permanently attached to the bed or there is insufficient room to get behind the bed, massage the face and head from the patient's side.

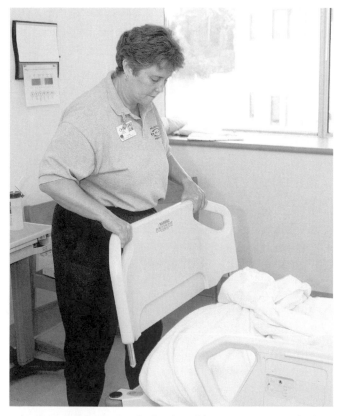

FIGURE 11-4 ■ Removing the footboard for easing access to the feet. (Photo by Don Hamilton.)

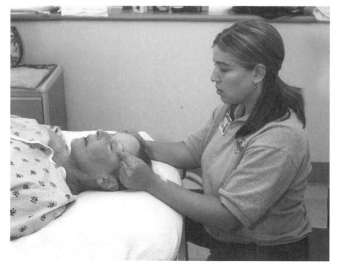

FIGURE 11-5 ■ Massaging from a chair. Notice that the patient is lying with her head at the foot of the bed. The therapist has removed the footboard to create comfortable body mechanics. (Photo by Don Hamilton.)

- Practitioners should place their body close to the bed so as to avoid reaching. Do not hesitate to ask patients to move closer to the side of the bed if they are able. If they are unable to move without minimal assistance or without causing pain, work with them where they are. Sometimes sitting on a chair or stool will put the therapist in closer proximity to the person (Fig. 11-5).
- If the patient has given permission for the therapist to sit on the bed, this can be a comfortable way for some touch practitioners to work, especially when massaging the hands.
- Use the bed for support by leaning against it.
- When massaging the seriously ill, therapists will find themselves standing in one place more often. Taking time out during longer sessions to move the body and reestablish blood flow to the feet is important.

TOUCH MODALITIES FOR THE MEDICALLY FRAIL

A handful of bodywork techniques are commonly used in massaging the seriously ill—gentle effleurage and petrissage, as well as modalities such as Reiki, Therapeutic Touch, cranialsacral therapies, or Jin Shin Jyutsu®. With the proper adjustment, many other touch therapies can be administered. By using a broad hand with gentle force, shiatsu could be applied along meridian lines; Trager Psychosocial Integration® could be used for some patients by decreasing the vigorousness of the jostling motion; and trigger-point or fascial-release therapies could be used by decreasing the effort and shortening the time applied.

The following lists of techniques are grouped into two categories. List 1 presents examples of modalities that can be administered without pressure modification. However, care should still be taken when employing them. Despite

being gentle, they are also potent. List 2 is composed of therapies that can be used if the appropriate pressure adjustments are made.

List 1: Techniques Requiring No Pressure Modification

The following are examples of techniques that can be administered with no pressure modification. However, they can be very potent, and care should still be taken not to create a demand on the patient:

Bowen Technique
Compassionate Touch®
Cranialsacral therapies
Healing Touch
Jin Shin Jyutsu®
Polarity therapy
Reiki
Rosen Method
SHEN
Therapeutic Touch

List 2: Techniques Requiring Pressure Adjustments

The following are examples of techniques that nearly always require pressure modification from their typical use, but can be administered if the level of pressure and demand on the body is reduced:

Acupressure
Amma
Bindegewebsmassage
Esalen Massage
Jin Shin Do
Kripalu Bodywork
Lomilomi (gentle aspects only)
Myofascial release
Neuromuscular therapy
Reflexology
Russian massage
Shiatsu
Swedish massage
Trager Psychosocial Integration®
Trigger-point therapy
Zero Balancing®

Learn your techniques well but be prepared to drop them when you touch the human soul.

C. G. Jung

The need for bodywork that is undemanding cannot be emphasized enough. Many times, a massage session feels good in the moment, but later that night or the following day, the patient feels unwell, often for several days. The person may feel fatigued, nauseous, chilled, or fevered.

Bodyworkers often believe that intention and intuition provide sufficient guidance toward performance of safe touch-therapy sessions, but patients have stories to the contrary. Intention must be combined with intuition AND knowledge. Heart and head are required when working with medically fragile individuals. If a conflict develops between the therapist's intuition and knowledge, knowledge should be given the deciding vote. Caution should always win out in cases of indecision.

It is not always prudent to depend solely on patients' feedback. As the story, "The Day After," in the box shows, a massage can feel wonderful in the moment, only to leave the person feeling worse later in the day. Healthier clients, too, may be sore the day following a massage. But this is less of a concern than with people who are ill. People in poor health are already feeling vulnerable and are in pain or discomfort; the confidence in their body is low. If a

therapy such as massage makes them feel worse, they will abandon it more readily than healthy people, which means the opportunity to support them and ease their way is lost. Although the man in story was not deterred by the negative side effects of massage, many who suffer discomfort after a massage lose trust in it altogether.

LENGTH OF THE SESSION

Sessions given in medical settings or with the ill tend to be shorter. Even if patients have a long history of receiving massage before their illness, there is no way for them to predict how they will respond to bodywork during an episode of poor health. It is prudent to modify the length of the session at the start to assess patients' reactions. If they respond well to that amount of time and want to increase it for the next session, the practitioner should make a cautious increase. Inching forward, rather than taking leaps and bounds, is the best approach.

A FEW GENERAL SUGGESTIONS

- Evenings are a good time for hospital patients to receive massage. The day shift in a hospital is anything but soothing and restful. Bodywork sessions often are cut short, interrupted, late in starting, or unable to be scheduled at all because of lab tests, physical therapy, pastoral visits, or consults with the doctor. Not only are there fewer intrusions in the evening, but it helps the patient to relax before going to sleep. Although patients tend to have more visitors in the evening, this can be viewed as an opportunity to teach family and friends how to give attentive touch.

A THERAPIST'S JOURNAL
The Day After

A doctor referred a man with colon cancer to me; the client had been treated with surgery three months prior and was presently receiving chemotherapy. For the past couple of months, the client has made an appointment every other week at the cancer support center to receive a full-body massage. My intention when I work with him is not to fix anything, but to provide comforting, soothing sessions. I felt that the most important aspect of my work was to be a companion in a process that seemed as much emotional and existential as physical. I always allow him to guide me with regard to the length of the session and the amount of pressure, which was a little less than a healthy person. However, I also use my intuition as a backup to his feedback. Each time, the client reported how much he enjoyed the massage.

After the fourth massage, I had reason to contact him the next day. I asked how he felt, and he commented that he felt flu-like. "But," he said, "that is how I usually feel for a couple of days following the massage. By the third day," he reported, "I always feel much better." This feedback was news to me, as I had never spoken with him the day following the massage. The client didn't seem upset about the side effects of the massage, but I was. It had been my intention to make this man feel better, not worse. The flu-like symptoms didn't dissuade him from coming for his regular massage, but I realized the level of ignorance with which I was working. I thought that the intuitive care and gentler pressure that I used was enough to avoid the risk of causing clients any discomfort. It wasn't.

—Jackie M. RN, LMT
Toledo, Ohio

☞ TIP: Immediate Follow-Up

Private practitioners who work with medically fragile clients should follow up with them within 48 hours of the massage. Inquire if they had any extra fatigue, flu-like sensations, or pain after the massage. Waiting until the next massage to inquire is too late to get accurate feedback because clients forget exactly how they felt. One therapist had gotten feedback in this way, and her client, who was in chemotherapy at the time, reported to her that he always felt great a couple of days after the session. When she started calling him the next day and asking specific questions, she discovered that he always experienced flu-like feelings after the massage. He had not put the two events together until being specifically questioned right after the massage. It is especially important to follow up with these private practice clients because they tend to want and receive massage that is more vigorous than hospitalized patients receive.

- Allow patients to do as much for themselves as they show an interest in. In sessions with healthier individuals, therapists usually encourage them to completely relax and be pampered. However, people who have had long-term health problems often feel guilty about the number of daily tasks that must be done for them. If patients show an interest in adjusting the bed or helping during draping, allow them to assist in these ways.

- Dawn Nelson, author of *From the Heart Through the Hands*, suggests avoiding "the temptation to do things for others that they may be able to do for themselves. Ask a person if he or she needs help getting into bed or getting a glass of water instead of assuming that help is needed." She also reminds therapists to talk directly to the patient instead of to family or other visitors in the room.[4]

- When speaking to patients who are in bed, stand in front of them rather than at their shoulder. This angle creates a more comfortable line of sight. When speaking, talk slowly, distinctly, and in short statements. People on medication or coming out of anesthesia can be temporarily confused or unalert.

- Most patients are able to carry on a conversation with those around them. Conversations are generally much like those with any other individual. Topics such as children, pets, the garden, and occupations are common subjects of discussion. Some patients openly talk about their illness, but many do not. Mostly, people want to be understood. The goal is not to "fix," but to appreciate what is happening. Talking with patients and family members is a dance—they lead; the therapist follows.

- Bodyworkers should communicate to the patient what they are doing just before the fact, such as raising the bed, leaving the room to speak to the nurse, undraping the body, or clearing a space around the room. Explain briefly why these actions are being taken.

- Check with the nurse if any uncertainties arise, such as an unreported skin condition, bruise, or swelling.

PATIENT SAFETY

It could be said that this entire book focuses on patient safety. This brief section, however, brings several other specific safety issues to the practitioner's attention.

- In an emergency, do not push the nurse's call button. Quickly secure the patient, bedrails up and bed down, and step out into the hall and call to whichever staff member is nearby. Pushing the call button many not get an immediate response. Patients may need immediate attention because their IV has become dislodged or they are having difficulty breathing. A patient who was very cachectic once became wedged in between the bedrail and the side of the bed and needed immediate help to be dislodged.

- When working in a home setting, know what to do in case of an emergency, and have access to emergency phone numbers.

- Patients may be at risk for falling and therefore listed as a "fall precaution." Weakness, disorientation, the side effects of medication, partial paralysis, poor balance due to deteriorating eyesight, dizziness, pain, or neuropathy are some of the reasons a person may be on this status. Actions taken to prevent them from falling include:

1. Allowing these patients out of bed only with the assistance of the nursing staff. Most likely, the hospital will want only those with special training to provide this assistance.
2. Returning the bed to the lowest position with the side rails up following the massage.
3. Never leaving the room with the person unattended if the bed is elevated and the side rails are down.

AFTER THE SESSION

The following tasks are usually performed more or less in the sequence listed:

1. Wash hands briefly to remove lotion or oil.
2. Lower the bed and raise the bedrails. These tasks **MUST** be done, even if the patient is a asleep! Failing to perform these two tasks is guaranteed to invoke the ire of nurses.
3. Replace the overbed table and telephone within reach.
4. Tidy the patient's bed.
5. See if the patient needs anything before you leave.
6. Have closure with the patient each time. Consider each session a one-time window of opportunity to be with that person. It is natural to say, "See you next week." However, there may be no next week. Patients may be discharged unexpectedly, they may take a turn for the worse and be transferred to intensive care, or they may die. Instead, you could say, "I enjoyed our time together," or wish them "All the best."
7. Remove the massage sign.
8. Thoroughly wash hands and forearms with soap and water after leaving the patient's room.[1,5]

SUMMARY

In *Close to the Bone*, Jean Shinoda Bolen describes illness as a descent into the underworld.[6] This subterranean place is hard for friends and family to enter. Those who are sick inhabit a different world than their healthier family and friends. Their days are indistinguishable from one another. Each day circles into the next, spinning a hazy cocoon around them. The one who is ill cannot come up to the surface; friends and family have trouble submerging. To journey with the person who is acutely sick or injured requires traveling between two worlds. The world of doing, moving, and productivity is left behind for a state of be-ing, stillness, and reflection.

Relationships often revolve around what people do together. When illness becomes a part of life, there must be a transition from "doing" to "being." New ways to relate must be found. Massage can bridge the gap between doing and be-ing and help family, friends, and caregivers enter into the world of the person who is below the surface. Through massage, the one who is sick and the one who is well can simultaneously come together, engaged in an experience that encompasses both "doing" and "being."

TEST YOURSELF

Create a massage plan:

Write a plan for a 30-minute touch session for the following patient using the bodywork modalities that you are trained in. Starting from the referral or request, write a narrative of your entire experience. In the narrative, include the following items:

1. The imaginary intake conversation you would have with the nurse

2. The patient's pressure, site, and position adjustments

3. The way in which you opened and closed the session

4. A description of the bodywork performed with the patient, including the positioning

Iris is 31 years old and was recently placed on the heart transplant list. She has congestive heart failure due to a congenital defect. Hospitalization is required until a heart is available because of the need for medications to maintain heart function and the need for constant monitoring.

Iris is in good spirits, fatigued but ambulatory, and has no difficulty breathing. She receives daily physical therapy and walks slowly for 10 minutes twice a day. Iris is on dopamine, a medication that supports the heart, and Lasix because of significant fluid retention. She is also on heparin but does not bruise easily. Two IV catheters have been placed: a Swan-Ganz catheter in the right side of the neck and a peripherally inserted central catheter (PICC) line in the left antecubital space. Several leads on her chest connect to a heart monitor. She is hemodynamically stable.

The patient requested massage through the heart transplant social worker. She would like her back massaged but is interested in having other areas massaged if there is time. The nurse has given the green light to whatever Iris wants as long as it is moderate or less pressure, and she should not lie on the side containing the Swan-Ganz catheter.

REFERENCES

1. Smith I. Bodywork for HIV Infected Persons. San Francisco, CA: Everflowing Handbooks, 1994.
2. Dunn T, Williams M. Massage Therapy Guidelines for Hospital and Home Care. 4th Ed. Olympia, WA: Information for People, 2000.
3. Rose MK. The Gift of Touch—Comfort Touch: Massage for the Elderly and the Chronically and Terminally Ill. Boulder, CO: Hospice of Boulder County, 1996.
4. Nelson D. From the Heart Through the Hands: The Power of Touch in Caregiving. Findhorn, Scotland: Findhorn Press, 2001.
5. MacDonald G. Medicine Hands: Massage Therapy for People With Cancer. Findhorn, Scotland: Findhorn Press, 1999.
6. Bolen JS. Close to the Bone. New York, NY: Scribner, 1996.

ADDITIONAL RESOURCES

Barnett L, Chambers M. Reiki Energy Medicine: Bringing Healing Touch Into Home, Hospital, and Hospice. Rochester, VT: Healing Arts Press, 1996.

Eos N. Reiki and Medicine. Grass Lakes, MI: White Feather Press, 1995.

Gordon R. Your Healing Hands: The Polarity Experience. Berkeley, CA: Wingbow Press, 1984.

Rose MK. The Gift of Touch: Comfort Touch: Massage for the Elderly and the Chronically and Terminally Ill. Available through the Hospice of Boulder County, 303-449-7740.

Schlossberg B. CranioSacral Therapy in the Medical Realm. Massage Mag 2003;105:46–49.

Smith I. Massage for the Ill in a Home Setting. Everflowing Handbooks. Available at 415-564-1750 or everflowing@earthlink.net.

Wager S. A Doctor's Guide to Therapeutic Touch. New York, NY: Perigee Books, 1996.

Holsters for lotion cups:

Soul Purpose Massage, Christine Moody, LMT. Available at 828-253-5336 or soulpurposemassage@webtv.net.

DOCUMENTATION

Massage given in healthcare settings is complicated by a number of factors. Side effects from drugs, medical devices, and procedures all contribute to the complexity. And yet, other aspects, such as the actual massage strokes or draping, are surprisingly simple. Documentation is also relatively simple in these circumstances because of the focus on comfort-oriented touch. This chapter presents the information needed to document accurately, concisely, and legally in the patient chart. Information, however, is not presented on insurance documentation, coding, or billing or on documentation for treatment-oriented interventions.

Massage therapists are hands-on people, and record keeping is not usually something they look forward to. The value of charting too often gets lost in a tangle of legal fears and obligations. However, by highlighting the simplicity of hospital record keeping and focusing on the important functions served by documentation, this chapter will hopefully enable bodyworkers to more readily embrace this task. Documenting patient care fulfills the following purposes:

- Apprises team members of what others are doing or observing.
- Provides continuity of care to the patient.
- Provides practitioners with time to reflect on the care given and bring closure to the session.
- Provides a place to plan and organize patient care such as orders for physical therapy, labs, or diagnostic procedures.
- Allows for accurate treatment assessment.
- Assesses costs and other aspects of patient care.
- Provides an educational and research document. Research is sometimes performed retrospectively. In other words, the researchers obtain their data by reviewing the chart after the fact. (An example is the study cited in Chapter 2 of Lively, et al.)

TYPES OF CHARTS

Therapists working in healthcare facilities will encounter three different charts, each with its own function—the Kardex, the bedside chart, and the medical chart.

> **TIP: Learn Medical Terminology**
>
> Community colleges offer courses in "Medical Terminology" and "Reading the Medical Record." Touch therapists new to health care should consider taking one of these courses as a way to speed up their process.

THE KARDEX

Nurses refer to the Kardex as their "cheat sheet" because information for each patient is boiled down to just a few pages. It is a single binder, or sometimes two, that contains basic data about all of the patients on a unit—the diagnosis, plan of care, family contact information, assessment of condition, and some lab results. The pages in this chart are not legal documents and are not part of the medical record. When the patient is discharged, Kardex materials are shredded.

THE BEDSIDE CHART

The bedside chart, which once hung on the footboard of the patient's bed, is now usually found just outside the patient's room in a wall frame. The forms in this binder are usually for the purpose of tracking vital signs, instructions for activities of daily living, or in some cases daily lab results. The forms in the bedside chart are considered by the nursing staff to be "working documents." Like the Kardex, the bedside chart is not a legal document.

THE MEDICAL CHART

The medical chart is located at the nurses' station and contains doctors' orders, the medication administration record, progress notes, lab and procedure results, and medical history. It is part of the patient's legal medical record. Because of its legal status, some hospitals do not allow the massage team, especially massage students, to have access to it.

GUIDELINES FOR CHARTING IN THE MEDICAL RECORD

The following charting policies are common to most healthcare facilities. Figure 12-1 illustrates the guidelines in use.

- Record legibly in black, permanent ink.
- Record the date and time care was given. Use military time.
- Do not leave a space between entries. This ensures that nothing else can be inadvertently inserted into the space by another care provider.
- If a line is left partially filled, draw a line through the remainder of the unused space.
- If the entry must be continued onto another page, write the word "continued" at the start of that portion of the entry, and then continue with the documentation.
- If a new page is added to the chart, be certain that the patient's name is on it. This is usually done with a card stamp or a self-adhesive strip containing the patient's name, medical number, and other information.
- If an error is made, cross out the incorrect part of the entry with a single line, and write the word "error" above it and initial. Do not scribble out the incorrect words. It is important to ensure that nothing appears to be covered up in the documentation, especially if legal action were ever threatened.
- If documentation is made in the wrong chart, cross out the entry using a single line, and write the word "error" above it.
- Use the accepted institutional terminology and abbreviations.
- Use the accepted charting style of the institution. In some facilities, a narrative style may be used; in others, the SOAP format may be the preferred way.
- Use terminology that will be understood by non–massage therapy care providers, such as nurses, physical therapists, social workers, and physicians.
- The use of sentence fragments is permissible.
- Enter the documentation in a timely manner, always before the end of the shift. If the entry is late, identify it as such. Use the phrase "late entry" at the beginning of the entry. Be certain to list the time that the massage was given, not the time the documentation is entered into the chart.

👉 TIP: Disposing of Documents

Pieces of paper or notes containing patient information or names should be placed in the shredding bin before the therapist leaves the hospital. There will be a multitude of these bins throughout the healthcare facility.

👉 TIP: Practice Makes Perfect

When first learning to document in the medical chart, do a trial run of the entry on another piece of paper. This will minimize beginner's mistakes.

STYLES OF DOCUMENTING

There is no one way of documenting patient care. Each institution establishes its own policies. This text can only present some of the common methods of charting that have been designed by other hospital massage programs; it cannot make definitive suggestions on how this should occur. Healthcare facilities have an employee who specializes in documentation. This person can assist massage therapists as they create document forms or establish charting protocols. Individual medical centers or health systems will have to make decisions about some of the following questions.

- Should massage therapists record in the medical record or document sessions on their own forms?
- Should massage therapists record in the medical record as well as maintain their own personal records?
- If massage therapists are to maintain their own charts, where should they be kept and for how long?

Massage documentation is performed in a variety of ways. One of the most common methods is to record in the Nursing Progress Notes. This is a logical place since massage historically has been part of a nurse's duties. When the notations are made in the "progress notes," a narrative style is usually used, although there is no reason the SOAP or other formats, which are discussed later, cannot be employed.

NARRATIVE STYLE

Include the following information when using the narrative style. Figure 12-1 illustrates the use of this recording style in the Nursing Progress Notes.

1. If nurses are allowed to give massage approval, enter a statement of authorization that includes the nurse's name. If approval is recorded in the chart by the physician or via verbal orders, the statement of authorization is not necessary.
2. Date and time of session.
3. Patient requests or complaints.
4. Action taken, including the parts of the body massaged. Always include a description of the amount of pressure used. Most often, words such as "light," "gentle," or "moderate" should be used to describe the amount of pressure.
5. Whose lotion was used: the hospital's, the patient's, the therapist's? If any skin problems develop fol-

Hospitals and Clinics

**ADULT ACUTE CARE
FOCUS NOTES**

Page 1 of 1

Instructions:
- Date and time first column for each entry made.
- List the main focus or problem the note is addressing in the "Focus Column."
- Describe the significant findings and actions taken.
- Initial all entries to match initials and signature on "Signature Page."

Date/Time	Focus/Problem	Notes: Significant Findings and Actions Taken
8/26/03 17:30	admit	46 yr. old admitted c̄ a hx of lung cancer. He is admitted for chemotherapy. This patient was here 1 month ago for treatment. He had severe bouts of nausea and vomiting controlled with antiemetics (see old chart for specific meds). He developed ~~some month~~ *error DK* diarrhea also. No known allergies. Currently he is using oxygen. Provide chemo teaching as needed. Plaza, RN
8/26/03 19:45	massage	Nurse (Donna) requested foot massage for pt. Pt. was agreeable. ↓ fatigue and nausea. Massaged feet for 30 min. using ~~pt.~~ *error GM* lotion. Strokes were light to moderate pressure. Reported to Donna that there were cracks in the skin between the toes. Pt. reported less nausea. Commented: "I didn't realize this would feel so good." Gayle MacDonell, Massage Therapy — Correction: Used hospital lotion. ———

FIGURE 12-1 ■ Sample of narrative style of documentation in the Nursing Progress Notes.

lowing the session, the lotion source will be on record in case follow-up is necessary.

6. Length of session.
7. Any unusual observations or findings about the patient. Document that the information was given to the patient's nurse.
8. Patient response.
9. Signature of touch therapist.

Hannah Thomassen gives two examples of narrative charting in her article, "Charting Massage in the Patient Record." The first set of entries exemplifies the use of unapproved terminology and abbreviations and the inclusion of opinions by the touch practitioner.

Example 1:
Craniosacral therapy—induced stillpoint from ASIS in flexion (internal rotation). Induced stillpoint from feet in ex- *tension (external rotation) to relieve pain from spinal tap and chronic pressure on nerve in lumbar area. Trager Psychophysical Integration—ROM—Neck and shoulder and cranial release. Atlas—R hip—sphenoid R side bend rotation.*

The following week, the bodyworker made the following entry about the same patient:
Craniosacral therapy—direction of energy from L ASIS to L knee and L foot—almost ended in normal syndronus (flexion/extension) internal and external rotation. Patient reported many transient jabbing pains (typical of this level of need).

Besides using abbreviations and terminology that were not on the hospital's approved list or that the staff wouldn't know, such as ASIS, stillpoint, craniosacral therapy, and Trager®, the therapist offered subjective judgments about the source of pain being a result of the spinal tap and chronic pressure on a nerve in the lumbar area.

These opinions are not within a bodyworker's purview. Also, the entries left the impression that physical therapy had been done without doctor's orders, and there was the sense that the "jabbing pain" experienced by the patient resulted from the massage. Follow-up of the pain should have occurred and been noted in the chart.

Example 2:

This example illustrates a simple, clear, and objective entry.

Patient complained of pain in R arm, stated she has had trouble sleeping on her arm. Gentle massage to right shoulder and arm. Patient very tender to touch, even very light touch. Pain level rated as 5 on a scale of 1–10 before massage remained unchanged after the massage session. Vital signs unaffected.

The above entry used easily understood terminology. The touch is described simply as "gentle massage." Responses from the patient, such as pain-level rating, are reported objectively without the practitioner's personal inferences.

Thomassen recounts that the patient in this scenario, who had been angry throughout her hospitalization, reported to her nurse that the massage therapist had performed "chiropractic manipulation" to her right shoulder and arm, which caused lingering pain. The patient's complaint was referred to the Director of Nursing, who investigated the situation. Review of the chart clearly indicated that the practitioner had administered gentle massage and that the pain level was unchanged following the session. Any formal complaint by the patient would have been proved invalid based on the therapist's documentation.[1]

DOCUMENTING IN SOAP FORMAT

The SOAP format provides a common framework for record keeping. Because many therapists are taught this method of documentation in school, it easily carries over to the hospital setting. In her book, *Hands Heal*, Diana Thompson describes the four components in the following way:[2]

- Subjective—data provided by the patient
- Objective—practitioner findings
- Assessment—functional outcomes and diagnoses
- Plan—treatment recommendations

However, when using the SOAP format in the hospital, it makes sense to slightly alter it from normal usage. Because the focus is on comfort rather than treatment, the "Assessment" component as normally used with healthy clients is irrelevant. By replacing "Assessment" with "Action," the SOAP acronym can still be used. Also, since the average patient does not remain in the hospital long enough to be seen frequently by the massage therapist, the "Plan" component needs to be altered. Instead, "Progress" can be substituted.

It is suggested that for hospital use, the four SOAP categories be as follows. The reader will notice that the Subjective and Objective aspects remain the same. Changes are made in the Assessment and Plan components.

- Subjective—data provided by the patient
- Objective—practitioner findings
- Action—a description of the massage session
- Progress—patient responses, including nonverbal ones

Subjective Data

Information given by the patient, who is also referred to as the subject, is recorded in this section. Examples of common information reported by patients are:

- Physical complaints, such as back discomfort, sleeplessness, or pain.
- Emotional information such as boredom, frustration, or feeling fragmented.
- The Subjective section is also the place to note outcomes the patient hopes to receive from the massage, such as relaxation or wholeness.

Objective Data

Objective data is based on the factual observations of the bodyworker rather than opinion or guesses. Examples of objective information are:

- Skin is well hydrated and intact.
- The right shoulder was tender to the touch.
- Skin coloring was pale.
- Patient spoke very little.

The following statements stray from the goal of making factual observations and should not appear in documentation unless they are direct comments from the patient:

- The patient appears very anxious about her upcoming procedure.
- Skin is dry from chemotherapy and insufficient water intake.
- Neck is sore from lengthy procedure this morning.

Action

In this section, the therapist records what was performed during the touch session or any suggestions offered to the patient. As when using the narrative style, the description should include:

- The body parts massaged.
- The types of strokes, using easily understood terminology.
- The amount of pressure used. Most often, descriptive words such as "light," "gentle," or "moderate" are most appropriate.
- Length of session.

Progress

The final section is reserved for patient responses, which will hopefully indicate some short-term progress that was made during the session. However, the massage therapist should also document patient complaints that remain unchanged or any new complaints. Examples are:

- Comments, such as "I didn't know that would feel so good," "I feel whole again," or "I am going to sleep well tonight," are often-heard reactions.
- Objective changes, such as a drop on the pain-rating scale, slower breathing, sleep, pinker cheeks, or a brighter affect, for example.

SOAP Charting Examples

Look back to Example 2 on page 160. Originally, it was written in narrative fashion. If it were documented in SOAP format, it would read as follows:

S—*Patient complained of pain in R arm. Stated she has had trouble sleeping on her arm.*
O—*The R arm and shoulder were tender to the touch, even very light touch. Pain level rated as 5 on scale of 1–10.*
A—*Applied gentle massage to the R arm and shoulder.*
P—*Pain level rating remained unchanged. Vital signs unaffected.*

The Massage Patient Data Form has been seen throughout various chapters. Figure 12-2 illustrates the entire Massage Patient Data Form for the first time. The reader will notice it can be employed for both the intake process and SOAP noting. After the form has been filled out, it may be placed in the back of the medical chart under a special section specifically for massage or complementary therapies. One hospital has a tab at the back of the medical chart titled "Complementary Therapies." In it, the music therapist, hypnotherapist, aromatherapist, and massage therapist place their documentation forms.

If massage therapists are not allowed access to the chart, the Massage Patient Data Form is ideal for the massage therapy department to use when creating its own system of tracking patient care. It can be placed in a large three-ring binder that is kept in the massage office or at the nurses' station. Most important is that the collection of documents is kept in a secured place away from public access.

To illustrate the use of the SOAP charting part of the form, the patient in Figure 10-3—a 32-year-old woman who had, a few hours earlier, given birth via a C-section—is used.

CARE NOTES

CARE Notes, developed by Mary Kathleen Rose, are an alternative to the SOAP format (Fig 12-3).[3] This framework is easily applied in the hospital setting or with any clients who are medically frail and is especially useful if the massage therapists are unable to document in the Nursing Progress Notes. The CARE acronym stands for:

- **C**ondition
- **A**ction taken
- **R**esponse of the patient
- **E**valuation

Condition

The following is included in this portion:

- Current medical condition, including emotional state
- A concise summary of other relevant medical information
- Patient complaints, such as areas of discomfort, pain, or tension
- The patient's massage request, including goals or intentions for the session

Action taken

Record the following in this section:

- Type of massage strokes administered
- Length of session
- Positions used
- Parts of the body massaged

Response of the patient

Possible information to document includes:

- Observed physiological changes (i.e., breathing, coloring, posture, tonicity, fascial expression)
- Lack of change, if none
- Patient's verbal responses
- Outcomes of comfort survey (e.g., pain rating, nausea)

Evaluation

Rose points out that the Evaluation section is optional. This is especially true in acute care facilities in which people may only be seen once by the touch therapist before discharge. This space can be used to record:

- Recommendations
- Questions that arose from the session
- Plans or expectations for subsequent sessions

CARP NOTES

Another system similar to SOAP or CARE notes is the CARP framework. This acronym stands for: **C**omplaint, **A**ction, **R**esponse, and **P**lan. It is especially straightforward and simple. Figure 12-4 exemplifies the use of the CARP format to document a patient massage session.

OB/GYN Massage Patient Data Form

PART A: (Nurse)

Patient Name _Anna Kim_   DOB _11/20/75_

Unit _MBU_   Room _42_   Nurse _Kathy_   Today's Date _1/5/04_

Dx _____   Dx Procedure _____

Surgery _C-Section_   Date of Surgery _1/5/04_

SENSORY IMPAIRMENT: ☐ blind   ☐ HOH   ☐ Speech

PRESSURE RESTRICTIONS: Ⓨ   N

☐ DVT   ☐ phlebitis   ☐ varicose veins   ☐ long-term bedrest   ☐ easy bruising   ☒ recent surgery

SITE RESTRICTIONS: Ⓨ   N   **POSITION RESTRICTIONS:**   Ⓨ   N

_____ skin condition   _____ epidural   ☐ no walking   ☐ lay flat

Abd. incision   _____ diagnostic monitor   ☒ no prone   ☐ no side-lying

_____ infection   _____ labor stim points   _____ elevate extremity or head

Ⓛ _wrist_ IV site   _____ severe varicosity   _____

_____

GLOVING REQUIRED: Y   Ⓝ

☐ open wound (patient or LMT)   ☐ skin condition   ☐ presence of body fluids

CHECK IF THE PATIENT HAS ANY OF THE FOLLOWING CONDITIONS:

☐ hepatitis   ☐ herpes   ☐ other contagious disease   ☐ allergy to lotion

other: _On pain meds_

PART B: (Patient)

Has the patient ever received a professional massage?   Y   Ⓝ

What would the patient like from the massage session?

Subjective – _Relief from headache and fatigue. Relaxation._

PART C: SOAP NOTES (Therapist)

Objective – _Flat facial expression. Untalkative._
Restricted movement in neck. Trapezius
and levators tight on both sides.

Action – _Semi-reclining position: Moderate pressure effleurage_
and petrissage to upper back, neck, & occiput.
Effleurage and acupressure to face & scalp.

Progress – _Began smiling half way through. Pain rating_
dropped from 7 to 2.

Therapist's Name _Monica Southwell_   Length of session _30 min._

FIGURE 12-2 ■ Sample SOAP notes. Developed by Gayle MacDonald for use at Oregon Health and Science University.

C.A.R.E. NOTES for Massage Therapy

Therapist Name _John Moe_   Date _8 / 01 / 03_

Client Name _Clara Doe_   Age _48_

Setting _University Hosp - 5A56_

Condition of Client:
(medical condition, physical discomfort or areas of pain or tension, emotional state, etc.)

End stage liver disease related to alcohol abuse & hepatitis C. Admitted c̄ SOB and ascites. Hx of renal disease and cardiomyopathy. Plt. level - 50,000, ↓ RBC & hematocrit. Edema in legs, on bedrest 5 days, minimal ambulation. Emotionally depressed. Meds: Lasix

Before session: _8_ physical pain or discomfort *(0 = none 10 = highest level)*
_7_ emotional pain or discomfort *(0 = none 10 = highest level)*

Action taken:
(massage strokes performed, parts of body massaged, length of session, etc.)

40 min. session, semi-reclining. Used static holds, gentle effleurage and acupressure for the purpose of comfort. Static hold starting c̄ feet and progressing up the leg c̄ hold at each joint — ankle/knee, knee/hip, hip/shoulder, shoulder/wrist. Gentle acupressure to head & face. Light effleurage c̄ hosp. lotion to neck & shoulders.

Response of Client:
(physiological changes noted during and after the session, nonverbal feedback, verbal feedback, etc.)

Pt. reported ↓ anxiety, physically greater comfort, and improved sleep during the night.

After session: _3_ physical pain or discomfort *(0 = none 10 = highest level)*
_2_ emotional pain or discomfort *(0 = none 10 = highest level)*

Evaluation:
(expectations or plan for next session, recommendations to client, suggestions to other caregivers, etc.)

Dr. ordered massage 3x/week before bed.

FIGURE 12-3 ■ Sample CARE notes. Copyright © 2003 Mary Kathleen Rose.

MASSAGE THERAPY PROGRESS NOTES

Patient Name: <u>Jane Jones</u>   **MR#:** <u>23331491-2</u> **Date:** <u>8/10/03</u>

Complaint: <u>C/o lower back pain and tightness on (L) side of neck and head. Feet are stiff and painful.</u>

Action: <u>Side-lying: Moderate pressure effleurage, fascial release, & trigger point to back, head, neck. Supine: Effleurage to arms, neck, shoulders; gentle reflexolgy to feet. Used pt. lotion. 60 min.</u>

Response: <u>Pt. reported increased comfort in back, neck, and head. Feet are still painful.</u>

Plan: <u>Twice weekly massages during hospitalization.</u>

FIGURE 12-4 ■ Sample CARP notes. Developed for use at Stonybrook University Hospital.

SUMMARY

Documentation is part of the healthcare culture. Everyone involved with patient care must record his or her actions and observations. The massage therapist who has previously found charting to be a difficult habit to establish will find it easier in this atmosphere.

TEST YOURSELF

Part A:

Use the case history below to practice charting. Record the information relevant to the massage session in narrative form. Refer to Figure 12-1 for an example. A sample narrative can be found in Appendix D.

Date: 8/23/03 Time: 13:10–13:50

Mr. A, 62 years old, has a history of multiple myocardial infarctions. He was admitted to the hospital with congestive heart failure. When the massage therapist asked the charge nurse which patient she would like to refer for massage, she immediately suggested Mr. A because he was having severe neck pain. Morphine had been administered and a hot pack applied to his neck without success. The patient was eager to try massage.

Besides morphine, Mr. A was on dopamine to support the heart, as well as a low therapeutic dose of heparin. His nurse (Avril) reported that he was not at risk for easy bruising. A PICC line had been placed in his left arm and a Swan catheter into the left side of his neck. The patient commented that he thought the procedure to place the Swan catheter had irritated a degenerating disk and was the cause of the neck pain. Oxygen was being delivered through a nasal cannula.

Mr. A asked for massage to his neck, shoulders, and back. The nurse requested he not be positioned on his left side, front, or in a totally flat, supine position. She approved the use of moderate pressure to the areas the patient requested. The therapist started the massage with the patient in the position she found him—semireclining. From this position, the therapist, using effleurage and acupressure, gently massaged the neck, being careful not to disturb the Swan catheter. The pressure to the shoulders was increased to a moderate force.

The patient wanted to try lying on his right side to facilitate back massage. The head of the bed was positioned slightly lower to make the side-lying position more comfortable. The practitioner applied moderate effleurage and acupressure to the back and posterior neck.

The pain in Mr. A's neck diminished greatly from the massage. He also commented that he "felt like a new man!"

Part B:

Now, choose one of the other frameworks, SOAP, CARE, or CARP, and document the same case history in that form.

REFERENCES

1. Thomassen H. Charting Massage in the Patient Record. Hospital-Based Massage Network Newsletter. Winter 2000:4–5.
2. Thompson D. Hands Heal: Communication, Documentation, and Insurance Billing for Manual Therapists. 2nd Ed. Philadelphia, PA: Lippincott Williams & Wilkins, 2002.
3. Rose MK. The Art of the Chart: Documenting Massage Therapy With CARE Notes. Massage Bodywork April/May 2003:80–88.

ADDITIONAL RESOURCES

CARE NOTES: Documenting Massage Therapy. Available from Mary Kathleen Rose, PO Box 17313, Boulder, CO 80308; 303-449-3945; or Rosevine@comforttouch.com.

13

BLAZING NEW TRAILS

*With contributions by Jan Locke, Adela Basayne,
Patti Cadolino, and Lee Daniel Erman*

Massage programs are common on obstetrical, oncology, general medicine, surgical, and cardiac units. Other hospital units or groups of patients, such as the emergency room, the intensive care unit (ICU) waiting room, apheresis, pediatrics, or psychiatric units, seldom or never receive massage services. This chapter presents the voices of massage therapists who have experience working with the above specialties, as well as other unique populations. Jan Locke recounts her work in the emergency room, Adela Basayne contributes material on massaging pediatric patients hospitalized for eating disorders, Patti Cadolino writes about teaching parents to provide nurturing touch to their premature infants, and Lee Erman shares the experience of massage therapists who assist during conscious brain surgery. Charlotte Versagi and Toni Kline generously give of their time to share about their work with people diagnosed with psychiatric disorders, and Nicholas Kasovac, Diane Charmley, and Marybetts Sinclair speak about pediatric massage. Other sections in this chapter are the result of my own experience.

The work of these practitioners has blazed a trail for the massage community. Each therapist could have written many pages about their work. Unfortunately, space confines them to a few pages. In that small amount of space, they have tried to give basic guidelines and benefits to readers interested in expanding their massage service to other groups of patients or to new parts within the medical setting.

THE EMERGENCY ROOM

by Jan Locke, LMT, McKenzie-Willamette
Medical Center[a]

Bringing massage into this constantly changing, fast-paced environment can be thrilling, challenging, frustrating, and poignant. As with other units in the hospital, most referrals are for comfort-oriented massage. However, massage therapists also encounter situations in the emergency department (ED) that are not typical of other areas

in the hospital. For instance, they work with patients at the beginning of their medical process, so they may not have a clear idea of the patient's medical status. Obtaining information about the patient can be difficult due to the constant fluctuation and movement of the doctors and nurses as they treat ongoing emergencies. Another difference is the increased risk of exposure to body fluids, requiring practitioners to more frequently use gloves.

Assessment by the ED staff is brief and specific to the patient's immediate complaints. Except for allergies, the massage therapist may not have a very complete medical or physical history. In light of having only minimal information and because patients' stress levels are so high, it is important to keep contact gentle and comforting. ED patients are rarely in touch with their bodies, much less their pain receptors, impairing their capacity to give accurate feedback about sensations. In addition, many patients in this setting are under the influence of recreational drugs, alcohol, or overmedicated with prescription drugs, further inhibiting their feedback ability.

In this urgent environment, it is important to be flexible and to get out of the way when necessary. Situations move quickly, and the staff needs a clear field in which to work. On the other hand, therapists should not be afraid to ask the staff questions. In most cases, the staff are happy to explain situations and precautions. This saves the patient in crisis from having to answer more questions after not only completing a series of forms in the lobby but also responding to a multitude of questions from the medical and nursing staff. Patients also may be confused, exhausted, and in pain, making their answers to massage intake questions incomplete and unreliable. It is, therefore, best to gain as much information as possible from the staff and the chart rather than from the patient.

There are, however, instances in which it is appropriate to question the patient regarding past injuries, especially if the staff has requested that the practitioner perform deeper bodywork to specific muscle groups. For instance, a male patient arrived complaining of back spasms. The doctor asked the bodywork practitioner if she would give the patient a back massage before muscle relaxants were prescribed. Before starting that particular session, the therapist, as would be appropriate, asked the man about his medical history, especially related to the musculoskeletal system. (And because of the massage, the patient was able to leave without medication.)

Being fully grounded and present is critical when working in this environment. Therapists must be able to regroup and recenter while on the fly. They must maintain flexibility and be ready for anything from disclosure of physical abuse, which may or may not have been shared with the nurses or doctor, to questions concerning life and death. Jan Locke recounted the time she was asked to keep an elderly female patient company while staff was diverted to another situation. The frail woman was exhausted, fearful, and in pain. While the woman waited for diagnostic testing to see if she had a bowel blockage, Jan stroked her brow and gently massaged her shoulders. Partway through the session, the patient quietly asked, "Should I pray to live or to die?"

The opportunities for massage in an emergency room are varied. The comfort of tender touch and some guided breathing may be sought while a finger or forehead is being sutured or while a patient waits for radiology to take them for x-rays. Light touch and soothing words can be a great gift for someone with a migraine, an elderly person waiting for family to arrive, or a mentally ill person who is confused and disoriented. Therapists may be asked to work with patients being evaluated for possible bone fractures or symptoms of stroke or heart attack. In any of these situations, it is important to help the patient stay calm and still. In the cases of potential stroke or heart attack, it's best to use caution and extremely light touch, staying away from the neck due to the possibility of carotid artery involvement.

There can be many interruptions as doctors and nurses continue to evaluate the patient's situation. But there also can be lengthy, uninterrupted time while the patient waits for test results or family to arrive. Massage is a powerful tool in this environment and can bring that one moment of connection and loving touch that can make a profound difference to the patient who is navigating the difficult waters of pain and confusion. Many times, simply holding a hand or lightly stroking the brow or scalp is all that is required to create comfort in the midst of chaos. For the therapist, too, giving massage in the ED is a rewarding experience. It can influence his or her personal growth, creating greater flexibility, insight, and compassion.

ICU FAMILY WAITING ROOM

A loved one has fallen from a roof, smashed a motorcycle at 70 mph, been accidentally shot during hunting season, or an aneurysm has burst. The person is rushed to a critical care unit, where he hovers between worlds. Friends and family arrive from every corner of the country to hold vigil, to be near the loved one who lies injured or critically ill. The ICU waiting room becomes part chapel, part en-

campment. Family and friends bide their time there, frequently for days, often for weeks, and sometimes for months. They sleep on couches, live on cafeteria food, and breathe only indoor air. Backs hurt from stress and too much sitting, hearts are broken, and hope is stretched beyond endurance. No matter, they want to be nearby in case the medical condition changes, the patient wakes, or a decision must be made.

The room is a jumble of emotions. One family is ebullient because their loved one opened his eyes, another is grief-stricken because they have just had to make the decision to withdraw life support. Others hold their breath, living in a state of limbo.

Life is a roller coaster in an ICU waiting room. One day the news is good; the next day the loved one has been taken back to surgery. One step forward, four back. Fifteen minutes of neck, shoulder, and back massage can be a godsend during this time.

A THERAPIST'S JOURNAL
Are You Really Giving A Massage?

Edna and her two daughters had already had a few bad days when the massage therapist first met them. Edna eyed the therapist as she set up her massage chair in the corner of the room. Someone always does. Often they know what it's for and ask, "Are you REALLY giving massage?" The question breaks the ice, and the practitioner has her first client. After that, it's a matter of keeping up with the multitude of requests.

Edna's husband was in need of a liver transplant and had just been transferred from a community hospital to the university medical center where patients with complicated medical conditions can receive advanced care. Not only was the man gravely ill, but the wife and daughters were small-town residents who found the city to be stressful. The daughters were particularly upset that day because their father's toxicity levels were so high that he did not recognize them and was behaving in a bizarre, antagonistic way.

As with most family members, these three women were frozen with fear. The therapist approached them gently, careful not to be intrusive. They were tired from the preceding days, nerves stretched tight, thoughts in chaos. Edna, though, didn't have to think more than a moment before accepting the offer of a back and neck massage. The touch practitioner began, as always, by asking Edna about her own health (Box 13-1) and then settled her hands gently onto Edna's shoulders, maintaining an extra-soft presence, hands accepting and noninvasive.

—Gayle MacDonald, MS, LMT

Of Special Interest

GENERAL SEATED MASSAGE INTAKE

Performance of a health intake before the massage is vital, even for just a 15-minute shoulder massage. A number of the patients in a critical care unit are in advanced years, which means that many family members are older and have a variety of medical problems. It is not uncommon to encounter such conditions as diabetes, prior cancer treatment, breathing disorders, fibromyalgia, or even mild congestive heart failure. Just as with collecting information about hospital patients, questions should be to the point, not vague. Remember, it is the therapist's professional duty to elicit the information from the client, not the client's responsibility to guess what the therapist needs to know. Inquire about the following:

- How the client is feeling at the moment
- General energy level
- Health of the neck and spine
- Treatment of any medical conditions
- Easy bruising
- Pregnancy
- Use of pain or anti-inflammatory medications
- Skin health in the area to be massaged
- Lymph node removal and/or radiation[e]

[e]Asking about lymph node removal is a gentle but direct way to gather the information the practitioner needs instead of inquiring if the person has a history of cancer. Because there are so many women who have a prior history of breast cancer treatment, it is imperative to ask this question. Breast cancer treatment nearly always involves either the removal of lymph nodes or radiation to them. Either intervention puts them at risk for lymphedema, which can be triggered by a short shoulder massage. Lymph nodes may be taken out for other reasons. One nurse had some removed when they swelled after a flu shot. Another had some removed for a biopsy. One woman had lymph nodes damaged by a bacterial infection when she was young. The outcome was lymphedema in one arm.

When working in this setting, bodyworkers should have no expectation that people will let go and completely relax. Family and friends have literally been holding themselves together to get through the crisis and are afraid to let go. The therapist should never tell them to "relax." In that way, the massage recipients never feel that they are failing at the massage if they can't relax. It is best to say nothing, allowing the massage to do its work.

For family and friends who have been at their loved one's side for an extended period, massage becomes a time to rest, a respite. People tend to be quieter than normal massage recipients. There is no extra energy for idle chit-chat. The touch practitioner should follow their lead if conversation arises, allowing them the space to share their situation or withhold it.

In her piece on massage in the emergency room, Jan Locke points out the need to regroup and become grounded quickly. The same is true in the ICU waiting room. One recipient may be cheerful and wanting to laugh; the next is somber and quiet. The therapist must keep her antenna up at all times, remain centered, and be able to switch gears at a moment's notice.

One day, circumstances dictated that the therapist do many of the massages in the regular waiting room chairs, even though she had her massage chair set up. She approached a woman who appeared to be simple and unaccustomed to attention. Her pregnant daughter had been shot a few days earlier in a drive-by shooting. The bullet entered the right side of the belly and came out the opposite side, missing the baby. The woman's nephew, a severely retarded teenager, was in the waiting room with her. When the therapist inquired whether she would like a massage, the woman looked at the massage chair hesitantly and then spoke about not wanting to leave her nephew. With the help of the waiting room receptionist, the mother was convinced that it would be OK to stay where she was to receive a massage. This was the key to allowing her to try this new experience, which she was ultimately grateful for.

The next woman eagerly sat down in the massage chair. As the touch therapist worked, the woman talked about her sister-in-law, who was sitting across the room, her eyes red and face blotchy from crying, staring off into the distance. Her husband wasn't going to survive and had been put back on the ventilator to keep him alive until their daughters could travel 2 hours to get to the hospital. The woman asked the practitioner if she would offer a massage to her sister-in-law, whose neck had been painful for days.

The therapist approached the grieving woman gingerly. She looked unable to move. It was clear to the touch therapist that the only way the wife would accept the massage was if it was given there in the waiting room chair. To the practitioner's amazement, the distraught woman agreed.

Families need to be supported when loved ones are in the hospital, especially when they are in the ICU. But even on regular hospital units, family and friends benefit from a short neck and shoulder massage (Fig. 13-1). These are often spur-of-the-moment events performed while the massage therapist waits to speak to a nurse or while the family member waits for the loved one to return

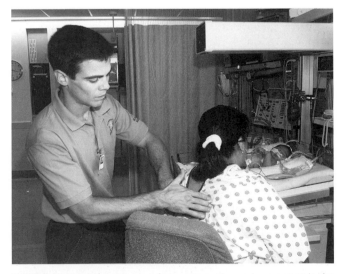

FIGURE 13-1 ■ Mother pauses for a moment to receive massage in the NICU; this allows her to stay at the baby's side. (Photo by Don Hamilton.)

from a procedure. The massage might take place in the patient's room, an exam room, or the nurse's conference room. It might be only 5 minutes, but 5 minutes of rest is an oasis in the middle of such stress.

PATIENTS WITH PSYCHIATRIC DIAGNOSES

Massage can also work its magic on those diagnosed with a psychiatric illness. However, a new set of precautions must be taken into account. Most important is the willingness of practitioners to set aside their agenda, to move even slower and gentler into the relationship with an emphasis on building trust.

People with a psychiatric diagnosis come in all shapes and sizes and with a variety of influencing factors. Like all others receiving medical treatment, no two are alike. One person's condition may be drug-induced, another's associated with trauma or abuse, while a third person may have a chemical imbalance. Despite the differences, there are some common concepts therapists can apply when massaging people diagnosed with psychiatric or mental health disorders. This section will focus on those commonalities.

In this arena, touch therapists will work more closely with the referring healthcare provider—psychiatrist, nurse practitioner, clinical nurse specialist, or psychotherapist—than with the care providers of nonpsychiatric patients. Psychiatric practitioners touch their patients with more forethought than is given to other patients. The decision to integrate massage therapy into a psychiatric patient's treatment plan will undergo even more scrutiny. Bodyworkers can expect a team approach that includes frequent communication about the bodywork sessions and the patient's response.

These patients, on the whole, are disconnected from their bodies, so it is necessary to proceed slowly. They are unaware of how their bodies feel, including pain levels. Toni Kline, a nurse massage therapist who specializes in adult psychiatry and mental health, tells of a patient who had had a hip fracture for some time. After a number of touch-therapy treatments, he was able to feel his body again and the pain in it. This allowed him to communicate about the pain to the doctor and receive treatment for it. Others have presented in the ED unaware of pain due to diabetic complications, cigarette burns, or cancer-related pain. Clients who are detached from their bodies cannot give the massage therapist accurate feedback and will sometimes allow invasive bodywork to be administered. Skilled, respectful touch helps these patients reconnect with their bodies.

As body awareness increases, so, too, do memories stored in the tissues. This is one of the reasons it is imperative that massage therapists work closely with the referring practitioner. This phenomenon also makes it essential that bodyworkers stay within their scope of practice. It is important with all clients, but it is even more vital with psychiatric patients. The temptation is to step

into the role of counselor or social worker, to encourage people to talk about their fears or grief, to offer advice. Both Kline and Charlotte Versagi, a massage therapist who specializes in psychiatric care, are emphatic about the necessity of avoiding this pitfall. They advise being an active listener rather than trying to play analyst. Become skillful at just listening without interruption, providing a nonjudgmental space in which people can talk, and at asking questions only to clarify meaning. But refer psychological issues to the psychological experts.

At the start of the therapeutic bodywork relationship, building trust is the only goal. For many with psychiatric disorders, touch has been associated with abuse or trauma, and relearning the experience of safe touch is invariably slow. Versagi tells of spending weeks massaging just the feet of a woman who had been physically abused. Both tibias of another woman had been broken with the butt of a gun. At first she wouldn't allow her legs to be touched. Even the idea of having them touched was intolerable. Bit by bit, with the client's permission, the therapist was able to extend the strokes from the feet up the legs. This client is now walking without a cane, her gait nearly normal.

Kline likes to start her mental health patients with Therapeutic Touch (TT), a modality that works in the person's energy field rather than directly on the skin. In this way, the therapist doesn't have to enter into such close proximity with the patient, which, if done too quickly, can sometimes exacerbate the symptoms. She recounts the story of a woman being treated for multiple personality disorder. After receiving TT a number of times, the patient felt ready for direct touch. Kline began with massage to only the hands, spending many sessions with just that area. Slowly, over a period of months, they progressed to the elbow and then eventually to the shoul-

A THERAPIST'S JOURNAL
The Doctor's Appointment

A woman who had psychosomatic seizures whenever she had a doctor's appointment also benefited from TT. One day when she was due for an appointment, the physician arranged for the TT practitioner to be in attendance. When the patient started seizing, the practitioner went down onto the floor with her and administered TT. Afterward, the patient remembered nothing of the seizure experience except a memory of someone combing her hair. She said it was like her mother used to do when she was a child. The remarkable part of this experience was that this was the only memory the patient had during the time she was seizing. Usually, patients don't remember anything. From then on, a touch session was scheduled before her doctor's appointments, with the end result being fewer seizures and less medication.

—Toni Kline, RN, LMT

der. The hand, Kline believes, is a good starting place when beginning to apply direct touch. As the hand opens, the heart opens, and then the whole body.

The medications taken for psychiatric disorders cause a number of unwelcome side effects, such as pacing, leg shaking, tongue rolling, hand clenching, muscular rigidity, and a flat affect. Touch therapies can calm these motor activities. According to Kline, some people are eager to get off of or cut down on their medications, not only because of the **dyskinetic** effects mentioned above, but also because some cause sluggishness or agitation. She believes massage helps during the process of tapering off or reducing medications.

Kline, who also conducts group therapy for people who are **bipolar, schizophrenic,** severely depressed, or anxious, finds that touch therapy given before an individual counseling or group session promotes increased disclosure, making for a more effective session. One afternoon, she was late to "group." Her usual way of beginning was to administer a brief TT session to each person. When she arrived that day, they had already begun, mimicking with each other what she did in TT sessions at the beginning of each group meeting. They were moving their hands above the body in the energy field like they had seen her do. That one spontaneous interaction did more to change the group's dynamic than anything they had ever done, creating deep bonds between one another.

Until patients have confidence in the massage experience, they may have special needs that the bodyworker must honor. People may need to keep their eyes open during the session so that they can see the therapist. Others may not be able to lie prone on the massage table for fear of what is going on behind them. One man with posttraumatic stress disorder was afraid to lie prone because he invariably fell asleep in that position. Falling asleep triggered flashbacks, causing the man to thrash severely. He was afraid of falling off the table during a thrashing episode. Another man who received TT in a regular chair would not let the therapist work behind him. The face cradle, too, may provoke a similar psychological discomfort, requiring the therapist to work on the client from supine and side-lying positions. (Personal interviews with Charlotte Versagi, LMT, on June 15, 2003, and Toni Kline, RN, LMT, on June 18, 2003.)

Other adjustments that are necessary when massaging patients with a history of mental health problems are:

- The application of a firm but light touch. However, the pressure should not be too light. Ultra-light touch may be misinterpreted, or the person may be too vulnerable for touch that is so intimate. Trust must be built before administering modalities that involve light touch, such as Reiki.
- Avoidance of percussive strokes such as tapotement or techniques that involve prodding or digging. Rocking may be appropriate.
- Work each area of the body for a longer duration before moving onto the next.

- Asking for the patient's permission every time you move to a new body part.
- Being aware of the body parts involved in trauma cases. They may need to be avoided indefinitely or for a prolonged period. For instance, someone who has been raped should not be touched on the buttocks, inner thigh, or chest.

PEDIATRIC AND ADOLESCENT EATING DISORDERS

by Adela Basayne, LMT, Legacy Emanuel Medical Center[b]

Massage therapy is gaining acceptance in pediatric and adolescent eating disorder units due to the study of its effects on those with **anorexia nervosa** and **bulimia nervosa** by the Touch Research Institute.[1,2] It can be a key intervention for people whose illness has caused them to fixate on their appearance while simultaneously disconnecting from their bodily sensations. Skilled touch is a way of increasing body awareness and relaxation and decreasing anxiety and depression. For one young woman, receiving massage was the only time she felt beautiful.

The majority of eating disorder patients are female. Most commonly, they are diagnosed with anorexia or bulimia. A few others have disorders such as food or choking phobias. As of yet, the root cause of these conditions is not understood. There may be a psychosocial component, a genetic connection with an environmental trigger, or a viral connection; or it may be the result of a brain disorder similar to **obsessive-compulsive disorder.**

Generally, eating disorder patients are hospitalized or put into day treatment against their will. People with anorexia exhibit physical symptoms of prolonged starvation—orthostatic hypotension, **bradycardia,** low potassium and phosphorus levels, **osteopenia** or osteoporosis, hypothermia, menstrual dysfunction, cachexia, hair loss, and diminished cognitive function. People with bulimia, while generally of normal body weight, are affected by cardiovascular and electrolyte dysfunction. Emotionally, all are depressed, anxious, angry, or suicidal.

Treatment includes reintroduction to ordered eating behavior; weight restoration by slowly increasing calories (fast reintroduction stresses the heart); family, individual, and group therapy; and medications. Generally, the individual is on an antidepressant and a **neuroleptic** such as Zyprexa, Geodon, or Risperdal. Neuroleptics are given to reduce anxiety about weight gain. People with bulimia may also be on a drug called Topamax, which has been shown to reduce the desire to binge. Typically, a course of medications is quite short. Exercise is kept to a minimum, and activities, such as bathroom use, meals, and exercise, are supervised. Those who are a suicide risk will have a 24-hour "sitter."

People with an eating disorder focus obsessively on the body, its size, and its appearance. There is an unrelenting drive for thinness, causing them to hide food, exercise in secret (including isometric exercises on the massage table), to wear weights, and to load up on water. One young woman was so obsessed that she would exercise every possible moment. Rather than sitting on a chair, she would squat above it. And, the first time the massage therapist worked with her, the practitioner discovered weights taped to her ankles. All of these actions were to increase the burden on her muscles in order to lose weight.

These massage recipients may try to entice the therapist into responding to questions such as, "Do I look fat?" "Is my back fat?" "Don't you think this food is disgusting?" They may also constantly attempt to get permission to exercise or to get information regarding their weight. It is important that practitioners not engage in conversations about appropriate body size or nutrition, no matter what their personal beliefs are.

Touch therapy must proceed slowly, obtaining permission at each step. The approach should be gentle and nurturing for a number of reasons. Patients with eating disorders are often unable to give accurate feedback about pressure due to the habitual disregard of body signals. In addition, cachexia and osteopenia or osteoporosis demand gentle touch due to fragile tissue or bones. Easy bruising is common to a number of patients, and the skin is generally dry and sometimes loose. A curious symptom called **lanugo** can develop; it causes the growth of fine hair on the back, such as occurs with newborns.

As with other psychiatric patients, patients with an eating disorder will be more comfortable if the massage is allowed to unfold at a slower pace. Sessions are frequently given over clothing because patients are uncomfortable disrobing. Those in day treatment can often have sessions of an hour, but hospitalized patients are weak and easily overstimulated, requiring a shortened duration, usually 15 to 30 minutes. For example, one prepubescent girl who was only 60% of her normal weight had become cognitively impaired from her disease, seeming dim and unreactive. Massage was the only activity she responded to. The therapist gave her 20-minute sessions for the first week of the girl's hospitalization but then stopped on the girl's request. The touch therapy triggered overwhelming emotion related to a prior traumatic event. It wasn't until the patient was well enough to be admitted to day treatment that the bodywork sessions could continue.

Other factors may influence the bodywork session. Patients who are unwilling or unable to feed themselves will have a nasogastric tube. Some may have an intravenous (IV) catheter if potassium or phosphorus must be administered. Additionally, attention must be paid to the degree of warmth applied because the patient's body temperature is often low.

PEDIATRIC MASSAGE

Most of the clinical adjustments necessary for massaging hospitalized or medically frail children are similar to those for adults. However, the way of relating is much different. As Marybetts Sinclair points out in her book *Pediatric Massage Therapy*,[3] children are not miniature adults; they require an approach that involves playfulness, imagination, singing, and games.

The way in which touch therapists build rapport is dependent on the youngster's age and level of development. Toys or stuffed animals often facilitate the connection with children, as does the style of communicating. When talking with a toddler or preschooler, the language should be playful and imaginative. Relaxed muscles become "blobs of Jell-o." Tense arms and legs are "sticks." Taking a deep breath becomes "filling the body like a balloon." Pretending games can give the child a sense of how the body feels when it's relaxed versus tense. "Pretend you are a cat lying in the sun; pretend you just saw a scary bug."

Children enjoy relating through role-playing. Massage might be introduced with the help of a teddy bear or doll. The therapist and child could rub the bear's back together. A demonstration and role-playing with the parent can also serve to familiarize the child with massage.

An introductory conversation about massage with school-age children might include questions and statements such as:

- I'm a massage therapist. Do you know what that is?
- Do you know anyone who has ever had a massage?
- What did they tell you about it?
- Has your mom or dad ever rubbed your back?
- Do you have any parts of your body that hurt?
- What do you think might make it feel better?
- We could start by showing you how massage feels on your hand.

Building on their interests, such as dance, sport, music, or theater, will help establish rapport with older children. One 15-year-old young man waiting in the hospital for a heart transplant had a stack of martial arts videos in his room, a poster of Bruce Lee on the wall, and was wearing a Kung Fu T-shirt. The massage therapist noticed his interests as soon as she entered the room. The patient's involvement with martial arts made it easy to talk about concepts such as centering and the use of the breath.

Nicholas Kasovac, a pediatric massage specialist, tells the story of a 9-year-old girl admitted to the pediatric pain clinic for chronic headaches. He discovered she liked to perform voices and characters from stories and movies. While working on her feet the first time, he started playing "This Little Piggy." With each toe, Kasovac used a different dramatic voice. When he moved to the second foot, the therapist suggested to the girl that she supply the voices for each toe, which she eagerly did.

The single most important factor in working with children is the establishment of trust. Like adult patients, hospitalized children have had painful procedures, placement of medical devices, and surgeries, but lack the ability to fully understand the experience. Those who have experienced unusual amounts of pain during early childhood may exhibit greater anxiety about potential pain. They may also be apprehensive about adults they don't know. Massage therapists must establish their role as someone who provides pleasurable touch.

Integral to the establishment of trust is obtaining permission to touch the child and honoring his boundaries. Even babies will communicate their permission through eye contact, maintaining loose muscles and a relaxed state. This can be seen in the infant in Figure 13-2. Turning or pulling away, agitation, crying, and no eye contact are signs that the baby does not want to be touched.

Kasovac is mindful of the way in which he carries his body and how he enters the child's space. When walking

---

A THERAPIST'S JOURNAL
Eddie

Eddie was an 8-month-old patient in the pediatric intensive care unit. Born prematurely with cardiac defects, he needed to have open-heart surgery but was too small and fragile to withstand its demands. Eddie was so weak that his heart was not able to adequately pump blood through his scrawny, baby-bird body, and he required mechanical ventilation to the lungs because his own were unable to sustain his life force.

His parents were unable to be with him much of the time. Most days, Eddie did not have someone to love and care for him at the bedside. It was never clear if the parents' absence was because of the mother's mental health issues, finances, or lack of transportation, or if it was the only way they could cope with having an ill baby being in an intensive care unit (ICU) on the brink of death. One thing was always clear: Despite not being there all of the time, these two people loved Eddie. Their choices may not have been what others would have done, but the parents cared very deeply for their child, doing what they thought was the right thing.

One of Eddie's biggest problems was the inability to sleep or rest. He was constantly agitated and restless, tossing, twisting, turning and fighting, using up what little amount of energy his body had. The nurses dutifully reported their assessments to the doctors, asking for more medication to calm him down and induce sleep. Sleep and rest were critically important because Eddie needed to gain weight and strength to withstand the rigors of open-heart surgery.

The day came when Eddie was being given the maximum amount of medication, Ativan and Versed, to calm him. The doctors could not prescribe any more without serious medical consequences. They were at the end of their rope. More accurately, Eddie was at the end of HIS rope. I decided to step in and try something no one had yet tried, unsure if it would even make a difference. At this point, no one had anything to lose, least of all Eddie.

I walked to the head of his ICU bed. Both his arms were in restraints, pulling them away from his chest, almost as if he were being crucified on the bed. At the same time, he was throwing his head back and forth, back and forth, as if emphatically gesturing "NO." (This scene may appear disturbing and cruel, but it was clinically necessary for Eddie to be restrained to maintain his airway.) The nurse gave me permission to untie one of his arm restraints. After untying the restraint, I eased my index finger underneath the tense and curled fingers of Eddie's hand. He quickly grasped it with unusual strength that did not let up. I gently bounced his little "chicken" arm up and down, using a small amount of space, but just enough for him to feel the movement in his body. With the middle finger of my other hand, I began to gently stroke Eddie's forehead very lightly in one direction just above his eyebrows. Slowly and methodically, I stroked his forehead while humming a lullaby close to his ear. Within 5 minutes or less, Eddie had stopped struggling and fighting and had fallen asleep. Carefully, I released my index finger and returned to work, surprised and pleased at my accomplishment.

Later in the day, the attending physician came by to check on Eddie, knowing that he was at the maximum doses for the sedating drugs. The nurse reported to the physician that he had been sleeping for the past 45 minutes, the longest he had slept or rested in the previous 3 days. She also mentioned my interaction with Eddie, to which the physician replied half-kidding, half-serious, "Can you stop by and see my other patients too?"

I don't know if Eddie ever got his heart surgery, but to be able to give him calm, peaceful relief during a difficult and stressful time was truly a gift, not just to him but to me as well.

Nicholas Kasovac, MA, LMT, Mesa, Arizona

---

into the young patient's room, Kasovac never walks directly into the child's space; he moves slowly, stopping at the foot of the bed to introduce himself. Diane Charmley, a nurse massage therapist, enters with a quiet mind, aware of the interaction between the child's energy field and her own.

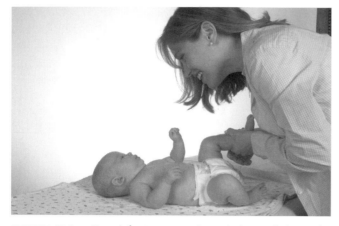

FIGURE 13-2 ■ Even infants communicate their permission to be touched through eye contact, loose muscles, and maintaining a relaxed state. (Reprinted by permission of Stonybrook University Hospital Medical Photography Department. Photo by Jeanne Neville.)

A THERAPIST'S JOURNAL
Joel

The nurses at Stanford Children's Hospital asked me to see Joel, a 14-year-old boy with cystic fibrosis. He was in a room with three other teenage boys. At night, Joel had leg cramps that were so painful he would cry, and his crying woke up his roommates. The nurses considered putting him in a room by himself, but they didn't want to humiliate or isolate him. At that age, kids need to be around other kids, and the nurses were afraid that Joel would feel ashamed to be put into a room by himself because of his crying. They asked me if I thought massage would help.

My experience with leg cramps is that once a cramp starts, massage doesn't do very much for it. I have found in many cases, however, that leg cramps can be prevented by a careful massage late in the day or just before bedtime. I went to Joel in the evenings at about 7 p.m. and massaged his legs and feet. What a difference it made! On the nights I was there, he did not wake up with leg cramps.

One night, I was massaging Joel when his father came in. He was a healthy-looking man with a florid complexion. He looked so unlike his son that I found it hard to believe they were related. The boy was so thin and pale with the narrow shoulders and hips of a cystic fibrosis child. He looked much younger than his 14 years.

The father sat down as he always did, nodded to the boy, and opened up his Wall Street Journal. I wondered about this. "Why does he come here if he's just going to read a paper all evening? Why doesn't he talk to the boy? Why does he even bother to come if this is what he's going to do every time?" As I got to know the boy better, I realized that his energy level was too low for conversation and that all he wanted was his father's loving presence.

That night, as I was working on Joel's legs and feet, I noticed the father lower the paper and watch me over the top edge. After a few minutes out of the corner of my eye, I saw him abruptly fold up the paper and put it down beside him. He said to me, "Could I do that? Is that something I could learn? Will you show me how?" I explained to him the reason for doing it and that it was easy to learn. I had him bring his chair over and put it beside mine so that we could work together. I continued to massage his son's left foot and instructed him to follow along on the right foot. I also showed him how to massage Joel's legs and hips and then how to turn his son onto the side to massage the back, shoulders, and scalp. That was the last time I had to go to Joel's room. His father, who had been coming every night anyway, now gave his son the massage.

The following Monday afternoon, I was at the hospital again. As I walked by Joel's room, I noticed two little girls beside him, one on each side of the bed. They were massaging him in exactly the way I had showed Joel's father. I went to the nurses' station to ask whom the little girls were and was told they were his sisters. Joel's father had gone home and said to his wife and daughters, "There's something we can all learn to do that will help Joel get through the night without any leg cramps." And so he taught his wife and daughters to massage Joel.

The mother brought the two girls after school, and she and her husband came together in the evening. One evening as I walked past the room, I saw father and mother massaging the boy. They sometimes would look up at each other and smile. From what the nurses had told me, the massage had given them a language with which they could talk to each other. The father, in teaching his wife, had demonstrated on her by rubbing her back and shoulders, forming a reconnection between them. For so long, they had felt sad and heavy, making it harder and harder to talk about the fact that Joel was dying. If you can't talk to the person you are married to about the most overwhelming sorrow that has ever come into your life, it is difficult to talk about anything else except in a perfunctory way. The communication between them had broken down.

The daughters, ages 9 and 11, had come to feel neglected. The mother had kept the house going, putting three meals a day on the table and keeping up with the laundry. But in a family in which one child has a catastrophic illness, it is very hard for the parents to be emotionally available to the healthy *children. Now the massage had become a family activity—something they could all do together.*

Teaching family and friends to give massage is one of the most valuable things a bodyworker can do for a patient. Massage is often better than conversation. It becomes a language through which family can express their love, a language that requires no reply. By helping loved ones be part of the patient's care, they feel empowered. To the patient, it makes the hospital seem like a far less alien place, and it gives the loved ones a way of expressing their love for the patient in a situation in which the sorrow is too profound for words. Giving massage is a way of siphoning off some of the terrible frustration families and friends feel when they are standing beside the bed unable to do anything for the person who is ill. Massage becomes the giving and receiving of love.

Helen M. Campbell, December 3, 1921, to April 22, 1999, hospital and hospice massage pioneer in the San Francisco Bay area

Massage is helpful to young patients in a variety of ways. Given by a family member, it becomes a bonding and empowering activity. Before an invasive procedure, massage can relax a child and teach her strategies for coping with the discomfort. Skilled touch can calm the youngster who is fearful during an asthma attack or is anxious about being tapered off pain medications. And, as with adults, children can benefit from gentle bodywork, which can dissipate some of the physical guarding brought on by the hospital experience.[3]

One of Patti Cadolino's patients was a cocaine-addicted baby who was also born HIV positive. He had been brought into the clinic by his foster mother, who was trying hard to do everything right. When the therapist undressed the infant, the child was stiff as a board, one of the side effects of neurological damage. The therapist pointed this out to the foster mother, who had not been aware of it. She started to cry vigorously. However, with a month of massage coaching from Cadolino and many more months of applying the touch techniques, the infant made a total turnaround. Much to the surprise of the physicians and physical therapists, the child is now running and moving like a normal kid.

The following are other general guidelines for massaging pediatric patients:

- Make it clear that children can leave some or all of their clothes on.
- Using simple language, explain to the child what you are doing as the massage unfolds.
- Start with the extremities.

- If a particular area hurts, start with an area that doesn't. This gives the child a chance to experience massage as a pleasurable sensation.
- If the patient has to consistently endure procedures in the same part of the body, begin the touch session in a different place. For instance, premature infants in the neonatal intensive care unit (NICU) frequently have their legs grabbed to be given a heel stick. If the massage therapist begins by grasping a baby's legs, it may trigger an agitated response.
- Ask permission before moving to the next body part. Not only does this impart control to the youngster, but it gives him many opportunities to say he is ready to stop.
- Adjust the length of the session for the attention span of the child. Often, the younger the child, the shorter the session.
- Use slow, gentle touch, especially with babies. Their immature nervous system is easily overstimulated.
- Children's muscle tissue is less dense than adult's and, therefore, requires less pressure. Children are not fragile, however, and can tolerate and enjoy firm pressure if it's medically appropriate.
- Younger children do not easily verbalize their feelings. The therapist needs to be mindful of nonverbal cues of resistance or discomfort, such as flinching, holding the breath, grimacing, or tensing other body parts.

(Personal interviews with Diane Charmley, RN, LMT, on September 3, 2003, Nicholas Kasovac, MA, LMT, on September 8, 2003, and Patti Cadolino on October 11, 2003.)

TEACHING NURTURING TOUCH TO PARENTS IN THE NEONATAL INTENSIVE CARE UNIT

by Patti Cadolino, LMT, Certified Infant Massage Instructor, Stonybrook University Hospital[c]

In the 1980s, standard care for neonates did not include significant amounts of positive touch. Signs were even hung in some NICUs warning staff and parents to not touch the infants. Slowly, this atmosphere is eroding, but there is still uncertainty about employing touch in this arena. Despite the research, which is beginning to paint a clearer picture showing that skillful touch can reduce the stress behaviors and increase weight gain in neonates, this practice remains on the cutting edge.

This section should **NOT** be considered instruction in the massage of preterm babies. It is merely an overview and introduction to the topic. Because these tiny patients are so medically unstable, the massage therapist wishing to pursue this work should find training that includes supervised massage experience. While touch can be immensely

[c]Copyright © 2004 Patti Cadolino

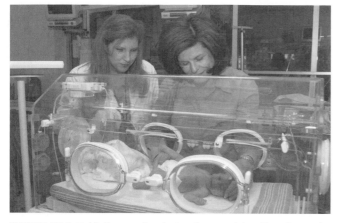

FIGURE 13-3 ■ Mother receives instruction on giving "hand containment" to her baby. (Reprinted by permission of Stonybrook University Hospital Medical Photography Department. Photo by Jeanne Neville.)

beneficial, even the slightest touch interaction can create changes to blood pressure, heart rate, respiration, or oxygen saturation levels that can endanger the infant. Given in an unskilled manner, touch has the potential to be harmful. It is, therefore, essential that therapists who work in this arena have knowledge about infant physiology as well as stress and behavorial cues, and have well-developed assessment skills. Premature infants are neurologically underdeveloped, and touch can be too stimulating.

Infants in a NICU are subjected to a highly stressful environment—bright lights, continuous noise, and endless medical interventions, some of which are excruciatingly painful. These interruptions interfere with the infant's healing process as well as having a negative impact on growth and development, disrupting sleep/wake states, and affecting parental bonding.

Skilled, nurturing touch can provide a safe and warm environment for the baby and at the same time empower the parents. Patti Cadolino's program at Stonybrook

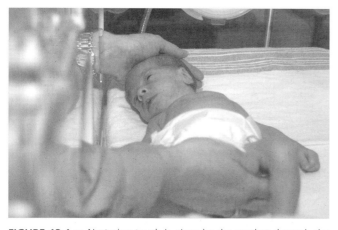

FIGURE 13-4 ■ Nurturing touch is given by the mother through the portholes of the baby's isolette. (Reprinted by permission of Stonybrook University Hospital Medical Photography Department. Photo by Jeanne Neville.)

University Hospital starts by teaching parents stress-reduction techniques, such as breathing exercises, that will induce a state of relaxation before they come into contact with their infant. Some parents are so frightened to touch their babies that they literally tremble. French studies have found that parents who were under immense stress passed the stress onto their babies, thereby affecting the infants' stress hormone levels. By learning to be in a relaxed state, parents are able to hold their babies in such a way that the infants melt into their parents' arms. Cadolino emphasizes to the parents that touch is not going to cure the baby. The goal is to provide a way for them to connect with their baby in a positive way, even if it is a short-term situation because the infant is expected to pass away.

The Nurturing Touch program at Stonybrook has three phases. Before instructing the parents in the art of touching their fragile infant, each baby is evaluated for medical complications, and parents are also assessed for stability and responsiveness. The first phase involves infants who are unable to be taken out of the isolette to be held. In this instance, parents are shown how to do hand containment through the portholes (Figures 13-3 and 13-4).

The next phase involves "skin-to-skin" contact. This method of connection is literally the parent's skin touching the infant's skin, chest-to-chest, heart-to-heart. Neonatologists discovered the power of this type of contact in the 1970s in Bogota, Colombia. The electricity that powered the medical machinery failed, meaning that the premature babies in isolettes would freeze to death. The doctors instructed the mothers to open their shirts and put the babies inside to keep them warm. To everyone's astonishment, the infants thrived.

Cadolino tells the story of a baby that the neonatologists had given up on. The mother was told the baby was going to die and that she should hold it. The ventilator was removed, and the mother spent the next 8 hours holding her baby skin-to-skin. Eventually, that tiny patient was discharged, and today it is a normal, healthy child.

Phase three of the Stonybrook program, "nuturing touch," is for infants who have reached 1,000 grams in weight and are, for the most part, medically stable. This type of touch involves holds; compression; strokes that use a moderate, relaxed pressure; and light stretching. The reader may recall from Chapter 2 that the research performed by the Touch Research Institute found that babies seem to prefer firmer pressure. In her book, *Touch Therapy*, Tiffany Field writes that "…most studies that preceded ours were ineffective, most likely because they used light stroking, which was like a tickle stimulus and was aversive to the infants. We used deeper pressure because the infants behaved as if they preferred deeper pressure."[4]

Touch is a silent but potent language. It is the medium through which parent and infant communicate and bond. Touch nurtures psychological growth, stimulates physical and mental development, enhances body awareness, and can even boost the immune system. Neonates can thrive without hearing, vision, or smell, but depriving them of touch can prove fatal. Scientists acknowledge that babies who don't receive adequate touch, such as occurs in some orphanages, can suffer from a range of neurological damage. Fredrick Leboyer, the author of *Birth Without Violence*, states that, "Being touched and caressed, being massaged is food for the infant, food as necessary as minerals, vitamins, and proteins."

MASSAGE DURING CONSCIOUS BRAIN SURGERY

by Lee Daniel Erman, NCTMB, Stanford Hospital and Clinics[d]

Parkinson's disease (PD) is a progressive brain disorder that causes tremors and lack of motor control. It is usually treated with levodopa ("L-dopa") and other drugs. These medications eventually become less effective and produce disabling side effects. Since the late 1980s, a surgical procedure known as deep brain stimulation (DBS) has been increasingly used for advanced PD. In DBS, a tiny electrode is implanted in the subthalamic nucleus deep in the brain. The electrode is connected by a wire that runs to the surface of the skull, then under the skin, to a pacemaker-like sending unit implanted in the patient's chest. The unit, which can be externally programmed, produces precise amounts and frequencies of electrical stimulation. This can provide significant relief from symptoms of advanced PD, necessitating much less medication. DBS is usually done bilaterally, with an electrode and sending unit on each side.

DBS requires exquisitely precise placement of the electrode. The team at Stanford Hospital and Clinics (Palo Alto, California), led by neurosurgeon Gary Heit, PhD, MD, achieves excellent success using a combination of methods, including presurgery magnetic resonance imaging (MRI) and, during the surgery, x-rays and a physiological mapping technique in which the doctors listen to the nerve cells' responses as the patient moves, speaks, and is passively moved. The mapping requires that the patient be awake and alert, be off all their PD medications, and have the absolute minimum of anesthesia. During the conscious portion of the procedure, which typically takes 5 hours, the patient's head is held rigidly in place by a metal "halo."

The length of the procedure, use of minimal PD medication and anesthesia, and the physical restraints can cause such discomfort at times that the surgery must be aborted. Since 2000, massage therapists at Stanford have assisted patients as they undergo this event. The massage therapists are recruited from those working in Stanford's in-patient massage program, administered by the Office of Community and Patient Relations, and from Stanford's (out-patient) Center for Integrative Medicine.

Patients have reported that massage helps them through the experience. One patient wrote: "[Without the massage therapist,] I would have never lasted to complete the procedure." Another wrote: "[The massage therapist] used his expertise to provide pain relief to my rigid muscles. ... Not only did he provide comfort through his healing touch, but he also provided comfort by his presence."

Three hours into her first surgery, a 62-year-old woman reported increasing low back pain. The touch therapist used gentle traction, rocking, direct massage, and coaching the patient's breathing to alleviate her pain. Without these interventions, anesthesia would probably have been administered. However, because the use of anesthesia might impair the mapping, it is best if it is not used.

Although all the other 20 or so people in the operating room serve the patient, they have duties that require their attention to be focused mainly on monitors, equipment, or narrow aspects of the patient's condition. The massage therapist's only task is to be "with" the patient. Even with all of the equipment around the patient, the need for access by the doctors, and the cautions of the sterile field, the massage therapist is able to get excellent access to the patient, including most of the body from the mouth to the feet. A variety of approaches are used, including careful positioning of the patient, movement, and direct soft-tissue work. In addition, the practitioner also provides valuable support for the patient, both verbally and, of course, through the power of compassionate touch.

The Stanford team does four to six DBS surgeries per month. With increasing enthusiasm and recommendation by the surgeon, patients are now requesting massage more than 75% of the time. Dr. Heit says: "Massage therapy has become an integral part of the procedure for many patients. It allows them the extra perseverance to get through a long case. It is the standard of care in many European operating rooms, and I am happy we are able to provide the service here at Stanford."

MASSAGE DURING APHERESIS

No doubt by now, the reader understands that nearly everyone, despite his or her medical condition, can receive touch therapy. This includes the person undergoing apheresis, a procedure unfamiliar to many therapists. The apheresis process could be compared to that of a high-tech creamer. A creamer is an old-fashioned piece of farming machinery that spins milk in a centrifuge, separating the cream from the milk. Similarly, during apheresis, the blood is pulled from a central IV catheter into the apheresis machine, where it is mixed with an anticoagulant medication to prevent the blood from clotting. The machine centrifugally separates the blood into fluid and

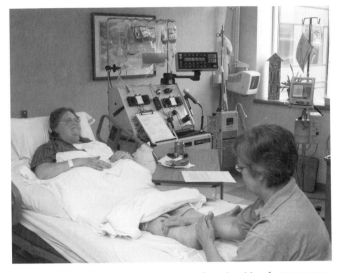

FIGURE 13-5 ■ Patient relaxes during apheresis with a foot massage. (Photo by Don Hamilton.)

cellular components. Each type of blood cell has a certain weight and resides in a specific layer according to its weight. Red blood cells are the heaviest and, therefore, are on the bottom, white cells are in the middle layer, and plasma is on the top. After the desired blood component has been removed, the remaining components are returned to the patient via the IV catheter's second lumen.

Apheresis is sometimes performed on an outpatient basis in a specialized room, or in the case of an emergency, it is done at the bedside. Patients undergo apheresis for a variety of medical reasons. Plasma apheresis is performed on people affected by platelet disorders, such as **thrombotic thrombocytopenic purpura** (TTP). It is used to harvest peripheral blood stem cells, which are located in the same layer as the white blood cells. The stem cells are then transplanted back to the patient at a later time as part of certain cancer treatments or other blood disorders. People with severely high cholesterol levels (i.e., 900 or higher), have the cholesterol removed through the apheresis process. Other conditions, such as **thalassemia** and **antiphospholipid syndrome,** are treated in the apheresis clinic.

This process can take hours. Massage is a welcome and pleasant distraction (Figure 13-5). However, there are a number of potential complications relative to touch therapy. As with hemodialysis, apheresis patients can become medically unstable in a short period of time due to the decrease of blood volume combined with the centrifuging of the blood. Also, the ability of the blood cells to function is affected after being whirled through the machine. **Hypocalcemia** can be caused due to the drugs that are mixed in with the blood to prevent it from coagulating in the machine. Signs of this are tingling around the mouth, fatigue, dizziness, and cramps in the extremities. Heparin is also used to avoid coagulation of the blood. Easy bleeding and bruising is a side effect of this, especially when the

blood is returned to the body. Certain apheresis procedures remove the platelets, which further causes easy bruising or bleeding. And finally, the central line puts patients at increased risk for phlebitis, infection, and thrombosis. (Personal interview with Patti Wyman, RN, on September 2, 2003.)

Bodywork given during and shortly after this process should be very light and undemanding. The area around the catheter should not be directly touched, and the limb on the catheter side should only be touched with extra gentleness due to the risk of clot formation. For the most part, patients need to remain supine or semireclining. Foot, head, neck, shoulder, and hand massage are particularly appropriate in this setting. Because of the potential for patients to become medically unstable, the nurse-to-patient ratio is very low in an apheresis unit. There will always be someone nearby to answer the massage therapist's questions.

MASSAGE FOR BONE MARROW AND STEM CELL TRANSPLANT PATIENTS

This form of treatment is most commonly associated with cancer care and could have been included in Chapter 6. However, because the side effects from a bone marrow or stem cell transplant are unique and much more severe than typical cancer treatment, the decision was made to present it in this chapter.

Blood **stem cells** are immature or primitive blood cells that grow into red blood cells, white blood cells, and platelets. In the past, these stem cells were obtained almost exclusively from the bone marrow, the collection of which is painful. Although some stem cells also circulate in the blood, their numbers are generally not sufficient for a full transplant. However, the creation of new drugs, such as Neupogen and Leukine, that stimulate white blood cell growth, has allowed stem cells to be harvested from the blood. This is a significantly more comfortable process than bone marrow collection. Because most centers no longer collect stem cells from the bone marrow and for the sake of ease, this procedure will be referred to as stem cell transplantation from this point forward, even though some bone marrow transplants still take place.

Stem cell transplantation is most often known for its function in treating certain cancers, particularly bone marrow–related ones, such as leukemias, lymphomas, and multiple myeloma. This process allows for the administration of higher-than-normal doses of chemotherapy, which increases the likelihood of curing the patient's disease. In the past, these high doses were often fatal because the patient receiving high-dose chemo has no immune system for 5 to 6 weeks. Today, however, with a stem cell transplantation, the transplanted cells "rescue" the immune system.

The role of stem cell transplantation in treating solid malignancies, such as testicular, lung, brain, and ovarian, is still being investigated. However, some nonmalignant diseases, such as aplastic anemia, myelodysplasia syndrome, and myelofibrosis, in which the bone marrow is defective, respond to transplantation with healthy stem cells from another donor. Also, research is being conducted into the effectiveness of stem cell transplantation on a variety of conditions, including multiple sclerosis, lupus, thalassemia, and severe rheumatoid arthritis.

There are two main types of transplantation, **autologous** and **allogeneic.** The type used is dependent on the disease and its level of advancement, patient's age, and donor availability. In autologous transplantation, patients donate their own stem cells before treatment. An allogeneic transplant involves the cells of a donor whose tissue matches that of the patient as closely as possible, such as a sibling.

Stem cell recipients are admitted to the hospital up to 7 days before the transplant to undergo what is known as a "conditioning regimen." This protocol involves high-dose chemotherapy, total body irradiation (TBI), or both. It is for the purpose of killing remaining cancer cells, suppressing the immune system to prevent rejection of the new cells, and creating space in the bone marrow for the cells to engraft. The days before transplantation are referred to as Day -7, Day -6, Day -5, etc.

Stem cell transplantation is not a surgical procedure like an organ transplant. It takes place in the patient's room and is similar to a blood transfusion. The stem cells are contained in a blood products bag that is hung on an IV pole and fed into the patient's central IV catheter. The day of the transplant is known as Day 0.

There is no medical reason that gentle touch modalities cannot be administered during stem cell infusion. However, patients are sometimes are so anxious that they are not receptive to the idea. Also, the nursing staff is particularly attentive during this time in case patients have a reaction to the preservative the cells are stored in. Allogeneic patients in particular may experience side effects similar to those from a blood transfusion—shortness of breath, chills, fever, rash, chest pain, and hypotension.

Engraftment, which takes 2 to 4 weeks, is the process of the stem cells traveling to the bone marrow and producing new blood cells. Until this occurs, patients are severely neutropenic and thrombocytopenic. The white blood cell count usually drops to 0.1 (the norm is 4.5 to 10), and platelets plummet to 10,000 (150,000 to 450,000 is the normal range). This is a dangerous time because the immune system is greatly compromised, and the patient is at risk for spontaneous bleeding into the brain or retina. The risk of bleeding is so severe that patients aren't allowed to brush their teeth in case the gums bleed.

A number of other side effects occur. The kidneys and liver may go into failure, and the heart and lungs become

toxic, potentially fatal complications. Patients who have allogeneic transplants almost always suffer from some degree of graft-versus-host disease (GVHD). The new stem cells (the graft) see the body (the host) as an enemy and attack it. GVHD can affect the skin, gastrointestinal (GI) tract, and liver, resulting in skin rashes or discoloration, nausea, vomiting and diarrhea, an inability to absorb nutrients, and liver dysfunction.[5] Even massage lotion will not absorb into the skin of some people with GVHD.

Stem cell transplantation is an isolating experience for patients due to the need to protect them from infectious agents during immunosuppression. (Fresh food and flowers are not even allowed due to the bacteria and fungi that are on them.) Emotional problems can arise during this time. Further contributing to mood shifts are drug reactions or the patient's lack of preparation for the physical and emotional intensity of the treatment. Anxiety, depression, and panic are common.

So far, a highly clinical picture has been presented. But no words can truly describe the "healing hell" of stem cell transplantation, particularly an allogeneic one. People frequently have fevers, tremors from cyclosporine, and mouth and esophageal sores from **mucositis,** making eating and talking impossible. The skin of the hands and feet can peel off down to the dermal layer, and then there is the fatigue, which is fierce and unyielding.

Massage is highly beneficial during this time but must be performed with great mindfulness and care. Nurses are very protective of their thrombocytopenic patients because of the risk of bleeding or bruising. A bruise for one of these patients is potentially a serious event. The touch therapist must use only the amount of pressure required to spread the lotion or apply noninvasive modalities such as Reiki, polarity, or cranialsacral therapies. Amazingly, patients with low platelets are just like many massage clients; they want more pressure. BUT, no matter how much the patients try to talk the therapist into it, the practitioner absolutely must use only gentle pressure! Besides the risk for bruising and bleeding, a number of other complications demand the use of light pressure—organ toxicity, fatigue, and nausea.

A THERAPIST'S JOURNAL
How Comfort Massage Changed My Life

I was enjoying freshman year of college in September of 2000, with no idea of what I wanted to do with my life. Socializing and elective classes were great, but my major remained undeclared. In December, life came to a halt when I was diagnosed with chronic myeloid leukemia. However, despite visits to the doctor, constant blood draws at the lab, and chemotherapy, I managed to finish one more term of school.

The next spring, a bone marrow transplant was needed. It was a second chance at life and ultimately was my cure. I was on the transplant unit for about a month. The first 2 days, I received chemotherapy, followed by 4 days of radiation. Then came the actual transplant, which was more like a blood transfusion rather than surgery. I had a catheter in my chest with a line directly to the main arteries. This carried the new marrow into my bloodstream, which then found its way to my bones. It's a very confusing process that I let the doctors and God handle.

Each day ended with a massage from my mother. Not only was this soothing and comforting, but it was also a way to replenish my skin with moisture depleted by the medications, chemo, and radiation. The power of healing through touch was the best medication I could have received. After being poked and prodded all day by doctors and nurses, it was nice to be touched like a human being instead of a science project.

While in the hospital, visitors were limited to family and a few close friends. One afternoon, I had an unexpected visitor. I welcomed her, but with a sense of vulnerability. A local massage school had students on the cancer and bone marrow units to give massages to patients as well as their caregivers. I had never received a massage other than those my mother had given me. At first I was very scared, but who would pass up a free massage?

Once I let myself relax, I was amazed that I was able to let my mind wander, releasing the fear of someone I didn't know being so close to me. I was bald from chemo and had gained weight from prednisone, an antirejection medication. Letting someone other than family or friends touch me was difficult, but I was quickly able to get past this issue.

The road to recovery was not as easy as the transplant itself. Once out of the hospital, I needed a long healing period. This gave me time to think about my future. Finally, I made the decision to pursue massage therapy. Now, after just two terms in school, I know with confidence what I will do with the rest of my life. I don't yet know where I will go when massage school is finished. Maybe I will work with oncology patients, maybe with infants. But, I do know that massaging others is as helpful to me as it is to them, and what began as a devastating prognosis has turned into a new life with new horizons ahead.

Jessica Glade, massage student, Portland, Oregon

Patients are discharged when the blood counts have returned to certain levels, generally 15 to 30 days after transplant. However, they must remain within 20 to 30 minutes from the hospital for an extended period of time, usually 80 to 100 days. A medical crisis can develop quickly for stem cell recipients, and they must be able to get to the hospital rapidly if an emergency occurs.

The body, particularly the immune system, requires a lengthy period of time to recover from a stem cell transplant. Those who have undergone an autologous transplant recover more quickly; recovery from an allogeneic transplant may take up to 2 years. Some people never completely recover.

Following discharge from the hospital, transplant patients should continue receiving bodywork that is nondemanding, and therapists should strictly adhere to Standard Precautions. They should slowly work up to a firmer pressure over a long period of time as the patient's energy returns, remembering that less is better. Most patients experience some level of fatigue for an extended amount of time, often more than a year. GVHD can continue for years. One patient who is 9 years old still has bouts that cause a scleroderma-like hardening of the skin and GI problems. Another woman who received her own cells describes her energy level as only 80% of normal 18 months after transplantation and suffers from a form of GVHD that makes her joints and muscles ache. Many transplant patients are on prednisone, especially if they are affected by GVHD.

Practitioners are perhaps reading this section with wide eyes, wondering if they dare massage people affected by such grave complications. The answer is yes. Massage is one of the few pleasant sensations patients experience, especially during hospitalization. Massage gives them something to look forward to during the longs days of semi-isolation. It can temporarily reduce anxiety, pain, fatigue, nausea, and even neutropenic fevers. One person even told her therapist that massage gave her the will to live.[5-7]

MASSAGE ADJUSTMENTS NEEDED FOR ORGAN TRANSPLANT PATIENTS

What was once a novel treatment for organ failure has become almost commonplace. As of October 2003, almost 83,000 people were listed as transplant candidates. The majority of those, nearly 56,000, are waiting for a kidney to become available. More than 17,000 are listed for a liver, and 3,600 are waiting for a heart.[8]

Anecdotal evidence shows touch therapy and other complementary modalities to be extremely beneficial before and after transplantation. Julie Motz has even blazed a trail for the use of energy work in the operating room during transplantation. A description of this can be found in her book *Hands of Life*.[9]

PRETRANSPLANT

Organ transplantation is characterized by waiting. People not in crucial need of a new organ wait in their hometown with a beeper for word that an organ matching their tissue type and body size is available. Those who are medically unstable wait in the hospital, where they can receive the medications and care necessary to sustain their life. Sometimes the wait is weeks; sometimes, as with a heart, it can be many months.

Mark waited for 6 months in the hospital for a new heart. The old one had suffered numerous myocardial infarctions and the implantation of several pacemakers and portable defibrillators. When his kidneys stopped working, Mark was admitted to the hospital until a new heart could be found. His first massage was received several hours after "coding." Earlier in the day, his mother had received a massage in the ICU waiting room. A little later, she came back to ask if the touch practitioner would go into the ICU and massage her son, who had had a bad day. (Coding definitely qualifies as a bad day!)

The wait is longest for those needing a new kidney; often, it takes years. Unless a friend or family member is able and willing to donate a kidney, the person with severe renal disease frequently is kept alive by dialysis. In addition to the waiting, fatigue is part of the shared experience for those in organ failure, as well as hypertension and often depression or anxiety. However, each group displays specific side effects, depending on the organs involved.

Kidney Failure

Chronic kidney failure is often a result of multiple system disorders. Patients may be in congestive heart failure and often are on medications to control blood pressure. Sustained high blood pressure and diabetes are two of the root causes of scarring in the kidneys. Because the kidneys aren't processing the body's fluid, it may accumulate in the extremities, causing edema. Shortness of breath can also accompany the buildup of fluid, which pushes on the heart and lungs. Electrolyte levels can be affected, as the kidneys are an important factor in their regulation.[10] (Personal interview with Judy Schwarz, MSW, kidney transplant social worker, on October 2, 2003.)

Liver Failure

The person in liver failure will experience a buildup of fluid in the abdomen, referred to as ascites. Ammonia, one of the toxins metabolized by a healthy liver, accumulates, causing poor mental functioning, confusion, and irritability. Platelet levels drop due to coagulopathy, putting the person at risk for bleeding, and electrolytes can become unbalanced, causing severe muscle cramping. GI problems such as nausea, diarrhea, and constipation are common, as is significant weight loss. Bile salts are deposited on the skin, leading to severe itching, also known as pruri-

---

A THERAPIST'S JOURNAL
Preparing for Organ Donation

My partner generously donated a kidney to a friend who had been in renal failure for many years. No one enters into such a life-altering decision lightly. As a close observer and caregiver, I can offer insight into the process of both the donor and recipient. A combination of many things contributed to the successful outcome — massage, guided imagery, and antinausea herbs used postsurgically.

The donor, Priscilla, prepared physically, mentally, emotionally, and spiritually before the actual procedure. She lost weight, exercised, used guided-imagery tapes in preparation for surgery, received bodywork, increased her regular intake of supplements, asked for and received support, and took time to seriously grieve the permanent loss of a healthy body part.

Before the surgery, I did a combination of full-body general massage and foot reflexology to soft music. The bodywork provided a sense of support and nurturing . . . a way of preparing and sending the body off to do a very difficult task. We paid special attention to the left kidney, the one chosen to take up residence elsewhere, and expressed words of appreciation and well-being during the transition to a new body. We used the quiet and safety of the treatment to express sadness over the physical loss of such an extraordinary organ, which had worked a lifetime at keeping the body well. I would gently place my hands over the kidneys but did very little massage, mostly holding and just being with the area. Foot reflexology was the most requested modality and most comfortably given and received. We listened to Belleruth Naparstek's "Preparing For Surgery" CD for many nights until those safe and healing images became part of our consciousness. I used lavender oil to create a sense of well-being as well as for the universal healing benefit it provides. During the surgery to remove her kidney, Priscilla also listening to comforting music.

As the massage therapist and designated caregiver after the surgery, I made a concentrated effort to center myself and clear any negativity or fear that might have been present during the hands-on time. I chose to deal with my own personal feelings about the procedure at more appropriate times so as to create the most pure exchange possible. Being an active participant in such a profound experience requires a calm presence and the ability to make the donor the focus of good thoughts and positive energy.

Immediately after surgery, the only touch Priscilla wanted was very gentle work on the feet and gentle stroking *around the face and scalp. The nursing staff advised against massage to the legs until several weeks later to avoid any chance of blood clots. Foot reflexology provided a sense of grounding and support and allowed for some means of maintaining a physical connection during the hospitalization. Priscilla's nausea and pain required a modification in the type of touch provided. Some of the discomfort was caused by carbon dioxide gas in the abdominal and chest cavities. Again, foot reflexology proved to be the best modality to use since the areas in pain could not be directly touched. I also performed some Therapeutic Touch in the hospital, noticing some temperature differences while moving over the abdominal area postsurgery.*

Since returning home, chair massage for the neck and shoulder area has been very helpful because lying prone is not yet possible. The abdominal area is still a very vulnerable area, and touch there has been avoided. Foot reflexology is also being given, along with gentle stroking of the hands, arms, and face. As soon as the incision is totally healed, I intend to do some cross-fiber friction on the scars.

Massage therapists can play a significant role in the healing and recovery process with clients, family, and friends who are facing surgery. Simple touch can provide extraordinary results. When we touch skin, we touch the soul. I now have a greater sense of the power we have as massage therapists. I felt honored and humbled to have witnessed the courage of those undergoing such unbelievable procedures and in knowing that my touch played a role in helping to provide pain relief and support. This experience also opened my eyes to the extraordinary job our bodies do for us everyday. I now take time to express gratitude to my own organs.

A month later, both donor and recipient are doing well. The separated kidneys have been given names to identify who they belong to. They are now referred to as Thelma and Louise, with Priscilla keeping Thelma, and Lou receiving Louise.

Carol Weinert, LMT, Batavia, Ohio

tus. People in liver failure may be on diuretics, lactulose to counteract the ammonia buildup, antibiotics to suppress enteric bacteria, antiemetics, and pain medication.[11] (Personal interview with Kim Howell on September 26, 2003.)

Heart Failure

As with the need for a liver transplant, there is a sense of urgency about being placed on the heart transplant list.

The person needing a new heart can be sustained for a certain period of time on medications or a ventricular assist device, but not indefinitely. Fatigue, shortness of breath, edema, depression, and agitation are common symptoms. Those who require hospitalization, such as Iris in the Test Yourself feature of Chapter 11, may have a long, tedious wait. Hers was 8 months. A number of drugs may be used to support the heart, control blood pressure, thin the blood, expel excess fluids, and fight against the emotional side effects of the experience.

Massage Adjustments Before Transplantation

As with all medically fragile patients, touch therapy should place minimal demand on the body. It is impossible to give a blanket answer regarding the amount of pressure. Some people can easily tolerate a moderate amount of acupressure to sore muscles. Mark, for instance, the previously mentioned heart transplant patient, was a fairly fit individual before placement on the transplant list. He wanted, and coped well with, a limited amount of firm pressure. Others are so fragile that they should have no more pressure than it takes to apply lotion. Therapists should work with the healthcare staff to create a massage plan.

Each of these organ transplant groups can be affected by edema, pain medications, and antidepressants. Therapists also must be aware that those with liver disease have a tendency toward easy bleeding, and liver and kidney patients have particularly high levels of toxins. Other adjustments to the massage, such as positioning for breathing difficulties or elevation for edematous limbs, have been addressed in other parts of the book.

POSTTRANSPLANT

After transplantation, patients will be on immunosuppressive drugs, often cyclosporine, for the remainder of their lives to prevent rejection of the new organ. The majority of long-term complications are related to the immunosuppression caused by these medications. (Refer to the section on Immunosuppression in Chapter 7 for information and guidance.) For a few months, or less, following the surgery, patients also will be on a long list of other drugs such as antifungals, antivirals, antibacterials, corticosteroids, analgesics, diuretics, laxatives, and antianxiolytics. Often, blood pressure medications must be included.[12–14]

Massage Adjustments Following Transplantation

Touch therapy can be initiated immediately after surgery, gradually becoming firmer as the months unfold. Initially, adjustments must be made due to the risk for deep vein thrombosis, easy bruising or bleeding, pain medications, and fatigue. Positioning adjustments also will need to be made because of the incision. Mostly, this is a matter of common sense and can be guided by the patient. Those who have had a heart transplant will be unable to lie prone for many months due to the sternotomy, which requires a prolonged healing period. Even when the cardiac patient is able to lie facedown, no compression should be performed on the back until another few months at least. Administer shearing strokes on a horizontal plane to avoid causing discomfort to the sternum.

SUMMARY

Most touch practitioners feel an affinity for certain groups of patients. Sometimes a therapist will want to work with that group of people so much that she aches. Listening to that call and following it is important. That pull is showing therapists where their gift lies.

It is also essential to understand the need for training and supervised experience rather than just assuming that intuition and good intentions will be enough. This is especially true when working with certain groups such as psychiatric patients, those with eating disorders, or preterm infants. Therapists with sufficient experience may find it easy to cross over from oncology to organ transplantation or cardiology to general medicine. However, crossing over to certain other departments requires intense learning, well thought out protocols, and frequent communication with the staff.

TEST YOURSELF

Return to one of the following sections, apheresis, bone marrow and stem cell transplantation, organ transplantation, pediatric and adolescent eating disorders, or psychiatric diagnoses, and organize the precautions by pressure, site, and position adjustments.

REFERENCES

1. Hart S, Field T, Hernandez-Reif M, et al. Anorexia Nervosa Symptoms Are Reduced by Massage Therapy. Eat Disord 2001;9:289–299.
2. Field T, Schanberg S, Kuhn C, et al. Bulimic Adolescents Benefit From Massage Therapy. Adolescence 1998;33:555–563.
3. Sinclair M. Pediatric Massage Therapy. Philadelphia: Lippincott Williams & Wilkins, 2004.
4. Field T. Touch Therapy. Edinburgh, Scotland: Churchill Livingstone, 2000.
5. Randolph SR. Home Care of the Bone Marrow Transplant Recipient. Home Healthc Nurse 1993;11(1):24–28.
6. Maningo J. Peripheral Blood Stem Cell Transplant: Easier Than Getting Blood From a Bone. Nursing2002 2002;32(12):52–55.
7. Keller C. Bone Marrow and Stem Cell Transplantation in Oncology Nursing. 4th Ed. St. Louis, MO: Mosby, 2001.
8. The Organ Procurement and Transplantation Network. Data. Available at: www.optn.org/data/. Accessed October 3, 2003.
9. Motz J. Hands of Life: From the Operating Room to Your Home, An Energy Healer Reveals the Secrets of Using Your Body's Own Energy Medicine for Healing, Recovery, and Transformation. New York, NY: Bantam Books, 1998.
10. The Organ Procurement and Transplantation Network. Organ Datasource: Kidney. Available at: www.optn.org/organDatasource/about.asp?display=Kidney. Accessed October 3, 2003.
11. Nettina S. The Lippincott Manual of Nursing Practice. 7th Ed. Philadelphia, PA: Lippincott Williams & Wilkins, 2001.
12. University of Southern California Kidney Transplant Program. Long-Term Complications. Available at: www.kidneytransplant.org/longtermcomplications.html. Accessed October 3, 2003.
13. Outpatient Management of Adult Liver Transplant Recipients. Stanford University Liver Transplant Program. Available at: www.med.stanford.edu/shs/txp/livertxp/. Accessed October 3, 2003.
14. Health Alliance. Liver Transplant Timeline: Care and Concerns After Your Transplant. Available at: www.health-alliance.com/transplant/liver_time_post.html. Accessed October 3, 2003.

ADDITIONAL RESOURCES

DeVito M. Eating Disorders: Finding Balance Through Energy Work. Massage Bodywork February/March 2002:84–92.

Edwards D, Bruce G. For Cerebral Palsy Patients, Massage Makes Life Better. Massage Mag 2001;92:93–110.

Farlow P. Touch to Teach: Massage Helps Special Needs Children. Massage Mag 2000;88:106–116.

Foundation for Human Enrichment. A Naturalistic Approach in Healing Trauma: Somatic Experiencing® (training that addresses trauma issues), www.traumahealing.com.

Mines S. War and the Body: Serving the Survivors. Massage Bodywork August/September 2003:74–83.

The TARA Approach for the Resolution of Shock and Trauma, www.tara-approach.org.

United Network for Organ Sharing, www.unos.org.

COMMON ABBREVIATIONS

Healthcare facilities each have abbreviations that are specific to them and that they consider "official." Some of these shortened forms may be different than indicated here. The following, however, are common to many healthcare settings, especially hospitals. Many medical words and abbreviations have Latin origins. For instance, the abbreviation for "before" is $\bar{a}$, which comes from the Latin word "ante." Where the Latin derivation is known, it is indicated parenthetically.

The reader will notice that some abbreviations are in capital letters, others are in lowercase, and still others are a mixture. It is important that they be used in this way. For instance, while uppercase "CA" is the frequent abbreviation for "cancer," "Ca" is the shortened version of "calcium" and "cardiac arrest." Sometimes identical abbreviations will be found that stand for different phrases. CVA can indicate a "cerebrovascular accident" or "costal vertebral angle." The usage will be dependent on the context and field of specialization. And, bear in mind that each medical care facility may use abbreviations slightly differently.

This section is not meant to be all-inclusive. There are far too many abbreviations to list even half of them. The handful highlighted here is only meant to give bodyworkers a start so that they may better understand the language around them.

$\bar{a}$ (ante)	before
ac (ante cibum)	before meals
ADL	activities of daily living
A&P	anterior and posterior
bid (bis in die)	two times a day
BP	blood pressure
bpm	beats per minute
bs	breath sounds
Bx	biopsy
$\bar{c}$ (cum)	with
CA	cancer
CABG	coronary artery bypass graft
CBC	complete blood count
cc	chief complaint
CCU	coronary care unit; critical care unit
CHF	congestive heart failure
CNS	central nervous system
c/o	complains of
COPD	chronic obstructive pulmonary disease
CVA	cerebrovascular accident (stroke)
DVT	deep vein thrombosis
Dx	diagnosis
ECG	electrocardiogram
EEG	electroencephalogram
EMG	electromyogram
ENT	ear, nose, and throat
Fx	fracture
GI	gastrointestinal
GU	genitourinary
GYN	gynecology
H, hr	hour
H_2O	water
Hct, HCT	hematocrit
HIPAA	Health Insurance Portability and Accountability Act
h/o	history of
HOH	hard of hearing
HR	heart rate
hs (hora somni)	bedtime (hour of sleep)
Hx	history
ICU	intensive care unit
IM	intramuscular
inf	inferior
I&O	intake and output
IV	intravenous
JCAHO	Joint Commission on Accreditation of Healthcare Organizations
lat	lateral
Lt, L, Ⓛ	left
MI	myocardial infarction
MRI	magnetic resonance imaging
MRSA	methicillin-resistant *Staphylococcus aureus*
NG	nasogastric
NPO	nothing by mouth
NWB	non–weight bearing
O_2	oxygen
OSHA	Occupational Safety and Health Administration
OT	occupational therapy
$\bar{p}$	post
P	pulse
PACU	postanesthesia care unit (recovery room)
pc (post cibum)	after meals

PCA	patient-controlled analgesia	SOB	short of breath
PET	positron-emission tomography	stat	immediately
PICC	peripherally inserted central catheter	SVO_2	saturated venous oxygen
		Sx	symptom, sign
PO (per os)	by mouth	T	temperature
prn (pro re nata)	as needed	TIA	transient ischemic attack
pt	patient	tid (ter in die)	three times a day
PT	physical therapy	TPN	total parenteral nutrition
q (quaque)	every	Tx	treatment
qid (quater in die)	four times a day	UA	urinalysis
R	respiration	URI	upper respiratory infection
rt, R, Ⓡ	right	UTI	urinary tract infection
Rx	prescription	VRE	vancomycin-resistant enterococcus
s̄	without		
SaO_2	systemic arterial oxygen saturation	vs	vital signs
		WBC	white blood count

GLOSSARY OF TOUCH MODALITIES

Most touch modalities, even those with a reputation for being vigorous, such as Thai massage or myofascial release, can be adjusted for use with seriously ill people. Below are some of the techniques that are commonly used in healthcare settings or that can be used with minimal adjustment. Space considerations necessitate an abbreviated listing.

Acupressure has its roots in the Chinese medical system and is closely related to acupuncture. In this philosophy, the body contains hundreds of small energy centers, or acupoints, close to the surface arranged along energy channels referred to as meridians. Putting pressure on these points can either activate the "chi," which translates to "life-force energy," or drain excess chi. Disease is believed to be the result of a disturbance in the flow of chi, and reestablishing the flow stimulates the body's ability to heal itself. Acupressure practitioners use a gentle but deep finger pressure. Clients receive sessions while fully dressed, usually on a floor mat or massage table. Acupressure can, however, be adapted to the hospital bed. Recipients find these sessions to be both stimulating and relaxing, which can ease the fatigue that accompanies illness. Only a very light pressure should be used when patients are medically fragile. Also see "Shiatsu."

The **Bowen Technique** is the invention of Australian Tom Bowen. Mirka Knaster compares practitioners of his modality to piano tuners because of the way they gently pluck tendons, nerves, and muscle fascia. Joints are freed, muscles relaxed, the functioning of the blood and lymph systems improved, and the energy and organ systems balanced. None of the usual massage strokes, such as pounding, stroking, or pressing, are used. Sessions are given without oil. The clothes can be kept on. Because of its gentle nature, the Bowen Technique can be used at all stages of health. Many ailments respond to this style of work: Bell's palsy, bursitis, sports injuries, scoliosis, constipation, and colic, for example.[1]

Compassionate Touch®, developed by Dawn Nelson, is a therapeutic modality for relating to elderly and/or ill individuals. It combines one-on-one focused attention, gentle touch, and other relaxation techniques with communication skills such as active listening, reflective feedback, and position instruction. All patients would benefit from receiving this modality. Sessions can be received in a hospital bed, wheelchair, or on a massage table. Recipients can remain clothed or partially clothed or may completely disrobe.[2]

Cranialsacral therapies work to balance the flow of the cerebrospinal fluid to restore optimum functioning to the central nervous system and ultimately the entire body. The practitioner uses gentle compressions to realign bones and soft tissue in the skull, mouth, face, vertebral column, and sacrum, thereby allowing the cerebrospinal fluid to flow freely. While these therapies can be used to resolve specific maladies such as headaches, neck and back pain, or balance problems, they also are useful in freeing accumulated stress, which is beneficial to patients at any time. Sessions are received clothed in a bed or on a massage table.

Esalen Massage was developed by practitioners at the Esalen Institute in Big Sur, California. This technique aims to relax by blending the long, flowing, gliding strokes of Swedish massage with light rocking, passive joint movement, and deeper tissue work, if appropriate. Esalen Massage conveys a sense of being nurtured and supported and reunifies body, mind, and spirit. With modification, it can be administered at any stage of the illness experience, especially during treatment or any other time that requires a gentle modality. A lubricant is used, and sessions are performed with the client disrobed.

Jin Shin Jyutsu® is a Japanese modality that aims to balance the flow of chi, or life energy, by releasing energy that is blocked or redirecting it along the pathway. As with other Oriental systems, Jin Shin Jyutsu® is based on the idea that chi circulates in 12 major channels, or meridians. Practitioners "listen" to the 12 energy pulses at the wrist to determine where to place their hands. The body is not physically manipulated; instead, a light pressure is used along the energy pathways with the palms, fingertips, or back of the hand. Sessions are generally performed with the client clothed. This technique is ideally suited for those times a patient feels fragile.

Lomilomi was passed down from Hawaiian shaman, or kahunas, where it was performed as a spiritual practice. Known for using a deep pressure, particularly with the elbows and forearms, it also can include gentle strokes, pressing on special points, walking on the back, and rhythmical rocking. Historically, Hawaiians used Lomilomi in childbirth, for congestion, inflammation, circulatory problems, asthma, bronchitis, rheumatism, and musculoskeletal conditions. It is believed to stimulate the life force, or mana. Sessions are given using oil. The client is unclothed. It goes without saying that only gentle strokes should be used if the patient is medically fragile.

Lymph drainage techniques use "light, slow, repetitive strokes specifically designed to boost the circulation of the lymphatic system."[3] This assists the body in removing excess fluids, toxins, and substances such as proteins, immune cells, and fatty acids. Lymph drainage therapies, of which there are many versions, are especially helpful for postmastectomy patients in relieving pain, fibrosis, and edema and in regenerating scarred tissue. In addition, headaches, insomnia, chronic fatigue syndrome and fibromyalgia, acne, eczema, and allergies respond well to these techniques. Clients receive sessions unclothed on a massage table or in a hospital bed.

Myofascial release frees tension in the connective tissue, or fascia, that surrounds and supports muscles, bones, and organs. This allows the body to regain proper structural alignment, relieves pain associated with adhesions, increases range of motion and function, and can release emotional trauma. A sustained pressure is used with the fingers, hand, forearms, and elbows to apply "long, slow, gliding strokes to stretch . . . the fascia."[3] Practitioners of myofascial release have reported improvement in such conditions as fibromyalgia, temporomandibular joint (TMJ) syndrome, headaches, birth trauma, sports injuries, and neurological and movement dysfunctions. Patients may find this technique useful to work out adhesions that develop from surgical incisions or fibrosis from radiation. Only implement gentle myofascial release during illness.

Neuromuscular Therapy. See "Trigger-point therapy."

Polarity therapy combines Western and Eastern principles of healing. The aim is to balance negative and positive poles of electrical energy in the body. Dr. Randolph Stone, the originator of polarity therapy, believed that "universal energy" flowed in specific patterns between negative and positive electrical poles both inside and outside the body. These patterns consist of five vertical currents, as well as horizontal zones, that are positive, neutral, and negatively charged. Polarity therapy works to restore the flow in places where it has become blocked or to dissipate energy in areas where there is too much. Generally, this technique is gentle, noninvasive, and nurturing. However, deeper pressure may be called for at times. Sessions can be performed in a chair, in a bed, or on a massage table. The client may be clothed or unclothed. In addition to being useful when the patient feels fragile, this system of healing also provides a way to affect areas of the body that cannot be touched directly, such as an incision or an abdomen that is painful due to blocked bowels. By working above and below the site, energy flow can be reestablished without touching the area.

Reflexology is administered primarily to the feet and sometimes to the hands. This modality operates under the principle that every part of the body is associated with a corresponding place on the foot. By stimulating a specific point on the foot, positive effects can be realized to the reciprocal part of the body. For instance, an area at the base of the big toe corresponds with the thyroid gland. By pressing this point, energy will be activated that can "reflex" to the thyroid, thus helping it function better. Reflexologists apply a deep pressure with the thumbs. Modification in pressure may be needed for people who are seriously ill. Reflexology is especially useful for conditions in which massage directly to an area is inadvisable or not tolerated by the patient, such as constipation or a surgical site.

Reiki is a Japanese word that roughly translated means "universal life force." It is a method of natural healing designed to strengthen a person's absorption of universal life energy (similar to chi). This technique is nonmanipulative and works with or without touch, as necessary. It balances and aligns the body's energy and energy field, systematically teaches people how to access and use universal energy for stress management and personal growth, and helps the body, mind, emotions, and spirit regain balance. Practitioners serve as a conduit to universal life energy and may transmit it directly to clients by giving hands-on treatments or by conducting it through "distance healing." One way to describe the hands-on sessions is "sacred touch." Sessions are given with the recipient being clothed and consist of a series of hand positions that begin at the head and systematically work toward the feet. A pressureless touch with no movement or stroking is used. Recipients find the sessions to be calming, nurturing, and undemanding. Reiki is an excellent modality for people who are medically fragile, following surgery, or at times when it is inadvisable to apply strokes that increase circulation or use pressure, such as with thrombocytopenia or deep vein thrombosis. In addition to being useful as a hands-on technique, Reiki also can be beneficial for situations in which the practitioner is unable to be with the patient, such as in the operating room, during procedures, or if the practitioner lives in another city. This "distance healing," which some liken to prayer, is useful during these times. Another feature of Reiki is that it can be self-administered and is extremely simple. Anyone can learn to be a practitioner, even children. Many other systems have been formed around the Reiki modality, such as The Radiance Technique and Mariel.

Russian massage (Kurashova Method) is a common, well-accepted form of treatment in Russian hospitals, clinics, and wellness resorts. The strokes administered in this technique look similar to those used in Swedish massage. The focus, however, is not on the anatomical structure as with most bodywork therapies, but is on the body's physiology. According to Zhenya Wine of the Kurashova Institute, Russian massage is based on the idea that the body is its own best healer and "that massage can teach the body how to heal itself." Soviet physicians developed this form of treatment to solve post WWII health problems and have performed 80% of the world's massage research. The Kurashova Method is used to treat many dysfunctions such as neuralgia, scoliosis, arthritis, fractures, and tendon or ligament damage. In many cases, patients are able to replace drugs with these massage techniques. It is also given for relaxation, to enhance athletic performance, and to energize the body.[4] The strokes, which are painless and non-invasive, can be applied gently or deeply, as needed, and therefore can be adapted to any stage of illness. Sessions can be given on a massage table or hospital bed, generally with the client unclothed.

Seated chair massage, also known as "on-site massage," generally focuses on the recipient's head, neck, back, and arms. The client sits/kneels on a padded chair specially designed to support the face, chest, and arms. The massage is usually 10 to 20 minutes in length and is given through the clothing, using such techniques as compression, acupressure, kneading, and stretching. Chair massage is especially helpful in the hospital for family caregivers.

Shiatsu is a cousin of acupressure. In Japanese, it means "finger pressure." However, the hands, elbows, or knees may also be used on the acupoints along the meridians if the patient's health level is sufficient. This technique aims to balance the flow of vital life energy, or ki. (Ki is the Japanese word for chi.) Shiatsu is a synthesis of modern information from Western anatomy and physiology and the principles of traditional Japanese massage. Its purpose is not just relaxation, but as a tool to treat disease. Different styles of Shiatsu are practiced, each with its own emphasis. Some focus on the meridians, others on the neuromuscular system. Buddhist philosophy, breathing practices, and exercises to stimulate ki are features in various schools of Shiatsu. Stretching and range of motion usually are involved. Sessions are generally performed on a floor mat with the client clothed but can also be administered in a hospital bed or on a massage table.

Swedish massage is the most commonly practiced bodywork modality in the West. Long, gliding strokes (effleurage) or rhythmical, kneading strokes (petrissage) form the basis of the sessions. Three other strokes are also included in this system: friction, vibration, and tapotement (tapping). Swedish massage sessions are designed to produce relaxation and increase circulation, which may help the body flush out toxins and bring fresh nutrients to the tissues. In addition, it can be used for stimulation, rehabilitation, and recovery from strains and trauma. Effleurage is one of the staples of a bodyworker who gives massage to the ill. This stroke can be modified to fit almost any situation. Swedish massage is applied directly to the skin. The body is draped with a towel or sheet; only the part being massaged will be exposed. Oil or lotion is applied to facilitate the rhythmical, gliding motion.

Therapeutic Touch (TT) is based on the idea that our energy extends beyond the skin into an "energy field" that surrounds and interpenetrates the body. Illness is believed to be influenced by imbalances or blockages in the energy field, also known as the aura. TT aims to assist the physical body by attuning the energy field around it. Practitioners generally do not touch the body, but work with the hands in the energy field. Reestablishing proper energy flow then allows the individual's own healing powers to take over.[5] Because this modality is not administered directly to the body, it can be given at all stages of illness and may be especially helpful for situations in which touch is not tolerated by the patient or is inadvisable, as in the case of bone metastases, incisions, or deep vein thrombosis.

Trager Psychophysical Integration® is the creation of Milton Trager, MD. Dr. Trager taught that the mind is the source of pain, rigid movement, and dysfunction, and that by releasing the body's holding patterns, the mind also will be liberated. These holding patterns may have developed as a reaction to emotional injury, surgery, an accident, or disease. The trademark of a Trager session is a gentle, steady, rhythmical rocking by the practitioner, which seeks to impart a sense of lightness and freedom to the client's unconscious mind. Deep relaxation, increased mobility, greater energy, and inner peace are created. The body is reminded of feeling open and free. Trager's work also includes a series of movement exercises called Mentastics, which the client performs at home to reinforce the feelings gained during the hands-on session. During his life, Dr. Trager was able to improve the health of people with a variety of neuromuscular disorders, such as multiple sclerosis, Parkinson's disease, polio, and stroke. With proper adaptation, Trager could be used with many patients who are in treatment or recovering from it. The gentle movements would help the patient let go of the fear accumulated in the body over months or years of treatment, improve functioning in areas affected by surgery, and increase energy and vitality.[6] Sessions can be conducted on a massage table or hospital bed and can be received clothed or unclothed.

Trigger-point therapy is a generic term for the variety of bodywork modalities used to release tender areas in the muscles that can be felt as lumps or knots. These sensitive areas are known as trigger points because they cause pain to radiate to other parts of the body. Trigger-point therapies, such as neuromuscular therapy and Bonnie Prudden's Myotherapy, use a deep, sustained pressure with the fingers. Stretching exercises are used following the release of a trigger point. Practitioners must be mindful of the amount of pressure applied to people who are seriously ill. Trigger-point modalities are used for muscle-related conditions such as headaches, whiplash, TMJ syndrome, sciatica, occupational and sports injuries, and carpal tunnel syndrome. Patients who have had to lie in contorted positions for an extended period of time during a procedure may find relief through this intervention. Treatments can be given on a massage table, seated massage chair, or in a hospital bed. A lubricant is not used so the treatment can be employed through clothing or on bare skin.

Zero Balancing® (ZB), created by Fritz Smith, MD, is a method of gentle touch used to align the body's skeletal structure with its flow of energy. Western concepts of anatomy, physiology, and kinesiology are brought together with Eastern concepts of energy currents, mechanisms of healing, and anatomy. The goal is not to fix or heal but to create a state within the body that will allow well-being and health to arise naturally. Contact with specific bony points is emphasized. One of the underlying beliefs is that bones contain the most dense and unconscious energy, and that one's deepest essence is carried within him. ZB does not diagnose illness nor claim to be a treatment for certain maladies. However, relief from physical and emotional symptoms may occur. In addition to gentle touch, pressing, lifting, pulling, twisting, stretching, and bending may be incorporated into the sessions if appropriate to the person's medical condition. Smith advises people with knee replacements to forego Zero Balancing®, and those with hip replacements to proceed with care.[7] With proper modification, ZB could be used for many ill people. During periods of fragility, it may be best to avoid the lifting, pulling, twisting, and bending, and apply only gentle touch and movements. Sessions are received clothed.

REFERENCES

1. Knaster M. Discovering the Body's Wisdom. New York: Bantam Books, 1996.
2. Nelson D. From the Heart Through the Hands. Findhorn, Scotland: Findhorn Press, 2001.
3. Claire T. Bodywork: What Type of Massage to Get—And How to Make the Most of It. New York: William Morrow, 1995.
4. Kurashova Institute brochure 1997.
5. Juhan D. The Trager Approach: Psychophysical Integration and Mentastics. Trager J Vol. II 1987.
6. Wager S. A Doctor's Guide to Therapeutic Touch. New York: Perigee Books, 1996.
7. Jerome T. Zero Balancing: Bodywork of Relationship. Massage Mag September/October 1997:35–43.

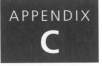

ADDITIONAL SAMPLE FORMS

Included in this section are a variety of forms contributed by other massage practitioners. All of the forms in this section are copyrighted. However, forms created by the author, C-1C, C-1D, and C-2B, can be used without permission. Other forms should not be copied; instead, therapists should use the ideas sparked by these samples to create a form specially tailored to their situation.

McKENZIE-WILLAMETTE HOSPITAL MASSAGE THERAPY REFERRAL

Patient Name _____ Room _____ Date _____

Massage Therapist _____ Referring RN _____

Note: MD order required in presence of: hemophilia, coagulopathy, bone mets, unstable spine, platelet count <20,000, **massage to legs post-op abdominal surgery** (feet do not need order).

Goal of Massage Therapy (check all that apply):

_____muscular tension in:

_____back _____shoulders _____neck _____head _____arms _____feet other_____

_____fatigue _____general relaxation _____anxiety _____stress

_____trouble sleeping _____instruction to family _____pain other _____

Current condition(s): _____

Medical diagnosis: _____

Secondary conditions: _____

Site of injury/surgery/procedure:

	Yes	No
Precautions:		
Fragile skin	____	____
Draining lesion	____	____
Infection	____	____
Deep vein thrombosis	____	____
Low platelet count	____	____
Osteoporosis	____	____
Neutropenia _____	____	____
Pain: Location _____	____	____
Edema: Location		

Postural limitations (check all that apply):

Cannot/should not lie: _____flat _____on back _____on abdomen _____on R side _____on L side

Cannot/should not: _____sit up _____walk Other:_____

O   T   H   E   R:

_____

_____

FIGURE C-1 ■ (A–D) Sample Intake Forms. (A) Reprinted with permission from McKenzie-Willamette Medical Center.

HOPES CHAIR MASSAGE PROGRAM

PATIENT NAME: _____

MGH ID #: _____

TODAY'S DATE: _____

PATIENT: Please check if you have any of the following conditions in YOUR HEAD, NECK OR ARM AREAS...

☐ Swelling
☐ Active Radiation Therapy
☐ Skin Reactions/Rashes
☐ Intravenous/Central Lines

PATIENT: Please read and sign the following statement...

I am requesting chair massage therapy, understanding that there is minimal risk of soft tissue injury and bruising. I have reported all health conditions that I am aware of and will inform my practitioner of any changes in my health.

Patient Signature _____ Date _____

_____

NURSE: Please complete the following checklist for the above identified patient...

☐ No evidence of Deep Vein Thrombosis within past 6 months

☐ Blood thinning medications for treatment other than line/port prophylaxis

☐ ANC greater than 1,000 (exceptions with approval from MD)

☐ Platelets greater than 50,000 (exceptions with approval from MD)

☐ No incisions or wounds in the massage fields

☐ No swelling/edema in the upper extremities

☐ No active infection that requires precautions (i.e. Shingles, Herpes, Chickenpox, respiratory)

☐ Patient has VRE or MRSA – use contact precautions

☐ No skin reactions/rashes in the massage field (exceptions with MD approval)

☐ Not receiving radiation therapy in the massage field

☐ No unstable medical conditions

☐ No central line in the massage field ** Note – if patient has central line in massage field, please alert massage therapist so that massage is not performed in that area

☐ No evidence of disease in the massage field

REVIEWED BY: _____
          (NURSE OR PHYSICIAN SIGNATURE)

FIGURE C-1 ■ (B) Reprinted with permission from Massachusetts General Hospital.

Massage Patient Data Form

PART A: (Nurse)

Patient Name _____ DOB _____ M   F

Unit _____   Room_____   Nurse _____ Today's Date _____

Dx _____   Secondary conditions _____

Surgery _____   Date of surgery _____

SENSORY IMPAIRMENT: ☐ Blind   ☐ HOH   ☐ speech   **FALL PRECAUTIONS:**   Y   N

PRESSURE RESTRICTIONS: Y   N   ☐ pain meds   ☐ edema   ☐ bone fragility

☐ DVT   ☐ bruises easily   ☐ extended bedrest   ☐ fatigue   ☐ nodal dissection   ☐ central line

SITE RESTRICTIONS: Y   N   **POSITION RESTRICTIONS:**   Y   N

_____ IV site   _____ skin condition   ☐ no walking   ☐ lay flat   ☐ logroll

_____ incision   _____ tumor   ☐ elevate extremity _____

_____ open wound   _____ infection   ☐ no prone   ☐ no sidelying

_____ ostomy   _____ pain   other: _____

other: _____

GLOVING REQUIRED: Y   N

☐ thiotepa or cytoxan (w/in 24 hrs)   ☐ open wound (pt or LMT)   ☐ skin condition   ☐ contact precaution

CHECK IF THE PATIENT HAS ANY OF THE FOLLOWING CONDITIONS:

☐ immunosuppressed   ☐ fever   ☐ contagious disease   ☐ allergy to lotion

other: _____

PART B: (Patient)

Has the patient ever received a professional massage?   Y   N
What would the patient like from the massage session?

Subjective –

PART C: SOAP NOTES (Therapist)

Objective –

Action –

Progress –

Therapist's Name_____   Length of session_____

FIGURE C-1 ■ (C) From Oregon Health and Science University.

Oncology Massage Patient Data Form

PART A: (Nurse)

Patient Name _____ DOB _____ Sex _____

Unit _____ Room _____ Nurse _____ Today's Date _____

Dx _____ Chemo: Y N   Hx of Radiation: Y N

Surgery_____ Date of surgery _____

SENSORY IMPAIRMENT: ☐ Blind   ☐ HOH   ☐ speech   **FALL PRECAUTIONS:** Y   N

PRESSURE RESTRICTIONS: Y   N

☐ DVT   ☐ heparin   ☐ ↓ plt   ☐ ↓ WBC   ☐ fatigue   ☐ nodal dissection   ☐ central line

SITE RESTRICTIONS: Y   N   **POSITION RESTRICTIONS:**   Y   N

_____ ostomy   _____ rash   ☐ no walking   ☐ lay flat   ☐ logroll

_____ incision   _____ tumor   _____ elevate extremity

_____ open wound   _____ infection   _____ posture limitations

_____ IV site   _____ drain   _____

GLOVING REQUIRED: Y   N

☐ thiotepa or cytoxan (within 24 hours)   ☐ open wound (patient or LMT)   ☐ skin condition

CHECK IF THE PATIENT HAS ANY OF THE FOLLOWING CONDITIONS:

☐ hepatitis   ☐ herpes   ☐ other contagious disease   ☐ allergy to lotion

other: _____

PART B: (Patient)

Has the patient ever received a professional massage?   Y   N

What would the patient like from the massage session?

Subjective —

PART C: SOAP NOTES (Therapist)

Objective —

Action —

Progress —

Therapist's Name _____ Length of session _____

FIGURE C-1 ■ (D) Sample of intake form specifically for oncology patients, from Oregon Health and Science University.

EVALUATION of
MASSAGE EXPERIENCE

The purpose of this form is to provide feedback to the massage students and therapists, which will assist them in their learning.

Patient: _____ Time of massage: _____

Massage Therapist: _____ Date: _____

BEFORE THE MASSAGE

Please circle the number that indicates your level of pain, physical and emotional comfort, and fatigue.

PAIN RATING:

No pain   0   1   2   3   4   5   6   7   8   9   10   Extreme pain

PHYSICAL COMFORT

| Extremely Comfortable | 1 | 2 | 3 | 4 | 5 | Extremely Uncomfortable |

EMOTIONAL COMFORT

| Extremely Comfortable | 1 | 2 | 3 | 4 | 5 | Extremely Uncomfortable |

FATIGUE

| No fatigue | 1 | 2 | 3 | 4 | 5 | Severe fatigue |

AFTER THE MASSAGE

List words that describe the sensations you noticed during the massage:

_____ _____ _____

PAIN RATING:

No pain   0   1   2   3   4   5   6   7   8   9   10   Extreme pain

PHYSICAL COMFORT

| Extremely Comfortable | 1 | 2 | 3 | 4 | 5 | Extremely Uncomfortable |

EMOTIONAL COMFORT

| Extremely Comfortable | 1 | 2 | 3 | 4 | 5 | Extremely Uncomfortable |

FATIGUE

| No fatigue | 1 | 2 | 3 | 4 | 5 | Severe fatigue |

THERAPIST FEEDBACK

Patient Responses: _____
_____
_____

Massage techniques used: _____
_____
_____

Length of session: _____ Time of rating: _____

Adapted from a Boulder Community Hospital feedback form developed by Karen Gibson.

FIGURE C-2 ■ (A–C) Patient Evaluation or Survey Forms. (A) From Oregon Health and Science University.

Date: _____

PLEASE CHECK ALL THAT APPLY:

<u>Your Gender:</u> ☐ Male ☐ Female   <u>Your Age:</u> ☐ under 35   ☐ 35–64   ☐ 65 and over

<u>Your Type of Cancer:</u>

☐ Brain   ☐ Head and Neck
☐ Breast   ☐ Hematology (lymphoma, leukemia etc)
☐ Connective Tissue (sarcomas etc.)   ☐ Melanoma
☐ Gastrointestinal (colon, pancreatic etc.)   ☐ Thoracic (lung, esophageal etc.)
☐ Genito-urinary (prostate, testicular etc.)   ☐ Other _____
☐ Gynecologic (ovarian, cervical etc.)

<u>Unit Where You Received Your Massage:</u>

☐ Bigelow 12 Infusion Unit   ☐ Blake 2 Infusion Unite
  Ellison 14   ☐ Radiation Oncology

---

1) AFTER MY CHAIR MASSAGE TODAY, I FEEL ....

	Strongly Agree	Agree	Neutral	Disagree	Strongly Disagree
Relaxed					
Anxious					
Calm					
Tense					
Energized					

2) Prior to this massage, how many chair massages have you had at MGH? _____

3) Have you had massages outside of the MGH?   ☐ Yes   ☐ No

4) Would you have a chair massage at MGH again?   ☐ Yes   ☐ No

5) I would recommend a chair massage to another patient.   ☐ Yes   ☐ No

Your comments (please feel free to use the back of this page as well):

_____

_____

_____

FIGURE C-2 ■ (B) Reprinted with permission from Massachusetts General Hospital.

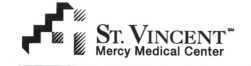

St. Vincent Mercy Medical Center
Integrative Medicine

Your opinion about Integrative Medicine Services is very important to us. Would you take a minute to complete the survey on the bottom of this card? Simply detach the survey once you have completed and drop it into the nearest mailbox. There is no postage required. Your answers will help us to provide the best treatment possible with the utmost in caring. To give you a better understanding of some of the services referred to in the survey, please refer to the definitions below. Thank you.

Services

1. **Massage Therapy:** Soft tissue manipulation that improves nutrition and circulation to the tissues while promoting a sense of well being.

2. **Guided Imagery:** Direct visualization that harnesses the power of the mind to help heal and alleviate symptoms such as pain, nausea, sleeplessness, and anxiety.

3. **Healing Touch & Reiki:** Both are forms of energy work that balance and restore the energy field of the body while promoting a deep sense of relaxation. These therapies are beneficial in controlling symptoms by using a very gentle form of touch. This could be quite useful to those patients who can only tolerate light touch.

— — — — — — — — — — — — — — — — DETACH HERE — — — — — — — — — — — — — — — —

For each of the following statements, indicate whether you would rate the service Poor, Fair, Good, Very Good, or Excellent by checking the box that best describes your feelings.

Amount of dignity and respect shown to you.
❏ Poor   ❏ Fair   ❏ Good   ❏ Very Good   ❏ Excellent

Compassion and understanding received from the therapist.
❏ Poor   ❏ Fair   ❏ Good   ❏ Very Good   ❏ Excellent

Amount of personal attention that you received.
❏ Poor   ❏ Fair   ❏ Good   ❏ Very Good   ❏ Excellent

Helpfulness of the treatment you received in reducing or eliminating pain.
❏ Poor   ❏ Fair   ❏ Good   ❏ Very Good   ❏ Excellent

Helpfulness of the treatment you received to promote or provide relaxation.
❏ Poor   ❏ Fair   ❏ Good   ❏ Very Good   ❏ Excellent

Overall quality of the treatment you received.
❏ Poor   ❏ Fair   ❏ Good   ❏ Very Good   ❏ Excellent

Would you be interested in receiving these services, i.e. massage therapy, energy work, guided imagery, as an outpatient?
❏ Yes   ❏ No

Additional comments about your experience with Integrative Medicine: _____

_____
_____
_____
_____
_____
_____

If you would like to comment further, please contact: Jeff Peterson, Executive V.P. & COO, St. Vincent Mercy Medical Center

FIGURE C-2 ■ (C) Reprinted with permission from St. Vincent Mercy Medical Center, Toledo, Ohio.

TEST YOURSELF ANSWERS

CHAPTER 3

1. No information should be divulged. Even the fact that the church member is in the hospital is confidential.
2. The therapist might answer, "I don't know anything about that patient. Masking, gloving, and gowning instructions are posted for a variety of reasons. Sometimes it's needed to protect patients whose immune system is suppressed. Other times it's to protect the nurses or the patient's family from a communicable situation."
3. "Only the patients themselves or designated family member can talk about the treatments being received at the hospital. Staff aren't allowed to share information with people outside the hospital for reasons of confidentiality."
4. No, even though in this case, the news was all good.
5. Only information that is relevant to a massage session should be shared with other touch therapists on the team. For instance, it would be relevant if the patient enjoys the sensation of pain and requests really deep massage from the therapists just for the sake of pain. Or, if the patient is prone to crossing boundaries with his comments, other therapists should be alerted so that they can be prepared.

CHAPTER 4

1. In which of the following situations should a massage therapist glove?
   A, C, E, F, G, and J
2. If a massage therapist is experiencing the following conditions, should she refrain from working with patients?
   A. No
   B. Yes
   C. Yes
   D. No
   E. Yes
3. True/False
   A. True
   B. False
   C. True
   D. True
   E. False

CHAPTER 5

1. A, B
2. A
3. A, B, C, D
4. B, D
5. A, B
6. A, B, D
7. A, B, D
8. A

CHAPTER 6

MR. WILLIAMS		
Pressure	**Site**	**Positioning**
infection	surgical site	elevation L foot
pain medication	L wrist	no prone
overall poor health	long-term insulin injection site	R side-lying OK
fragile skin		
neuropathy R foot		

MRS. JENNINGS		
Pressure	**Site**	**Positioning**
pain medications	abdomen	no prone
naproxen	L wrist	side-lying OK

CHAPTER 7

1. A, B, C
2. C, D
3. B, C, D
4. A, D
5. B, D
6. B
7. C, D
8. B
9. A
10. A, B, D

CHAPTER 8

MULTIPLE CHOICE

1. B, D
2. C
3. A, B
4. A, B, C
5. B, C
6. C
7. A, B
8. A, C, D

MATCHING

1. A
2. D
3. B
4. G
5. C
6. E
7. F

CHAPTER 9

1. D
2. B
3. A, B, C
4. A, B
5. C
6. A, B, D
7. D
8. C, D
9. B
10. A, D

CHAPTER 10

Massage Patient Data Form

PART A: (Nurse)

Patient Name _Katherine Sonora_ DOB _6/30/47_ M (F)

Unit _10A_ Room _12_ Nurse _Manny_ Today's Date _1/12/04_

Dx _____ Secondary conditions _____

Surgery _(L) Knee replacement_ Date of surgery _1/10/04_

SENSORY IMPAIRMENT: ☐ Blind ☐ HOH ☐ speech **FALL PRECAUTIONS:** (Y) N

PRESSURE RESTRICTIONS: (Y) N ☒ pain meds ☐ edema ☐ bone fragility

☒ DVT risk ☐ bruises easily ☒ extended bedrest ☐ fatigue ☐ nodal dissection ☐ central line

SITE RESTRICTIONS: (Y) N

(L) wrist IV site _____ skin condition
(L) knee incision _____ tumor
_____ open wound _____ infection
_____ ostomy (L) knee pain

other: _legs — no massage_

POSITION RESTRICTIONS: (Y) N

☒ no walking ☐ lay flat ☐ logroll
☒ elevate extremity (L) leg
☒ no prone ☐ no sidelying
other: _____

GLOVING REQUIRED: Y (N)

☐ thiotepa or cytoxan (w/in 24 hrs) ☐ open wound (pt or LMT) ☐ skin condition ☐ contact precaution

CHECK IF THE PATIENT HAS ANY OF THE FOLLOWING CONDITIONS:

☐ immunosuppressed ☐ fever ☐ contagious disease ☐ allergy to lotion

other: _Hx of stroke – 2001; (R) arm & shoulder ↓ sensation, ↑ weakness_

Oncology Massage Patient Data Form

PART A: (Nurse)

Patient Name ___Bill Nguyen_____ DOB _6/10/73_ Sex _M____

Unit _5A_____ Room _32_ Nurse _John_____ Today's Date _7/4/03_____

Dx _Testicular CA_____ Chemo: (Y) N   Hx of Radiation: Y (N)

Surgery (R) _testicle removed_____ Date of surgery _April 2003_

SENSORY IMPAIRMENT: ☐ Blind   ☐ HOH   ☐ speech   **FALL PRECAUTIONS:**   Y   (N)

PRESSURE RESTRICTIONS: (Y) N

☐ DVT   ☐ heparin   ☒ ↓ plt   ☒ ↓ WBC   ☒ fatigue   ☐ nodal dissection   ☒ central line

SITE RESTRICTIONS: (Y) N   **POSITION RESTRICTIONS:**   Y   (N)

_____ ostomy   _____ rash   ☐ no walking   ☐ lay flat   ☐ logroll

_____ incision   _____ tumor   _____ elevate extremity

_____ open wound _____ infection _____ posture limitations

(L) _arm_ IV site   _____ drain   _____

_herpes in pelvic area_____

GLOVING REQUIRED: (Y) N

☐ thiotepa or cytoxan (within 24 hours)   ☐ open wound (patient or LMT)   ☒ skin condition – _herpes_

CHECK IF THE PATIENT HAS ANY OF THE FOLLOWING CONDITIONS:

☐ hepatitis   ☒ herpes   ☐ other contagious disease   ☐ allergy to lotion

other: _____

CHAPTER 12

Part A: Sample of narrative documentation for Mr. A:
Nurse (Avril) requested massage for pt. due to neck pain. Last pain score was a 9. Pt. was eager to try and requested massage to neck, shoulders, and back. Nurse approved moderate pressure to those areas with pt. in semireclining and R side-lying positions. In semireclining position, using hospital lotion, gave light strokes and light compression with fingertips to the back and right side of neck; moderate pressure to shoulders. From R side-lying—moderate pressure to back and posterior neck using stroking and compression with fingertips. Pt. reported pain was a 3. Commented: "I feel like a new man!" Length of session—40 min.

GLOSSARY

Ablation To remove or destroy part of the body or its function. Common methods include surgery or electrode catheter.

Abruptio placentae Premature separation of the placenta from the uterus.

Abscess Localized collection of pus in any part of the body.

ACE inhibitors A group of medications that cause vasodilation.

Acquired Characteristic, disease, or abnormality that is not inherited.

Activities of daily living Self-care, communication, and mobility skills needed to live independently. Includes the unaided ability to perform six basic personal care activities: eating, toileting, dressing, bathing, transferring, and continence.

Acute care Health care that is given for a brief but severe episode of illness, usually in a hospital by specialized personnel.

Afferent Carrying impulses to a center, such as a nerve carrying an impulse to the brain.

Airborne transmission Transfer of a disease-causing organism through the air. Chicken pox is an example.

Alkylating Therapy that introduces an alkyl radical into a compound in place of a hydrogen atom interfering with cell metabolism and growth. These drugs are used in cancer treatment.

Allogeneic transplant Stem cells donated by someone other than the patient.

Ambulatory The ability to walk.

Amniotic Referring to the amnion, a thin transparent sac that holds the fetus suspended in fluid.

Analgesics Medications that relieve the normal sense of pain.

Anastomosis Connection of two tubular structures such as an artery and a vein by which the capillary bed is bypassed.

Anecdotal Information based on testimony.

Anesthesia Partial or complete loss of sensation due to disease, injury, or the administration of an agent usually by injection or inhalation.

Aneurysm An abnormal enlargement of a blood vessel, usually an artery, which causes weakening of the vessel wall.

Angina Severe pain around the heart caused by oxygen deficiency to the heart muscle.

Angiogram A radiographic record of the size, shape, and location of the heart and blood vessels.

Angiograph Machine used to record information pertaining to the heart and blood vessels.

Angiography The use of a contrasting dye and x-ray to examine the functioning of blood vessels.

Angioplasty Dilation of blood vessels by surgery or through the use of a balloon inside the lumen.

Ankylosing spondylitis Fixation and inflammation of one or more vertebrae.

Anorexia An aversion to food.

Anorexia nervosa A pathological aversion to food.

Antecubital In front of the elbow.

Anticholinergic An agent that blocks parasympathetic nerve impulses, such as an antidepressant.

Anticoagulant An agent that prevents or delays blood from clotting.

Antihypertensives A group of drugs that lower blood pressure.

Antimetabolites Drugs used against rapidly growing tumors.

Antipyretic Fever-reducing medication or treatment.

Anxiolytics A group of drugs that relieve anxiety.

Antiphospholipid syndrome An autoimmune disorder in which the immune system produces antibodies against its own phospholipids, a type of fat that contains phosphorus. This increases the risk of blood clots, strokes, and thrombocytopenia.

Apheresis A hemodialysis-type of procedure that separates and removes specific blood components.

Aplastic anemia Anemia caused by decreased red blood cell production as a result of a bone marrow disorder.

Aromatherapy massage Massage given with the use of essential oils in a carrier oil.

Arrhythmia Irregular heart rhythm.

Arteriograph A procedure using X-rays and a contrasting dye to study arteries.

Arteriosclerosis Hardening of the arteries.

Arthrectomy Removal of a joint.

Arthrograph Machine used to examine the joint by radiography.

Arthrography A radiographic report of a synovial joint after injecting a dye.

Arthroscope An endoscope for examining the inside of a joint.

Ascites A collection of fluid in the abdominal area often related to liver disease.

Aspiration The drawing in or out by suction, such as foreign bodies breathed into the lungs or the withdrawing of fluid from the body.

Asthma Breathing difficulty caused by bronchial spasm or swelling of the mucous membrane.

Ataxia The inability to coordinate voluntary muscle activity.

Atelectasis Collapse or airless condition of the lung.

Atherectomy Removal of fatty deposits from the inside of arterial walls.

Atherosclerosis Fatty deposits on the interior of arteries causing narrowing and fibrosis.

Autologous transplant Stem cells donated by the patient.

Autonomic Self-controlling, working independently. Physiological functions such as blood pressure and heart rate are autonomic.

Axillary Pertaining to the armpit.

Bell's palsy One or both sides of the face are suddenly paralyzed or distorted. Cause is unknown. Patient may have uncontrolled salivation and in severe cases may not be able to close the eye(s) on the affected side(s) of the face.

Benzodiazepines A group of drugs given to reduce anxiety or induce sleep.

Beta-blockers A group of drugs that relieve cardiac stress by slowing heart contractions, improving rhythm, and reducing blood vessel constriction.

Beta-cells Cells of the islets of Langerhans of the pancreas that secrete insulin.

Beta-receptor site A site in an autonomic nerve pathway where inhibitory responses occur due to the release of substances such as epinephrine and norepinephrine.

Biopsy Excision of a small piece of tissue for microscopic study.

Bipolar Pertaining to manic-depressive disorder.

Blood Stream Infection Precautions Protocols designed to reduce the risk of transmission of pathogens from moist body substances.

Brace Device used in orthopedics for holding joints or limbs in place.

Brachycardia Slow heartbeat, usually below 60 beats/minute.

Bradycardia See brachycardia.

Bulimia nervosa An eating disorder characterized by binge eating followed by self-induced vomiting, the use of laxatives or diuretics, fasting, or exercise.

Cachexia A state of health resulting in malnutrition and wasting noted in chronic disease such as cancer or AIDS.

Calcium channel blocker A group of vasodilating drugs that block the influx of calcium into smooth muscle cells. This causes the muscle tone in the vessel wall to relax.

Candida A yeast-like fungus that is naturally occurring in the human body but that can become pathogenic if the balance is disturbed.

Cardiac Pertaining to the heart.

Cardiology Study of the heart.

Cardiomyopathy Disease of the heart muscle.

Cataract Clouding in the lens of the eye.

Catecholamines Chemical substances derived from the amino acid tyrosine that has a marked effect on the nervous and cardiovascular systems, metabolic rate, temperature, and smooth muscle.

Catheter A tube passed through the body for the purpose of removing or injecting fluids into body cavities.

Catheterization The act of passing a tube through the body for the purpose of removing or injecting fluids into body cavities.

Cellulitis Inflammation of subcutaneous, loose connective tissue.

Central IV catheter A tube, also known as a central line, which is inserted into and kept in the vein for a lengthy period of time in order to inject drugs or extract fluids. Types are Groshong, Hickman, Quinton, and port.

Central line See Central IV catheter.

Central venous access device Another term for central IV catheter.

Cerebrospinal Referring to the brain and spinal cord.

Cerebrovascular accident (CVA) Caused by disruption of the brain's blood supply and commonly referred to as a "stroke."

Cesarean section Surgical delivery of a baby in which an incision is made into the uterus through the abdominal wall.

Cholecystitis Inflammation of the gallbladder.

Chronic bronchitis Long term inflammation of the bronchial tubes.

Chronic obstructive pulmonary disease (COPD) A group of lung diseases that cause decreased lung functioning, such as asthma, emphysema, and chronic bronchitis.

Coagulation Clotting, usually in reference to blood.

Coagulopathy Defect in the clotting ability of the blood.

Colitis Inflammation of the large intestine.

Colostomy The opening of some part of the colon onto the abdominal surface.

Colposcope An instrument used to examine the tissues of the vagina and cervix through a magnifying lens.

Commode A bedside toilet that can be used instead of a bedpan when the patient is able.

Complementary medicine Treatments or therapy performed along with or in addition to conventional medicine.

Computed tomography (CT) A diagnostic scan that images cross-sections of the body with x-rays.

Congestive heart failure The presence of an unusual amount of fluid in the tissues of the heart contributing to heart failure.

Conjunctivitis Inflammation of the membrane that lines the eyelids and covers the eyeball.

Contact Precautions Practices employed to protect healthcare workers, families, and other patients from infections that are transmitted by direct contact, such as VRE, herpes, or conjunctivitis. These precautions involve handwashing, gloving, and gowning.

Continuous passive motion device A mechanical device used to provide continuous movement through specific ranges of motion at selected joints. Used following surgery to reduce complications and promote recovery.

Continuous positive airway pressure The provision of positive airway pressure during both inhalation and exhalation.

Control group A group involved in a research project that does not receive the treatment being tested.

Coronary Referring to the heart, specifically the vessels that feed the heart.

Coronary bypass A surgical procedure routing blood from the aorta to a part of the coronary artery past the site of the blockage.

Corticosteroids Hormonal steroid substances produced in the cortex of the adrenal glands.

Cortisol A hormone secreted by the adrenal cortex. It is essential for carbohydrate metabolism and influences the growth and nutrition of connective tissue.

Cryptococcal meningitis Inflammation of the covering of the brain and spinal cord caused by a fungal infection.

Cutaneous diphtheria An acute infectious disease characterized by the development of a false membrane lesion on the skin.

Cyanosis Blue discoloration of the skin due to lack of oxygen and excess carbon dioxide in the blood.

Cystoscope Instrument used to examine the interior bladder and ureter.

Cytomegalovirus A herpes virus found in human salivary glands. The virus may produce infection during periods of immunosuppression.

Debridement The removal of foreign material and dead or damaged tissue.

Decubitus ulcer An open sore resulting from pressure on the body from the bed or chair.

Deep vein thrombosis A blood clot in the deep venous system of the upper or lower extremities usually resulting from certain surgical procedures and the inactivity of the patient.

Diastolic The period of relaxation after the heart contracts, during which time the chambers fill with blood. The pressure in arteries is at its lowest during this time.

Diphtheria A bacterial infection that most often affects children. Inflammation is caused in the nose, throat, and bronchial tubes. The toxins can damage peripheral nerves, heart muscle, and other tissue.

Diuretic An agent that increases the output of urine.

Diverticulitis Inflammation of the diverticulum, small pockets in the intestinal wall.

Double blind A method of scientific study in which neither the subject nor the investigator knows what treatment, if any, the subject is receiving.

Doula A person trained to give nonmedical support to women who are preparing for birth and to assist during and after the event.

Droplet infection Infection transferred by means of spray from the mouth or nose. An example is the common cold.

Dyskinesia Difficulty in performing voluntary movements.

Dysmenorrhea Menstrual pain caused by congestion, inflammation, or other causes.

Dysphoria Exaggerated feeling of depression and unrest without apparent cause.

Dyspnea Difficult breathing.

Dysrhythmias Abnormal, disordered, or disturbed rhythm, such as cardiac dysrhythmia.

E. coli. See *Escherichia coli.*

Eclampsia Coma and convulsive seizures occurring between the 20th week of pregnancy and the first week after the birth. The cause is still unknown. It occurs more often during first pregnancies. Preexisting high blood pressure and infections that damage the kidney contribute to the condition.

Edema A local or generalized condition in which the body tissues contain an excessive amount of fluid.

Effleurage A long, gliding massage stroke usually done with lubricant.

Electrocardiograph Device for recording changes in the electrical energy produced by the action of heart muscles.

Electrode A device placed on the skin to measure electrical current.

Electroencephalograph Device for recording changes in the electrical energy produced by the brain.

Electrolyte A compound that conducts electricity and is then decomposed by the electric current, such as bases, acids, and salts.

Electromagnetic energy Energy moving from an electrical source into the air such as electromagnetic fields produced by light, radio, and x-rays.

Embolism Obstruction of a blood vessel, usually by a blood clot or other foreign substance.

Emesis Material ejected from the stomach.

Emetic Nausea producing.

Emphysema A disease process of the lung in which the air sacs of the lung have increased in size.

Encephalitis Inflammation of the brain.

Encephalopathy Dysfunction of the brain due to disease.

Endoscope Device for examining the inside of a hollow organ or cavity.

Endoscopic Pertains to an examination of the internal organs or cavity by use of an endoscope.

Endotracheal Inside the trachea. Usually referring to a tube inserted into the trachea, which is then inflated to provide an airway. It also prevents aspiration of foreign material into the bronchus.

Engraftment The process of stem cells traveling to the bone marrow and producing new blood cells.

Enteric Pertaining to the small intestine.

Enterococcus Any species of streptococcus found in the intestine.

Epidural Located over or on the outer layer of the spinal cord or the brain, also known as the dura. Also refers to anesthesia placed in the epidural space.

Epiglottitis Inflammation of the leaf-like structure that covers the larynx when a person swallows.

Escherichia coli (*E. coli*) Usually a nonpathogenic bacterium present in the digestive tract of all humans. It will cause infection if it enters the urinary tract. If found in milk or water, it is an indication of fecal contamination. It is the chief cause of "traveler's diarrhea."

Euphoria An exaggerated feeling of well-being, mild elation.

Evidence-based practice The use of interventions that are scientifically proven.

Experimental A scientific procedure to gain further knowledge. Also refers to the group in an experiment that is receiving the trial intervention.

External fixators External devices, such as pins or screws, used to keep fractured bone segments in place.

Extubation Removal of a tube, such as an endotracheal tube.

Febrile Relating to fever.

Fetal Pertaining to the unborn child in the uterus from the third month until birth.

Fiberoptic Flexible materials used to transmit light by reflecting it from the side or wall of the fiber, such as the walls of an organ. Often used during endoscopic examinations.

Fibrillation Quivering, spontaneous, or incomplete contractions of individual muscle fibers, such as in the heart. Often seen in sudden cardiac arrest.

Fistula Abnormal tube-like passage from a normal cavity or tube to another surface opening or cavity, such as an arteriovenous fistula, which is created by connecting an artery and a vein.

Fixator Orthotic device that can be internal or external. It uses a combination of pins, nails, screws, and plates to hold bones together.

Flaccid paralysis Lack of muscle tone due to temporary or permanent loss of function of a muscle. It is due to the damage to special nerve cells in the brain and spinal cord.

Foley catheter A tube that is placed in the bladder to provide continuous urinary drainage.

Formulary A book that provides standards and specifications for drugs.

Fowler's position Semireclining position.

Gamma-aminobutyric acid (GABA) An amino acid that is the principal inhibitory neurotransmitter in the central nervous system.

Gangrene The death of tissue due to a lack of blood supply.

Gastroenterologist A specialist in the study of the stomach, intestines, and other digestive organs.

Gastrostomy Surgical creation of a gastric fistula (opening) through the abdominal wall.

Glycoprotein A compound consisting of a carbohydrate and protein.

Gout Acute pain and inflammation of joints, usually the feet or toes, caused by hyperuricemia (excess uric acid). Often associated with kidney stones.

Groshong A type of central IV catheter.

Guillain-Barré syndrome Acute, inflammatory destruction of the peripheral nerves' myelin sheath. Causes rapid and progressive loss of motor function. Believed to be an autoimmune response.

Gynecology The science of female reproductive organs.

Handrub Waterless antibacterial hand cleanser.

HELLP syndrome A complication of pregnancy-induced hypertension that causes low platelets and destruction of red blood cells.

Hematocrit Percentage of the blood volume occupied by cells.

Hematoma A collection of clotted blood in an organ, tissue, or space caused by a broken blood vessel.

Hemiparesis Partial paralysis.

Hemodialysis A method for providing the function of the kidneys by circulating blood through tubes made of semipermeable membranes. These dialyzing tubes are continually bathed by solutions that selectively remove unwanted material.

Hemodynamics A study of the forces involved in circulating the blood through the body.

Hep lock A peripheral IV catheter with a reservoir that permits intermittent infusion of medications. Heparin is used to keep the catheter open when not in use.

Hepatitis Inflammation of the liver.

Herpes A virus that can cause vesicles to erupt most commonly on the mouth, genitalia, thighs, or buttocks. Also, see Shingles.

Herpes simplex A type of herpes virus that erupts either on the lips or genitalia.

Hickman A type of central IV catheter.

Hirsutism Excessive body and face hair.

Histamine A substance produced from the amino acid histidine. It causes a reaction, such as swelling, redness, and rash, when released from injured cells. If injected, histamine stimulates gastric secretion and causes flushing of the skin, lowered blood pressure, and headache.

Homeostatic A state of equilibrium.

Hormone Chemical substances formed in organs or glands. They travel through the blood to other parts of the body, stimulating their function or the secretion of more hormones.

Hydrocephalus A condition in which an excessive amount of cerebrospinal fluid accumulates in the brain.

Hypercholesteremia Excess cholesterol in the blood.

Hypertension High blood pressure.

Hypnotics Sedatives, analgesics, anesthetics, and intoxicants. Drugs used to decrease pain and/or induce sleep.

Hypocalcemia Excessively low levels of calcium in the blood.

Hypoglycemic Low blood sugar level.

Hypotension Low blood pressure.

Hypothalamus A part of the brain located in the middle of the base of the brain. It is involved with the autonomic nervous system, endocrine mechanisms, and mood states.

Hypoxia Deficiency of oxygen in the blood.

Hysterectomy Removal of the uterus.

Ileostomy An opening into the ileum (lower intestine) by way of the abdominal surface. Fecal material drains into a bag worn on the abdomen.

Ileum The longest and final part of the small intestine before it leads into the colon.

Immunocompromised An immune system that is incapable of reacting to pathogens. The cause can be drug-induced, genetic, or disease-related.

Immunosuppressed Another term for immunocompromised.

Impetigo A contagious condition caused by streptococci or staphylococci bacteria in which the skin becomes inflamed and isolated pustules form. They eventually rupture and become crusted. The skin of the nose and mouth is the most often affected area.

Implanted defibrillator An electrical device implanted in the chest that produces a shock to reestablish the heart's normal rhythm.

Incontinence Inability to retain urine, semen, or feces due to loss of sphincter control or brain or spinal lesions.

Infarct Part of an organ in which the tissue has died due to lack of blood supply.

Inherited Characteristics or conditions with a genetic connection.

Interstitial Refers to spaces within a tissue or organ.

Intervention Taking action so as to modify the result. Examples are the use of medication, massage, physical therapy, or chiropractic treatments.

Intravenous (IV) catheter A catheter inserted into a vein to administer fluids or medications or to measure pressure.

Intubation Insertion of a tube into any hollow organ for entrance of air or to dilate a structure.

Ischemia Obstructed blood supply to a localized area.

Isolation cart A cart in the hallway outside a patient's room upon which protective equipment, such as gowns, masks, gloves, and disposable dishes, is found. These items assist staff in avoiding the transmission of an infectious disease from one patient to another or to themselves.

IV pole Equipment that supports a hanging IV bag.

Jackson-Pratt tube A type of drain.

Jejunostomy A surgical opening into the jejunum by way of the abdominal surface.

Jejunum The middle portion of the small intestine.

J-Pouch A bag attached at the site of a jejunostomy for the purpose of collecting intestinal contents.

J-Tube A catheter inserted into the jejunum used for feeding.

Jugular vein A blood vessel in the throat that runs superficial to the sternocleidomastoid muscle.

Kaposi's sarcoma Normally a rather benign skin malignancy characterized by purple lesions. In immunodepressed HIV patients, other organs are also affected.

Kinins General term for a group of polypeptides that have considerable biological activity. They influence smooth muscle contraction, induce hypotension, increase blood flow and permeability of small blood capillaries, and incite pain.

Lactation The secretion of milk from the mammary glands. Also refers to the period of suckling.

Lanugo Downy hair such as covers a fetus or that accompanies eating disorders.

Laparoscope Instrument used to examine the inside of the abdominal cavity.

Lesion A pathological change in tissue from an injury, infected patch, cyst, or a cancer.

Leukopenia Less than the normal number of leukocytes.

Liability Obliged by law.

Lice A type of parasitic insect.

Likert scale A written research tool that measures patient feedback on a scale of 1 to 5.

Lupus A chronic, progressive, usually ulcerating skin disease.

Lymphadenopathy Any disease affecting the lymph nodes.

Lymphedema A collection of lymphatic fluid due to a congenital defect, obstruction of the lymph vessels, or removal of lymph nodes.

Lymphocytes Cells found in the blood and the lymph glands. They are the main means of providing immunity for our body. They compose 20% to 40% of the body's white cells.

Magnetic resonance imaging (MRI) Use of magnetic fields and radio-frequency waves in combination with computer technology to view images of soft tissue in the body.

Mastectomy The surgical removal of part or all of the breast.

Maternity The department of the hospital that cares for the mother at the time of childbirth and supervises the baby care.

Mechanical ventilator Mechanical device for artificially oxygenating the lungs as well as monitoring the flow of air to the lungs.

Medical Related to the term "medicine," the art and science of diagnosing, treating, and preventing disease. Also, the treatment of disease through the use of drugs or other remedies that are nonsurgical. Physicians and nurse practitioners are involved in the medical side of health care.

Meningitis Inflammation of the membranes of the spinal cord and brain.

Metastases Secondary cancerous tumors that form at a distant site.

Metastasis The movement of bacteria or body cells, such as cancer cells, from one part of the body to another.

Mixed venous oxygen saturation (SVO$_2$) The concentration of saturated oxygen in the venous system.

MRSA (methicillin-resistant staphylococcus aureus) A bacteria that is resistant to the antibiotic methicillin.

Mucositis Inflammation of the mucosal lining, generally occurring in the mouth and esophagus.

MUGA (multiple gated acquisition) scan A diagnostic scan that employs nuclear technology to assess heart function.

Multiple myeloma Cancer of the plasma cells, a type of white blood cell found in the bone marrow. Plasma cells normally produce antibodies, which are used to attack viruses and bacteria, for the body's immune system.

Multiple sclerosis A disorder of the central nervous system caused by loss of the myelin sheath around nerve fibers.

Myalgia Muscle pain.

Myocardial infarction A condition caused by a partial or complete occlusion of one or more coronary arteries, which carry blood necessary to keep heart muscle alive. It is commonly referred to as a heart attack.

Narcotics Opiate-based drugs that depress the central nervous system, thereby relieving pain and inducing sleep.

Nasal cannula Tubing used to deliver oxygen. It extends approximately 1 cm into each nostril and is connected to a common tube, which is then connected to the oxygen source. It is used in situations such as cardiac disease in which a low-flow of oxygen is desired.

Nasogastric Relating to the nose and stomach. Usually pertains to intubation of the stomach via the nasal passage.

Neonatologist A physician who specializes in newborns.

Nephrolithiasis Kidney stones.

Nephroscope A scope that is inserted into the kidney or ureter.

Nephrostomy The formation of an artificial fistula into the renal pelvis.

Nephrotoxic Poison that damages kidney tissue.

Neuralgia Nerve pain.

Neuroleptic An agent or drug that modifies psychotic behavior.

Neuropathy A pathological condition of the nervous system that results in tingling, loss of feeling, and pins and needles of a body part.

Neurotransmitter A chemical substance that is released by a presynaptic neuron, which then travels across the synapse to act on the target cell to either inhibit or excite it. Norepinephrine and dopamine are examples.

Neutropenic Less than a normal number of neutrophils, a type of white blood cell. These cells are responsible for much of the body's defense against disease. Low levels increase the chance of infection.

Neutrophil A type of granulocytic white blood cell.

Non-Hodgkin's lymphoma A group of cancers, other than Hodgkin's disease, that affect lymphatic tissue.

Nosocomial Pertaining to the hospital or infirmary.

Nurse A healthcare provider who manages the patient's plan of care and assists the patient to perform activities that contribute to health or its recovery (or to a peaceful death). He or she is unable to diagnosis or prescribe treatment but acts under the orders of the doctor.

Nystagmus An involuntary condition that causes the eye to rapidly move up and down or right and left.

Obsessive-compulsive disorder A disorder characterized by the need to perform repetitive acts or ritualistic behavior to relieve anxiety.

Obstetrics The branch of medicine that cares for pregnant women before, during, and after birth.

Occlusion Blocking.

Oncologist A physician who specializes in cancer medicine.

Oncology The branch of medicine dealing with tumors.

Orogastric Refers to the mouth and stomach.

Orthopedic The branch of medicine that treats problems of the muscular and skeletal systems of the body.

Orthostatic hypotension Low blood pressure that occurs when a person rises from a lying to a standing position.

Orthotics The science pertaining to mechanical appliances used in the treatment of musculoskeletal problems.

Osteoarthritis A chronic disease of the joints resulting in the destruction of the cartilage intended to cushion the joints. It is often found in the aged population and is disabling.

Osteopenia A decrease in calcification or bone density due to inadequate synthesis of bone cells.

Osteoporosis A disease process that results in the reduction of bone mass. Fractures often occur where they would not normally. Vertebrae are most commonly affected.

Otitis media Inflammation in the middle ear.

Pacemaker An electrical device placed in the chest to regulate heart rhythm.

Parenteral Any route other than oral, such as IV, subcutaneous, intramuscular, or mucosal.

Pathogen A microorganism or substance that is capable of causing a disease.

Patient-controlled analgesia Pain medications that can be administered in measured doses by the patient.

Percutaneous Application of medication through the skin, such as an ointment or by injection.

Pericardial Pertaining to the double membranous sac surrounding the heart and the origin of the great vessels.

Peripheral line An IV catheter usually placed in the lower arm for temporary use.

Peripheral neuropathy Neuropathy that generally affects the hands, feet, or lower legs.

Peripherally inserted central catheter (PICC) A catheter that is placed into a central vein either in the antecubital space or the upper arm. It is for patients needing long-term care.

Peritoneal Pertaining to the serous membrane over the abdominal organs and the lining of the abdominal cavity.

Peritoneum The membrane that lines the abdominal cavity and covers the viscera.

Perma-cath A large bore catheter that remains in place on a long-term basis. Often used for hemodialysis.

Pertussis Commonly called whooping cough, an infectious disease characterized by a runny nose followed by a peculiar spasmodic cough ending in a whooping sound. It is preventable by immunization of infants at 3 months.

Petechiae Small purplish, hemorrhagic spots that appear on the skin or mucous membranes with certain severe fevers or as a side effects of drugs.

Pharmaceutical Pertaining to drugs or pharmacy.

Pharyngitis Inflammation of the throat.

Phlebitis Inflammation of a vein.

Physical therapy The use of heat, cold, exercise, electricity, and massage to improve motion, thereby allowing individuals to perform activities of daily living.

Placenta previa A condition in which the placenta implants in the lower part of the uterus.

Plaque Deposits on tissue. An example is deposits of fatty substance inside blood vessels.

Plasma The somewhat clear fluid of the blood that carries corpuscles and platelets. It consists of serum, protein, and chemical substances in aqueous solution. The chemical substances include electrolytes, glucose, proteins, enzymes, hormones, and fats.

Platelet A blood component necessary for coagulation.

Pleural Pertaining to the membrane that enfolds both lungs, lines the chest cavity, and covers the diaphragm.

Pleur-evac The brand name of a device that drains fluid in the lungs.

Pneumocystis carinii pneumonia Inflammation of the lung found in very "wasting" problems of immunodeficient patients.

Pneumonia Inflammation of the lung caused by bacteria or chemical irritants.

Port-A-Cath The brand name of a type of long-term central venous catheter that is surgically placed under the skin. Also known as a "port."

Positron emission tomography (PET) scan A nuclear scanning process that measures how quickly tissue absorbs radioactive isotopes. This is an indication of cellular metabolism.

Positrons A particle having the same mass as a negative electron but possessing a positive charge.

Postmortem After death.

Postpartum The period after childbirth.

Posttraumatic stress disorder Psychological damage caused by a traumatic event.

Preeclampsia A condition associated with pregnancy that causes hypertension with proteinuria or edema.

Preterm labor The premature start of pregnancy contractions.

Prophylactic Any agent or regimen that contributes to the prevention of infection or disease.

Prostaglandin Any of a group of fatty acid derivatives that are biologically very active. They affect a number of systems, such as the cardiovascular, gastrointestinal, and respiratory systems.

Protective isolation Another term for reverse isolation.

Prothrombin A coagulation factor synthesized by the liver that is converted to thrombin.

Pruritus Itching.

Psychosocial Pertaining to the emotional and social component of patient care.

Pulmonary Concerning the lungs.

Pulse oximeter An electronic device that is usually attached to the finger to determine the oxygen concentration in arterial blood.

Radioactive isotope One of a series of chemical elements that have nearly identical chemical properties but different atomic weights and electric charges. An isotope in which the nuclear composition is unstable.

Radiopharmaceutical A radioactive chemical used in testing the location, size, outline, or function of tissues, organs, vessels, or body fluids. The presence and location of radiopharmaceuticals in the body are detected by special methods or devices that record the radioactivity being emitted. They may also be used in the treatment of diseases such as prostate cancer.

Randomized A research method in which individuals are arbitrarily assigned to one of two groups, experimental or control.

Relaxin A hormone secreted during pregnancy.

Renal Pertaining to the kidneys.

Respiratory therapy Treatment to preserve or improve lung function.

Retroperitoneal Behind the peritoneum and outside the peritoneal cavity, such as the kidneys.

Reverse isolation Infection control practices that protect the patient from infections that might be transferred to them from healthcare staff and family. Also known as protective isolation.

Reye's syndrome A rare illness affecting children who have taken aspirin. Causes acute encephalopathy and fatty infiltration of the liver and possibly of the pancreas, heart, kidney, spleen, and lymph nodes. May involve the central nervous system to varying degrees.

Rheumatoid arthritis Inflammatory changes of joints and surrounding tissues resulting in crippling deformities.

Ringer's solution A solution of recently boiled distilled water containing 8.6 g sodium chloride, 0.3 g potassium chloride, and 0.33 g calcium chloride per liter. Also known as Ringer's irrigation.

Rubella Commonly known as German measles, an acute, short-lasting, infectious disease resembling both scarlet fever and measles but differing in the short course. The rash begins on the face and quickly spreads over the whole body but fades very rapidly. Serious fetal anomalies may result if the mother contracts the disease in the first trimester of pregnancy.

Rubeola Commonly known as measles, an acute contagious disease with fever, nonelevated rash found in patches, and a runny nose.

Scarlet fever A bacterial infection that is highly contagious. Characterized by a sore throat, red tongue, fever, and scarlet rash.

Schizophrenia A mental illness characterized by distorted perception and thoughts, hallucinations, and delusions.

Sedative A substance that produces a calming, soothing, or tranquilizing effect.

Self-limiting Limitations controlled by the patient.

Semireclining The body in a half-back lying position. Also known as Fowler's position.

Sepsis An infection caused by the presence of bacteria in the bloodstream.

Sequential compression device A device that is used to apply pressure in an alternating fashion, usually to the lower extremities to prevent clot formation.

Sheath A covering structure of connective tissue, such as a membrane (fascia) covering a muscle. Also refers to a tubular instrument inserted into a vessel during angiographic procedures when multiple catheter changes are anticipated or through which special cutting instruments can be passed.

Shingles (herpes zoster) Eruption of acute inflammatory herpes vesicles usually on the trunk of the body along a peripheral nerve.

Shunt An artificially constructed passage to divert flow from one main route to another.

Sigmoidoscope A tubular instrument for examination of the sigmoid colon.

Splint An apparatus used for the fixation, union, or protection of an injured part of the body. Construction may be of wood, plastic, plaster, or metal.

Sputum Substance discharged by coughing or clearing the throat.

Standard Precautions The practices used to protect against infection from all body fluids regardless of a person's diagnosis or presumed infectious status.

Staphylococcus A term used loosely for any disease-causing microscopic bacteria that appear in "grape-like" clusters during microscopic study.

Statistical significance After appropriate analysis of numerical data, it is decided that the results are not happening by chance.

Stem cell Primordial, all-purpose cells that can develop into any tissue in the body.

Stenosis The constriction or narrowing of a passage or orifice.

Stent Any material or device used to hold tissue in place or to provide a support for a graft or anastomosis while healing is taking place.

Sternal Related to the breastbone.

Sternotomy A procedure in which the sternum is cut through.

Sterol One of a group of substances, such as cholesterol, belonging to the lipids.

Streptococcal Relating to the streptococcus bacteria.

Stoma An artificial opening between two passages or body cavities or between the body's surface and a cavity or passage. The opening created by a colostomy is an example.

Subcutaneous Beneath the skin.

Subjective Information arising from individual opinion, not from research.

Supine Lying on the back with the face upward.

Supine hypotensive syndrome Low blood pressure when in a supine position.

Sutured Stitched or joined by surgical thread.

Swan-Ganz catheter A flexible catheter with a balloon near the tip that is used in testing or monitoring pressures in the lung and heart.

Synovial Pertaining to the lubricating fluids of the joints.

Systolic The period of cardiac contraction. Blood pressure is highest during this action.

Tachycardia An abnormally fast heartbeat, usually defined as a heart rate greater than 100 beats/minute in adults.

Tapotement A percussive massage stroke.

Telemetry The transmission of data electronically to a distant location.

Thalassemia A group of inherited hemoglobin disorders.

Therapeutic A healing agent having medicinal or healing properties or results obtained from treatment.

Thrombin A plasma protein substance used topically to control capillary bleeding during surgical procedures. A blood-clotting agent.

Thrombocytopenia An abnormal reduction in the blood platelets.

Thrombolytic The breaking up of a blood clot.

Thrombophlebitis Occurrence of a blood clot in conjunction with an inflamed vein.

Thrombosis Formulation or presence of a thrombus.

Thrombotic thrombocytopenic purpura A rare blood disorder in which platelets are rapidly consumed as a result of excessive clotting. Consequently, thrombi occur in small blood vessels in many organs.

Thrombus A blood clot that obstructs a blood vessel or cavity of the heart.

Thrush An infection of the mouth or throat caused by *Candida albicans.*

Toxoplasmosis A protozoa-caused disease that can be mild or can trigger swollen glands, muscle pain, and malaise. In more serious cases, nervous system damage, jaundice, and general lymphadenopathy can occur.

Tracheotomy Incision into the trachea through the skin and muscles of the neck.

Tracheotomy tube The tube inserted into the trachea following a tracheotomy to maintain the opening.

Traction Usually used to pull and align structures such as the vertebrae or a structure that has been fractured.

Transcutaneous electrical nerve stimulation (TENS) A system that delivers electric currents to the surface of the skin to relieve pain in underlying areas.

Transdermal patch A method of delivering medicine by placing it in a special gel-like matrix that is applied to the skin like a Band-Aid. The medicine is absorbed into the skin at a fixed rate.

Transfer The act of moving a person with limited function from one location to another.

Transmission-Based Precautions The protective practices employed when caring for patients known or suspected to be infected by specific pathogens.

Transmural Across the entire wall of an organ or structure.

Trend With regard to research, data that lean toward a certain outcome but are not statistically significant.

Trigeminal Pertaining to the trigeminus or fifth cranial nerve.

T-tube A t-shaped tube that is placed within another tube such as for the patient on a vent.

Tuberculosis Bacterial infection that most commonly affects the lungs.

Ulcer An open sore on the skin or mucous membrane accompanied by sloughing of inflamed dead tissue.

Ulceration Formation of an open sore or lesion of the skin or mucosal lining.

Ultrasound A test that bounces sound waves off tissue to detect density and elasticity in various tissues. The echoes are changed into pictures.

Universal Precautions The practices employed to protect against bloodborne pathogens, such as hand washing, gloving, and gowning.

Ureterotomy Formation of a permanent opening for drainage of a ureter.

Urinal A container into which one urinates.

Urostomy The redirection of urine outside the body after the bladder has been repaired or removed.

Urticaria A vascular reaction of the skin characterized by a sudden general eruption of pale evanescent wheals or papules, which are associated with severe itching. May be caused by contact with an irritant such as nettles, chemicals, insect bites, or allergens.

Varicella Commonly known as chicken pox, an acute, contagious disease with fever and vesicular eruption initially on the back and face.

Varicose veins Distended, swollen veins.

Varicosity See Varicose vein.

Vasculitis Inflammation of a blood or lymph vessel.

Vasoconstriction Narrowing of the blood vessels.

Vasodilation Widening of the blood vessels.

Vasodilator Any substance that widens blood vessels.

Venogram A procedure using X-rays and a contrasting dye to study veins.

Vent A shortened term for mechanical ventilator.

Vital signs Body temperature, heart rate, respiration, and blood pressure.

VRE (vancomycin-resistant enterococcus) A bacteria resistant to the antibiotic vancomycin.

Whooping cough The common name for pertussis.

INDEX

Page numbers in italics (set in italics) denote figures; those followed by a t denote tables.